PRINCIPLES OF NEUROLOGY

Fourth Edition

Companion Handbook

NOTICE

Medicine is an ever-changing science. As new research and clinical experience broaden our knowledge, changes in treatment and drug therapy are required. The authors and the publisher of this work have checked with sources believed to be reliable in their efforts to provide information that is complete and generally in accord with the standards accepted at the time of publication. However, in view of the possibility of human error or changes in medical sciences, neither the authors nor the publisher nor any other party who has been involved in the preparation or publication of this work warrants that the information contained herein is in every respect accurate or complete. Readers are encouraged to confirm the information contained herein with other sources. For example and in particular, readers are advised to check the product information sheet included in the package of each drug they plan to administer to be certain that the information contained in this book is accurate and that changes have not been made in the recommended dosages or in the contraindications for administration. This recommendation is of particular importance in connection with new or infrequently used drugs.

PRINCIPLES OF NEUROLOGY

Fourth Edition

Companion Handbook

RAYMOND D. ADAMS, M.D.

Bullard Professor of Neuropathology, Emeritus
Harvard Medical School
Senior Neurologist and Formerly Chief
of Neurology Service
Massachusetts General Hospital
Director Emeritus, Eunice K. Shriver Center
Boston, Massachusetts

MAURICE VICTOR, M.D.

Professor of Medicine and Neurology
Dartmouth Medical School
Hanover, New Hampshire
Distinguished Physician of the Veterans Administration
White River Junction, Vermont

McGRAW-HILL, INC.
Health Professions Division

New York St. Louis San Francisco Auckland Bogotá
Caracas Hamburg Lisbon London Madrid Mexico
Milan Montreal New Delhi Paris San Juan São Paulo
Singapore Sydney Tokyo Toronto

PRINCIPLES OF NEUROLOGY, FOURTH EDITION COMPANION HANDBOOK

International Edition 1991

4 5 6 7 8 9 0 KHL SW 9 8 7 6 5 4 3

This book was set in Times Roman by Monotype Composition Company, Inc. The editors were Edward M. Bolger, William Day, and Lester A. Sheinis; the production supervisor was Richard Ruzycka; the cover was designed by NSG Design, the index was prepared by Irving Tullar.

Library of Congress Cataloging-in-Publication Data

Adams, Raymond D. (Raymond Delacy), date
Principles of neurology, fourth edition, Companion handbook/ Raymond D. Adams, Maurice Victor,
p. cm.
Includes bibliographical references and index.
ISBN 0-07-000334-3
1. Nervous system – Diseases. 2. Neuropsychiatry. I. Victor Maurice,date. II Title.
(DNLM: 1. Nervous System Diseases-handbooks. WL100 A216p 1989 Suppl.)
RC346.A3 1991
616.8——dc20
DNLM/DLC
for Library of Congress 90–13653
CIP

When ordering this title use ISBN 0-07-100845-4

Printed in Singapore

CONTENTS

PREFACE

Diseases of the nervous system number in the hundreds and are too numerous and varied to be learned in their entirety; hence, the common practice in clinical work of subdividing them into categories—traumatic, neoplastic, infective, metabolic, degenerative, congenital, and so forth. In our textbook, *Principles of Neurology*, we have attempted to describe the various categories of neurologic disease and the main diseases that constitute each category, and to explain their clinical manifestations in terms of anatomy, physiology, and biochemistry; in other words, to provide the scientific and intellectual background of neurology. Although modest in scope, in comparison with the 44-volume *Handbook of Clinical Neurology*, edited by Vinken and Bruyn, our textbook is a readable reference without excessive detail.

With each succeeding edition of *Principles of Neurology* and the inevitable growth of its contents, there has been an increasing number of requests from our students and residents for a small companion to our text—a book that could be carried conveniently in a pocket or an instrument bag and provide a quick orientation to a clinical problem when the larger text is not immediately available. It is in response to these requests and with the encouragement of our publisher that we accepted the challenge of preparing this handbook.

Our objectives in writing this handbook are to provide some guidance in the logic of neurologic case study and the ways in which one reaches a physiologic, anatomic, and etiologic diagnosis; to present in outline form the clinical approach to each category of neurologic disease, with emphasis on the more frequent and treatable types and on neurologic emergencies; and to satisfy the practical needs of selecting and interpreting the procedures, laboratory tests, and drugs that are used in the investigation and treatment of neurologic disease.

Although this small volume is patterned after *Principles of Neurology*, the one should not be considered a substitute for the other. The handbook is intended to be a companion to the *Principles*, in the sense of satisfying the immediate practical needs of student and resident but turning them to the *Principles* for a more complete and fully referenced account of the problem at hand. The style of the smaller edition is intentionally elliptic, to expose the most facts with the fewest words. We hope that the reader will accept it with these restrictions in mind.

Raymond D. Adams
Maurice Victor

PRINCIPLES OF NEUROLOGY

Fourth Edition

Companion Handbook

I | APPROACH TO THE PATIENT WITH NEUROLOGIC DISEASE

1 Case Study in Neurology

Diagnosis of a disorder of the nervous system, like that of any other organ system, begins with a detailed history and a careful examination, appropriate to the problem at hand. The symptomatology of nervous system disease is much more varied than that of other organ systems, and the physical manifestations are far more numerous and informative. The reason for this diversity is that the nervous system consists not of a single system of uniform function, but of multiple systems, each one unique.

Once the symptoms and signs have been elicited, they need to be interpreted in terms of physiology and anatomy. This correlation permits *localization* of the disease process; i.e., it provides an *anatomic or topographic diagnosis*. For example, paralysis or weakness of the lower face, arm, and leg on one side, with retained or hyperactive tendon reflexes, incontrovertibly directs attention to the corticospinal tract above its decussation and above the pontine part of the brainstem. Symptoms of diabetes insipidus implicate the anterior hypothalamus and posterior pituitary. Obviously, this second step in case analysis demands a certain knowledge of anatomy and physiology. For this reason each of the following chapters dealing with the motor system, sensory system, and special senses are introduced in our *Principles of Neurology* with a review of the anatomic and physiologic facts that are necessary for understanding the clinical disorders.

The next step in case analysis, that of determining the cause of the lesion, requires information of a different order. Here, knowledge of where the lesion(s) lie, coupled with information as to the mode of onset and temporal course of the illness, relevant past and family histories, general medical findings (hypertension, auricular fibrillation, diabetes mellitus, etc.), and the results of appropriate laboratory tests, enables one to deduce the causative disease (*etiologic diagnosis*).

The steps in this clinical method are summarized in Fig. 1-1. Each step follows in logical sequence and if the first or second step is not secure, the later ones may be misdirected. Thus, if the symptoms or physical signs are misinterpreted—for example, if a localized tremor or choreoathetotic movement (dentato- or

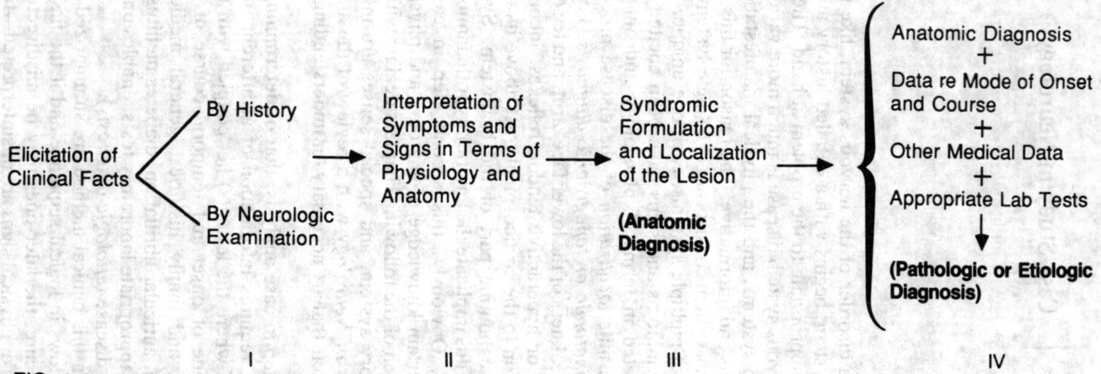

FIG. 1-1 Steps in the diagnosis of neurologic disease.

pallido-thalamic origin) is mistaken for partial continuous epilepsy (cerebral cortical origin)—one would place the lesion incorrectly. One of the most fascinating aspects of neurology is the evident effectiveness and logic of the clinical method in the diagnosis of many hundreds of diseases.

TAKING THE HISTORY

An intelligent, alert person should be able to give a coherent account of the problem that brings him* to the physician. There are, however, many circumstances that prevent him from doing so. He may have been unconscious when the symptoms occurred, e.g., from a seizure or a concussion. The patient's intellect may be impaired by the very disease under evaluation or by some other one dating from earlier life, i.e., by dementia or feeblemindedness. The lesion may have affected speech and language mechanisms, preventing communication. Or it may have impaired awareness of a specific neurologic defect, a condition to be described later, under *anosognosia*. Of course, infants and young children lack the ability to make observations concerning their own nervous functioning. A lack of knowledge of English poses yet another problem.

Under these many circumstances the neurologist must turn to a family member or other witness of an acute event or to a caretaker, parent, or translator. Their competence and degree of familiarity with the patient's problems are of critical importance in the first step of case study. *A lack of accurate knowledge of the mode of onset and evolution of the patient's symptoms deprives the physician of the most meaningful diagnostic informaton.*

THE NEUROLOGIC EXAMINATION

This is an integral part of the general physical examination. With most disease states, the neurologic examination is the last part; in a comatose patient, it follows immediately upon the recording of vital signs and the cardiopulmonary examination. The type and completeness of the neurologic examination is determined by the nature of the clinical problem. Obviously, it is not necessary to perform a detailed mental status exam in an alert patient with an acute compression of a peroneal nerve. Nevertheless, some assessment of the neurologic status should be part of every general medical examination. The following are

* Throughout this text we will follow the traditional English practice of using the pronouns *he, his,* or *him* in the generic sense whenever it is not intended to designate the specific gender of an individual.

suggestions as to the types of neurologic examinations that are pertinent to different medical situations.

1. The Medical or Surgical Patient Without Neurologic Symptoms

Although brevity is desirable, any test that is performed should be done carefully and recorded accurately in the patient's chart. Assuming that the patient is alert and of normal intelligence, a sufficient examination comprises the following: checking the pupils, ocular movements, visual and auditory acuity (by questioning), and movements of the face, tongue, larynx, and pharynx; observing the bare outstretched arms in the prone and supine postures and during movement (such as touching the nose with the index finger); inquiring about strength and subjective sensory disturbances; eliciting the supinator, biceps, and triceps tendon reflexes; inspecting the legs as the feet and toes are actively flexed and extended; eliciting the patellar, Achilles, and plantar reflexes; and testing vibratory and position senses of the fingers and toes. The entire procedure adds no more than 3 or 4 min to the medical examination and sometimes reveals diseases of which the patient is unaware. Recording these data, even negative ones, may be of value in relation to some future illness.

2. Examination of the Patient with a Neurologic Disease

Several guides to the examination of the nervous system are available (cf. Ross, Mancall, Staff Members of the Mayo Clinic). They describe innumerable tests in minute detail, but here only the relatively simple and most informative ones will be mentioned. Particular forms of testing are considered in subsequent chapters dealing with disorders of consciousness and mentation, cranial nerves, special senses, and motor, sensory, and autonomic functions.

a. *Testing of higher cerebral (cortical) functions* In the course of taking the history, one notes the patient's behavior, emotional state, speech, use of language, and capacity for sustained coherent thinking. Attentiveness, speed of response, and ability to remember events also lend themselves to straightforward observation. This is followed by a systematic inquiry into the patient's orientation, affect, and cognitive and conative functions, making due allowance for the patient's level of education and native intelligence. Useful bedside tests are repetition of digits in forward and reverse order, subtraction of 7's or 3's serially from 100, recall of a brief story or three test items after five mins, and the naming of the last six presidents. If there is any suggestion of a speech disorder, one notes the quality of articulation, the choice of words in conversation, and the ability to name the parts of a wristwatch, to follow two- and three-step commands, and to read and write. Bisecting a line, drawing a clockface, and copying figures are useful tests of visual-spatial and visual-motor functions. Tests of simple arithmetic may demonstrate an impaired ability to concentrate as well as to calculate. In the performance of these tests the examiner can note the presence or absence of apathy, depression, inattentiveness, and distractibility.

A more complete mental status examination is outlined on pp. 171–173.

b. ***Testing of cranial nerves and special senses*** Tests of smell are done if one suspects a lesion of the anterior cranial fossa. It suffices to determine if the odor of soap, coffee, tobacco, or vanilla can be detected in each nostril. Ammonia and similar pungent substances should not be used because they stimulate trigeminal and not olfactory nerves. The visual fields should be outlined by confrontation testing, and suspected abnormalities should be checked by perimetry and the Bjerrum screen. The size of the pupils and their reactivity to light and on accommodation and the range and quality of ocular movements should be observed and the optic fundi carefully inspected.

Sensation over the face is tested with a pin and wisp of cotton and the presence or absence of corneal reflexes noted. Strength of facial muscles is determined by asking the patient to wrinkle the forehead, show his teeth, and forcibly close his eyes and lips. Auditory perception is readily assessed by a number of tuning fork tests and most accurately by formal audiograms. Inspection of the tongue may disclose discoloration, loss of papillae, atrophy, and fasciculations. Testing of the jaw jerk and buccal and sucking reflexes should not be overlooked, particularly if there is a question of dysarthria and dysphagia.

Details of these test procedures are described in Chaps. 11 (olfaction and taste), 12 (vision), 13 (ocular movement and pupils), and 14 (hearing and vestibular function).

c. ***Testing of motor, sensory, and reflex functions*** A number of simple maneuvers will disclose the speed, strength, and coordination of movements: maintaining both arms or both legs against gravity; alternately touching the patient's nose and examiner's finger; making rapid alternating movements; buttoning clothes, opening and closing a safety pin, and handling common tools; standing on toes and heels; stepping onto and down from a chair and arising from a kneeling and squatting position without help; running the heel down the front of the shin; rhythmic tapping of heel on shin; touching and following the examiner's finger with the toe. No examination is complete without observing the patient's stance and gait and presence or absence of tremor, involuntary movements, and abnormalities of posture and muscle tone.

The testing of the biceps, triceps, supinator (radial-periosteal), patellar, Achilles, and cutaneous abdominal and plantar reflexes provides an adequate sampling of reflex activity of the spinal cord.

Additional items of the motor examination are considered in Chaps. 3 to 6, which deal with motor paralysis, abnormalities of movement and posture, and disorders of stance and gait, respectively. Particulars of *sensory testing,* the most difficult part of the neurologic examination, are described in the chapters on pain and other forms of somatic sensation (Chaps. 7 and 8). The assessment of bladder, bowel, and other autonomic functions are considered in Chap. 26 and of CSF circulation and meningeal reactions in Chap. 30.

3. Examination of the Comatose, Psychiatric, and Pediatric Patient

In each of these situations, the neurologic examination, though subject to obvious limitations, may yield considerable information concerning nervous system function. Adaptation of the neurologic examination to the *stuporous or comatose* patient is considered in Chap. 16.

In the examination of *psychiatric patients,* one cannot always rely on their cooperation and one must always be critical of their statements and opinions. The depressed patient, for example, may complain of weakness or impairment of memory when neither is present; or the sociopath may feign paralysis. Information from a person who knows the patient intimately is mandatory. The special methods of examination of *infants and small children* are summarized in Chap. 27.

For a more detailed discussion of this topic, see Adams and Victor: *Principles of Neurology,* 4th ed, pp. 3–9.

ADDITIONAL READING

André-Thomas, Chesni Y, Dargassies St-Anne S: *The Neurological Examination of the Infant*. London, National Spastics Society, 1960.

Holmes G: *Introduction to Clinical Neurology,* 3rd ed. Revised by Bryan Matthews. Baltimore, Williams & Wilkins, 1968.

Mancall EL: *Alpers and Mancall's Essentials of the Neurologic Examination,* 2nd ed. Philadelphia, Davis, 1981.
Mayo Clinic and Mayo Foundation: *Clinical Examinations in Neurology,* 6th ed. St. Louis, Mosby/Year Book Publishers, 1991.
Ross RT: *How to Examine the Nervous System,* 2nd ed. New York, Medical Examination Publishing Co., 1985.

2 Special Techniques for Neurologic Diagnosis

Clinical analysis alone may prove adequate for diagnosis, but more often it must be supplemented by one or more ancillary examinations. The frequency with which one resorts to the latter depends in large measure on the type of clinical problem and on the clinical experience and confidence of the neurologist. In turning to the laboratory for help the neurologist should choose the one or two procedures that are most likely to solve the problem and not blindly subject the patient to one test after another. The thoughtful selection of laboratory procedures is part of the strategy of case study and the intelligent use of medical resources.

Without question, the most significant advance in neurology and neurosurgery since the discovery of the Roentgen rays has been the development of computed tomography (CT) and magnetic resonance imaging (MRI). For the first time one can visualize all parts of the brain in a living patient and many of the lesions residing within it, and this can be accomplished with practically no risk to the patient. A new branch of medical science, *biopathology,* has been created. The older, painful, and potentially dangerous techniques of pneumoencephalography and ventriculography have been eliminated and the need for angiography has been greatly reduced; the latter procedure is now used mainly to expose vascular diseases or in planning an operation on a vascular tumor. Contrast myelography is in the process of being replaced by MRI and CT scans of the spine. Plain films of the skull are relied upon only to reveal fractures. Even cerebrospinal fluid (CSF) examinations and electroencephalograms (EEGs) are being done less frequently, the former being restricted largely to the diagnosis of infective and noninfective inflammations of the meninges and the latter to the study of seizures and toxic and metabolic disturbances.

The following laboratory procedures have application to a diversity of neurologic diseases. Procedures that are pertinent to a particular disease or category of diseases are discussed in the chapters dealing with those diseases.

COMPUTERIZED TOMOGRAPHY (CT SCANNING)

In this procedure the attenuation coefficients of the skull, CSF, cerebral gray and white matter, and blood vessels are measured, with computer assistance, by more than 30,000 beams of x-ray directed successively at several horizontal or coronal levels of the cranium. The differing densities of bone and the intracranial (or intraspinal) contents are distinguishable in the resulting picture. One can see hemorrhages, arteriovenous malformations, softened and edematous tissue, abscesses, and neoplasms as well as the precise size and position of the ventricles and changes in brain volume. The radiation exposure is equivalent to that from plain skull films.

The latest models of CT scanners yield pictures of great clarity. One can see the cerebral convolutions and sulci, caudate and lenticular nuclei, internal capsules, thalamus and hypothalamus, optic nerves and ocular muscles, and brainstem and cerebellum. Destructive and invasive lesions of these parts are readily localized.

MAGNETIC RESONANCE IMAGING (MRI)

Formerly referred to as nuclear magnetic resonance or NMR, MRI is the newest form of imaging. Like the CT scan, MRI provides images of thin slices of the brain in any plane but has the great advantage of using nonionizing energy.

MRI is accomplished by placing the patient within a powerful magnetic field, which causes the protons of the tissues and CSF to align themselves in the orientation of the magnetic field. Introducing a specific radio frequency (RF) into the field causes the protons to resonate and to change their axes of alignment. Removal of the RF pulse allows the protons to relax, so to speak, and to resume their original alignment. The RF energy which was absorbed and then emitted is subjected to computer analysis, from which an image is constructed.

The images generated by the latest MRI machines are truly remarkable. One can measure the size of all discrete nuclear structures, there being a high degree of contrast between white and gray matter. Deep lesions of the temporal lobe and structures in the posterior fossa and at the cervicomedullary junction are seen much better than with CT; the structures can be displayed in three planes and are unmarred by bony artefact. Demyelinative lesions stand out with clarity. Each of the products of disintegrated red blood corpuscles—methemoglobin, hemosiderin, and ferritin—can be recognized, and this enables one to follow the resolution of hemorrhages. Infarcts can be seen at an earlier stage than by CT. Unfortunately, at the moment, the scans often show alterations of periventricular and central white matter that are uninterpretable, but they will soon be better understood.

The investigation of developmental defects of the nervous system by MRI is a new and promising field.

ANGIOGRAPHY

The injection of contrast material into cranial arteries permits the visualization of narrowed or occluded arteries and veins, arterial dissecting aneurysms, angiitis, vascular malformations, and saccular aneurysms. Since the advent of CT and MRI, the use of angiography has been more or less limited to the diagnosis of these disorders. The procedure consists of placing a needle in the femoral or brachial artery under local anesthesia; a canula is threaded through the needle and then along the aorta and the arterial branch (carotid, vertebral) that needs to be visualized. Highly skilled arteriographers can also inject the collateral branches of the spinal arteries and visualize vascular malformations of the spinal cord.

A refined angiographic technique—*digital subtraction angiography (DSA)*—uses digital computer processing to produce images of the major cervical arteries. The great advantage of DSA is that the vessels can be visualized with small amounts of dye. The contrast medium can be injected intravenously, but this requires a large amount of diluent, so that the arterial route is preferred. The resulting picture does not attain the resolution of the standard angiogram but is less expensive and safer than the latter, which still causes an occasional fatality and a 2.5 percent morbidity, mainly in the form of a worsening of a pre-existent vascular lesion.

Noninvasive methods of studying carotid artery disease—Doppler techniques and ultrasound—are discussed in Chap. 32.

Magnetic resonance angiography is a new noninvasive technique for visualizing the main intracranial arteries. It promises to replace angiography.

RADIOPAQUE MYELOGRAPHY

By injecting 5 to 25 mL of a water-soluble dye (e.g., iopamadole) through a lumbar puncture needle and then tilting the patient, the entire spinal subarachnoid space can be visualized. The procedure is almost as harmless as a lumbar puncture. Pantopaque, a fat-soluble dye, is still approved by the FDA but is now rarely used; if left in the subarachnoid space, particularly in the presence of blood or inflammatory exudate, it may incite a severe arachnoiditis of the spinal cord and brain. The use of a self-absorbing water-soluble dye, in combination with CT scanning, is a particularly useful method for visualizing the cervical spinal canal. All of these procedures are gradually being replaced by MRI.

CRANIAL AND SPINAL BONE SCANS

These procedures are of value in visualizing inflammatory and neoplastic lesions of bone, Paget disease, and collapsed vertebrae from osteomalacia. They may reveal bone lesions not seen in plain films.

ELECTROENCEPHALOGRAPHY (EEG)

EEG is essential in the study of patients with epilepsy and those with suspected seizure disorders. It is also helpful in evaluating the cerebral effects of toxic and metabolic diseases and in the study of sleep disorders.

The EEG comprises 8 to 16 or more separate amplifying units capable of recording from many areas of the scalp at the same time. The brain rhythms passing through cranial bones and scalp can be amplified to the point where they are strong enough to move an ink writing pen, producing the waveform activity in the range of 0.5 to 30 Hz (cycles per second) on a paper moving at 3 cm/s. The resulting EEG, in reality a voltage-versus-time graph, appears as a number of parallel wavy lines, as many as there are amplifying units or "channels." Electrodes, which usually are solder or silver-silver chloride discs 0.5 cm in diameter, are attached to the scalp by means of an adhesive material such as bentonite or collodion, using ECG paste to improve contact. Patients are usually examined with their eyes closed and while relaxed in a comfortable chair or bed for 45 to 90 min.

In addition to the resting record, it is common practice to use the following activating procedures: hyperventilation for 3 min, stroboscopic retinal stimulation at frequencies of 1 to 20 per second, and induced drowsiness or sleep. Examples of the normal EEG, seizure discharges, both focal and generalized, hepatic coma with confusion, and brain death are presented in Fig. 2-1. EEGs in the different stages of sleep are described in Chap. 18.

Magnetoencephalography is a highly refined noninvasive technique that measures the magnetic fields generated by active groups of nerve cells in the brain. It is being developed in several centers in the United States, with the idea of obviating the need for depth electrodes in the precise localization of epileptogenic foci.

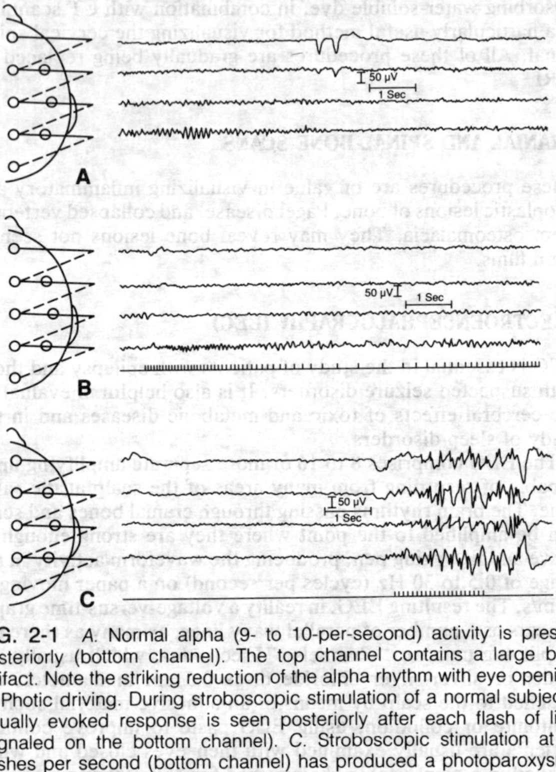

FIG. 2-1 *A.* Normal alpha (9- to 10-per-second) activity is present posteriorly (bottom channel). The top channel contains a large blink artifact. Note the striking reduction of the alpha rhythm with eye opening. *B.* Photic driving. During stroboscopic stimulation of a normal subject a visually evoked response is seen posteriorly after each flash of light (signaled on the bottom channel). *C.* Stroboscopic stimulation at 14 flashes per second (bottom channel) has produced a photoparoxysmal response in this epileptic patient, evidenced by the abnormal spike and slow-wave activity toward the end of the period of stimulation.

COMPUTERIZED EVOKED POTENTIALS

By the use of computers (instruments that have revolutionized neurology), one can summate the effects of several thousand visual, auditory, or tactile stimuli and trace them from the periphery to their cerebral terminations. This enables one to detect delays at several points along the course of these sensory systems even when there are no clinically manifest sensory symptoms. If visual, auditory, or tactile deficits are present, one can determine at what point the deficit lies. Recently it has been discovered that a single-pulse high-voltage stimulus applied to the vertex of the skull and over the cervical spine segments can

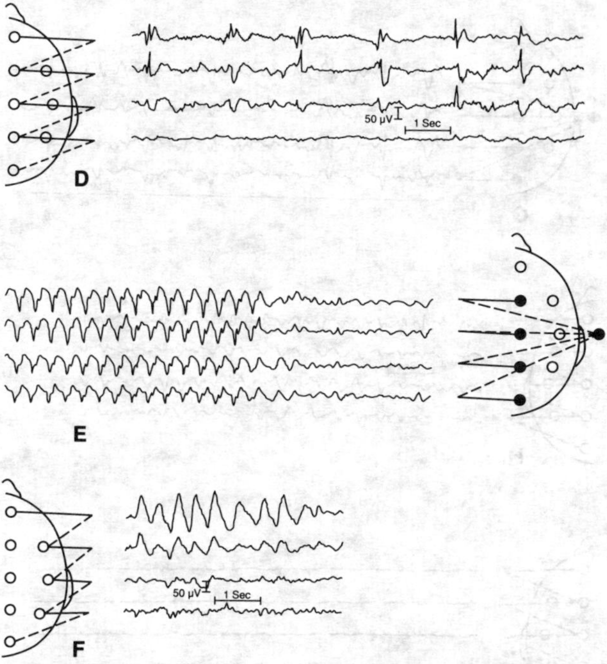

FIG. 2-1 (*continued*) *D.* EEG from patient with focal motor seizures of the left side. Note focal spike discharge in right frontal region (channels 1–3). The activity from the left hemisphere (not shown here) was relatively normal. *E.* Petit mal epilepsy, showing generalized 3-per-second spike-and-wave discharge. The abnormal activity ends abruptly and a normal background appears. *F.* Large, slow, irregular delta waves are seen in the right frontal region (channels 1 and 2). In this case a glioblastoma was found in the right cerebral hemisphere, but the EEG picture does not differ basically from that produced by a stroke, abscess, or contusion.

painlessly activate the motor cortex and corticospinal system and detect delays or lack of conduction in descending pathways.

LUMBAR PUNCTURE (LP) AND EXAMINATION OF CEREBROSPINAL FLUID (CSF)

The indications for an LP are as follows:

1. To obtain pressure measurements and to procure a sample of CSF for cellular, chemical, and bacteriologic examination.

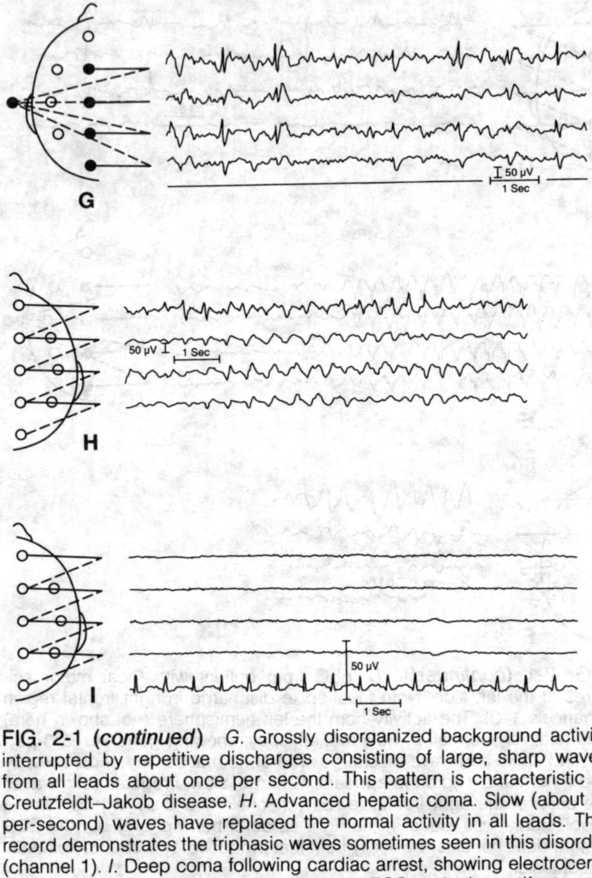

FIG. 2-1 (*continued*) *G.* Grossly disorganized background activity interrupted by repetitive discharges consisting of large, sharp waves from all leads about once per second. This pattern is characteristic of Creutzfeldt–Jakob disease. *H.* Advanced hepatic coma. Slow (about 2-per-second) waves have replaced the normal activity in all leads. This record demonstrates the triphasic waves sometimes seen in this disorder (channel 1). *I.* Deep coma following cardiac arrest, showing electrocerebral silence. With the highest amplification, ECG and other artifacts may be seen, so that the record is not truly "flat" or isoelectric. However, no cerebral rhythms are visible. Note the ECG (channel 5). *(Illustrations courtesy of Dr. Susan Chester.)*

2. To administer spinal anesthetics and antibiotic and antitumor medication.
3. To inject a radiopaque substance, as in myelography, or a radioactive agent, as in scintigraphic cisternography.

Lumbar puncture carries a risk of inducing or aggravating a temporal lobe or cerebellar herniation if the intracranial pressure (ICP) is very high. Therefore, if a high ICP is suspected, the LP should be preceded by CT or MRI, which with clinical data may yield sufficient diagnostic information to obviate the need for an LP.

Cisternal puncture and high cervical subarachnoid puncture are also safe procedures but should be done only by someone skilled in their performance.

The pressure of CSF should always be measured with the patient in a horizontal lateral decubitus position. Normally it ranges from 80 to 180 mmH_2O, and if the needle is properly placed, small pulse and respiratory excursions are seen. If the pressure is high (>400 mmH_2O), one should obtain the needed sample of fluid and then, according to the suspected disease and patient's condition, administer a unit of urea or mannitol and watch the pressure in the manometer until it falls. Dexamethasone should then be given in an intravenous dose of 10 mg.

The gross appearance of the CSF is noted, and samples are sent to the laboratory for some or all of the following tests: number and types of cells and presence of micro-organisms; protein and glucose content (with simultaneous blood glucose measurement); exfoliative cytology using a Millipore filtered or ultracentrifuged specimen; protein electrophoresis and immunoelectrophoresis for determination of gamma globulin, other protein fractions, oligoclonal bands, and the IgG-albumin index; biochemical tests for pigments, lactate, NH_3, pH, CO_2, enzymes, etc.; and bacteriologic cultures and virus isolation.

The CSF examination is essential in detecting meningeal inflammation, subarachnoid hemorrhage, and meningeal neoplasms. It carries essentially no risk if the CT and/or MRI shows no mass lesion and papilledema is absent.

ELECTROMYOGRAPHY AND NERVE CONDUCTION TESTS

These will be described in Chap. 43.

PERIMETRY, AUDIOMETRY, AND TESTS OF LABYRINTHINE FUNCTION

These tests will be described in Chaps. 12 and 14.

Biopsy of muscle and nerve is discussed in Chap. 43. Biopsies of skin, conjunctivum, and brain are sometimes diagnostic and will be mentioned in relation to the particular diseases in which they are indicated.

In addition to these many special laboratory techniques, one often obtains useful information about metabolic disorders of the brain by analysis of blood samples for O_2, CO_2, glucose, urea or NPN, NH_3, Na, K, Mg, Ca, thyroxin, cortisol, and amino acids.

For a more detailed discussion of this topic, see Adams and Victor: *Principles of Neurology*, 4th ed, pp 10–31.

ADDITIONAL READING

Brant-Zawadzki M, Norman D: *Magnetic Resonance Imaging of the Central Nervous System*. New York, Raven Press, 1987.

Chiappa KH: *Evoked Potentials in Clinical Neurology*. New York, Raven Press, 1983.

Fishman RA: *Cerebrospinal Fluid in Diseases of the Nervous System*. Philadelphia, Saunders, 1980.

Marsden CD, Merton PA, Morton HB: Direct electrical stimulation of corticospinal pathways through the intact scalp and in human subjects. *Adv Neurol* 39:387, 1983.

Niedermeyer E, Da Silva FL: *Electroencephalography*, 2nd ed. Baltimore, Urban and Schwarzenberg, 1987.

II CARDINAL MANIFESTATIONS OF NEUROLOGIC DISEASE

SECTION I
DISORDERS OF MOTILITY

A large part of the human nervous system is engaged in converting sensation, emotion, and thought into movement. The neural arrangements for motor control are to a considerable extent automatic and unconscious and are integrated at many levels, from the lowermost spinal cord to the cerebral cortex. In medical practice, disorders of motility are customarily subdivided, according to their anatomy and physiology, into several types: motor paralysis; abnormalities of movement and posture; tremor, myoclonus, spasms, and tics; and disorders of stance and gait. These disorders are the subject of the following four chapters.

3 | Motor Paralysis

The terms *paralysis, plegia,* and *palsy* are used interchangeably. Paresis refers to partial paralysis. On the basis of clinical examination and physiologic study, two types of paralysis can be recognized: (1) that due to affection of lower motor neurons and (2) that due to affection of the corticospinal system (upper motor neurons).

AFFECTION OF LOWER MOTOR NEURONS

Anatomic and Physiologic Considerations

The *lower motor neurons* include all the anterior horn cells (alpha neurons) of the spinal cord and the somatic motor neurons of the brainstem. By way of its axon, each motor neuron innervates from 20 to 1000 or more muscle fibers; together these elements constitute the *motor unit*, also called the *final common pathway*. All variations in force, range, and speed of movement are determined by the number and size of motor units and their rates of discharge. Destruction of the motor nerve cell or its axon paralyzes all the muscle fibers that it innervates regardless of whether they are engaged in reflex or voluntary activity. In some conditions (e.g., motor system disease, ventral root compression), the motor neuron becomes abnormally irritable, resulting in spontaneous contraction of all its muscle fibers. This is manifest clinically as a coarse twitch or *fasciculation* and, if many units are involved, as cramps or spasms. Fasciculations, which are often benign, differ from the smaller independent contractions of individual denervated muscle fibers, which are called fibrillations and are detectable only by electromyography.

The axons of many motor nerve cells form the anterior roots and motor cranial nerves, and many of the roots intermingle to form plexuses. From the latter emerge individual nerves wherein motor fibers are mixed with sensory and autonomic ones. Each large muscle is usually supplied by several adjacent roots but usually by only a single nerve. Therefore, the pattern of paralysis following disease of anterior horn cells and roots differs from that following interruption of individual nerves.

Any given movement requires the activity of many muscles, some acting as prime movers or agonists, others as antagonists, fixators, or synergists. These relationships are integrated in the spinal cord or brainstem, an arrangement known as *reciprocal innervation*. Complex motor activities such as the maintenance of posture, stance and gait, and the performance of voluntary and habitual actions depend on intersegmental spinal mechanisms and their integration with corticospinal and other suprasegmental systems.

The phasic, *myotatic or tendon reflex* depends on the sudden stretch-excitation of the muscle spindles which lie in parallel with muscle fibers (Fig. 3-1). The afferent volley of impulses is carried to the corresponding spinal segment and makes a direct (monosynaptic) connection with the alpha motor neurons. The gamma motor neurons keep the muscle fibers of the spindle in a proper state of tension. There are also inhibitory segmental mechanisms, mediated peripherally in muscle by Golgi tendon organs and in the spinal cord by Renshaw and other cells.

The nociceptive or flexor-withdrawal reflex is activated by the excitation of A-δ and C fibers; this excites polysynaptically many anterior horn cells (which flex the limb) and other motor neurons, which inhibit extensor antigravity muscles.

When all or practically all the peripheral motor fibers to a group of muscles are interrupted, all voluntary, postural, and reflex movements are lost. The paralyzed muscles become lax and soft and offer little or no resistance to passive stretching. This state, referred to as *flaccidity,* is due to a loss of normal

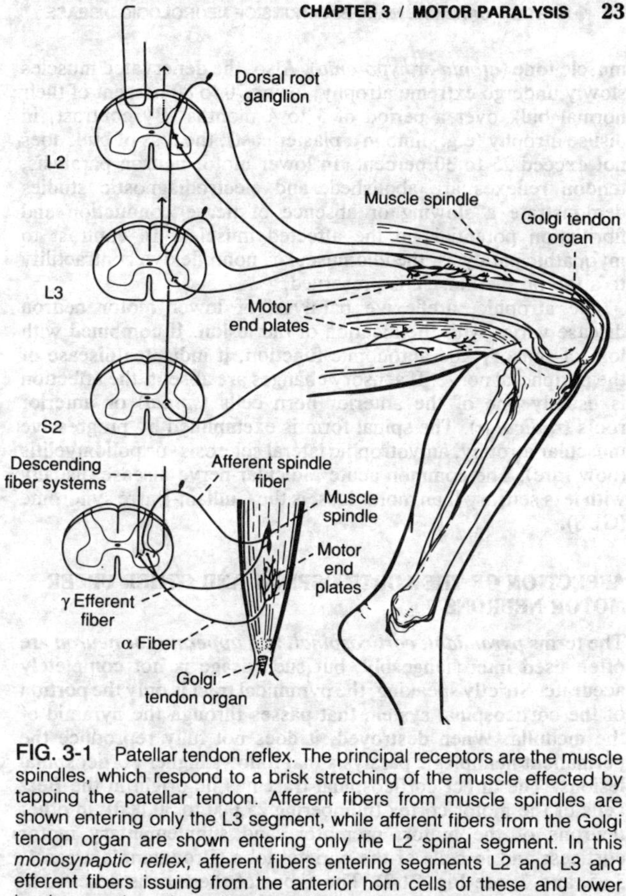

FIG. 3-1 Patellar tendon reflex. The principal receptors are the muscle spindles, which respond to a brisk stretching of the muscle effected by tapping the patellar tendon. Afferent fibers from muscle spindles are shown entering only the L3 segment, while afferent fibers from the Golgi tendon organ are shown entering only the L2 spinal segment. In this *monosynaptic reflex*, afferent fibers entering segments L2 and L3 and efferent fibers issuing from the anterior horn cells of these and lower levels complete the reflex arc. Motor fibers shown leaving the S2 spinal segment and passing to the hamstring muscles demonstrate the *disynaptic* pathway by which inhibitory influences are exerted upon an antagonistic muscle group.

The small diagram illustrates the gamma loop. Gamma efferent fibers pass to the muscle spindle. Contractions of the intrafusal fibers in the polar parts of the spindle stretch the nuclear bag region and cause an afferent impulse to be conducted centrally. The afferent fibers from the spindle synapse with many alpha motor neurons, the peripheral processes of which pass to extrafusal muscle fibers, thus completing the loop. Both alpha and gamma motor neurons are influenced by descending fiber systems from supraspinal levels. (*Redrawn from Carpenter and Sutin.*)

muscle tone (*atonia* or *hypotonia*). Also, the denervated muscles slowly undergo extreme atrophy, losing 70 to 80 percent of their normal bulk over a period of 3 to 4 months. By contrast, in disuse atrophy (e.g., limb in a plaster cast), the loss of bulk does not exceed 25 to 30 percent. In lower motor neuron paralysis, tendon reflexes are abolished, and electrodiagnostic studies demonstrate a slowing or absence of nerve conduction and fibrillation potentials in the affected muscles. In contrast to myopathic paralysis, the idiomuscular, nonreflexive contractility to a tap on the muscle is preserved.

The atrophic, areflexive paralysis of lower motor neuron disease varies with the location of the lesion. If combined with loss of sensory and autonomic function, it indicates disease of the peripheral nerve. If sensory changes are absent, the affection is usually one of the anterior horn cells (*spinal*) or anterior roots (*radicular*). The spinal form is exemplified by progressive muscular atrophy, amyotrophic lateral sclerosis, or poliomyelitis (now rare). The common acute radicular-nerve disease, usually with less sensory than motor loss, is the Guillain-Barré syndrome (GBS).

AFFECTION OF THE CORTICOSPINAL AND OTHER UPPER MOTOR NEURONS

The terms *pyramidal, corticospinal,* and *upper motor neuron* are often used interchangeably, but such usage is not completely accurate. Strictly speaking, the pyramidal tract is only the portion of the corticospinal system that passes through the pyramid of the medulla. When destroyed, it does not fully reproduce the permanent hemiplegic paralysis that follows higher corticospinal lesions. The direct corticospinal tract has its origin in the Betz cells of the motor cortex (numbering 25,000 to 30,000); in other neurons of the motor, premotor, and supplementary motor cortices; and in cells of the parietal lobe (Brodmann's areas 1, 3, 5, and 7; see Fig. 21-2). The axons of these cells descend in the corona radiata, posterior limb of the internal capsule, cerebral peduncle, basis pontis, and medullary pyramid (Fig. 3-2). At the junction of the medulla and spinal cord, the majority of these fibers decussate and descend as the crossed lateral corticospinal pathway, synapsing at various segmental levels of the spinal cord—the majority with internuncial neurons (which in turn project to anterior horn cells) and the remainder (20 to 25 percent) directly with anterior horn cells. A smaller contingent of direct corticospinal tract fibers does not decussate and descends as the uncrossed anterior and lateral corticospinal tracts.

In the brainstem, the corticospinal tracts are accompanied by

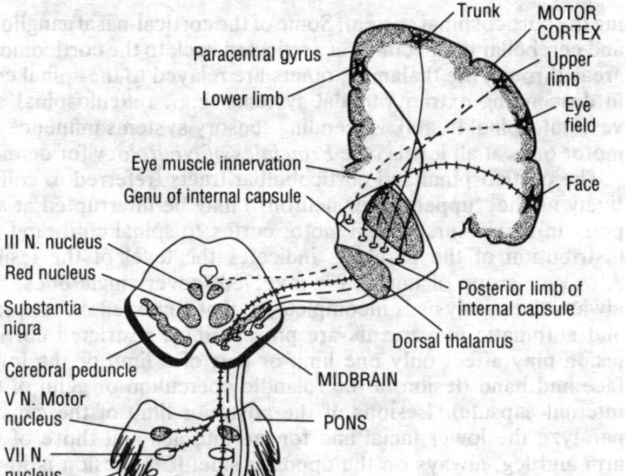

FIG. 3-2 The corticospinal and corticobulbar pathways, from their origin in the cerebral cortex to their nuclei of termination. Variable lines indicate the trajectories from particular parts of the cortex.

the corticobulbar tracts, which are distributed to the motor nuclei of the cranial nerves. Other offshoots of the corticospinal tracts are to the red nuclei, forming the corticorubrospinal tract, the reticular formations of the brainstem (corticoreticulospinal), the mesencephalic tectum (corticotectospinal), the vestibular nuclei (corticovestibulospinal), and the pontine nuclei and cerebellum (corticopontocerebellar). These descending corticobrainstem-spinal fibers are also involved in volitional movement, supplementing the corticospinal system. Some of the cortical-basal ganglionic and cerebellar connections are reflected back to the corticomotor areas through the thalamus; others are relayed to the spinal cord in descending extrapyramidal systems (e.g., reticulospinal and vestibulospinal tracts). Ascending sensory systems influence the motor ones at all levels (see *Principles of Neurology* for details).

The corticospinal and corticobulbar tracts (referred to collectively as the "upper motor neuron") may be interrupted at any point in their course, from motor cortex to spinal cord, and the distribution of the paralysis indicates the level of the lesion. Always a group of muscles is involved, never single ones, and always the paralysis is incomplete, in that some reflex, postural, and automatic movements are preserved. A restricted cortical lesion may affect only one limb or part of a limb or the lower face and hand (lesion in the rolandic operculum or genu of the internal capsule). Lesions of the posterior limb of the capsule paralyze the lower facial and tongue muscles and those of the arm and leg, always on the opposite side; if the lesion is in the left hemisphere, an aphasia may be added. Lesions at the lower pontine and medullary levels leave the face, tongue, and muscles of speech unaffected. The hand and arm are usually affected more severely than the foot and leg. Another general principle is that parts of the body most used for delicate individual movements, viz., the fingers and hand, suffer the most from purely corticospinal lesions. In a total suprasegmental hemiplegia, other corticobrainstem connections are interrupted as well. Muscles that are engaged in bilateral, automatic, and reflexive movements, such as respiration, are little, if at all, affected.

With lesions of the cerebrum and upper brainstem, *tone* of the paralyzed muscles is not altered in a consistent manner. The tendon reflexes, which at first are slightly reduced or unchanged, later become more active. Also there are *postural changes*. The arm gradually becomes flexed and adducted and the leg extended; and the limbs become spastic. The flexors of hip, leg, and foot and the extensors of arm, hand, and fingers are weaker than their opposing muscles. Attempts at voluntary movement of a hand or foot may increase the tone or cause involuntary contraction of an entire limb (synkinesia). With acute lesions of the cervical or thoracic spinal segments, muscle tone and tendon reflexes may be abolished in the legs for days or weeks, a condition known as "spinal shock" (see Chap. 34). Spasticity is revealed by the patient's attempts at active movement and by passive movement. In the latter, there is first a nonresistant "free interval" followed by a catch and rapidly increasing resistance, which gradually yields as the passive stretch is continued (clasp-knife phenomenon). In these ways spasticity differs from rigidity, which is described in the next chapter. The hyperreflexive state often gives rise to clonus, which is a series of rhythmic involuntary muscular contractions in response to an abruptly applied and sustained passive or active stretching of a muscle group. It is most easily evoked at the ankle, knee, and wrist. Its basis is a hyperexcitability of spinal motor neurons, which are released or disinhibited by the corticospinal lesions. The cutaneomuscular (abdominal and cremasteric) reflexes are abolished and nocifensive spinal reflexes, of which the Babinski sign is a part, are released. The latter sign is most consistently elicited by stroking the lateral side of the sole with a key or pin, but when the flexor reflexes are greatly enhanced, even pinching or touching any part of the foot or leg may evoke dorsiflexion of the toes and foot and flexion of the knee and hip. Usually, with an established corticospinal lesion, both a Babinski sign and heightened tendon reflexes are present; but since they depend on different mechanisms, they need not appear together or persist together in chronic paralysis. With bilateral cerebral lesions the cranial muscles may be paralyzed and their stretch reflexes exaggerated; i.e., jaw and buccal jerks are increased (pseudobulbar palsy, see below).

While convenient to think of motility in terms of upper and lower motor neurons, this is a gross simplification. All segments of the spinal cord are integrated in posture and movement, under control of the cerebellar, vestibular, and other brainstem systems, the basal ganglia, and the motor cortex. Even the simple act of scratching an insect bite with one hand involves a minimum of 19 limb muscles and 17 postural ones, most of them acting involuntarily. (See Chap. 34 for further discussion of brainstem-spinal mechanisms.)

Diagnosis of Paralytic States

The term *monoplegia* designates a paralysis of one limb; *hemiplegia,* paralysis of an arm and leg on the same side; *paraplegia* (sometimes referred to as *diplegia*), paralysis of both legs; and *quadriplegia* or *tetraplegia,* paralysis of all four extremities.

Bulbar palsy refers to weakness or paralysis of the muscles innervated by the motor nuclei of the lower brainstem, i.e., muscles of the face, tongue, larynx, and pharynx. The paralysis may be atrophic and flaccid (i.e., lower motor neuron in type), in which case it is most often due to a degeneration of the lower cranial motor nuclei, as occurs in amyotrophic lateral sclerosis. If both corticobulbar pathways are interrupted, voluntary movements of the bulbar musculature are paralyzed, whereas reflexive movements are retained or heightened; this state is referred to as *spastic bulbar* or *"pseudobulbar" palsy* (see also p. 199).

An *atrophic monoplegia* with loss of tendon reflexes points to a lesion of the anterior horn cells or to a lesion of the peripheral nerves if there are sensory or autonomic changes. Without atrophy or reflex loss, monoplegia suggests a unilateral spinal cord or, rarely, a cerebral cortical-subcortical lesion.

Hemiplegia with retained or heightened reflexes is the common manifestation of a lesion in the cerebral white matter, internal capsule, cerebral peduncle, basis pontis, or pyramid. Usually it is due to vascular disease, less often to trauma, tumor, or an infective or demyelinative process. If facial muscles are spared, the lesion is in the lower brainstem or high cervical cord. Since brainstem and cord lesions are often bilateral, other motor cranial nerve or nonmotor signs may be added and indicate the level of the corticospinal lesion.

Paraplegia with retained reflexes (except during the period of spinal shock) indicates involvement of the motor pathways in the thoracic or upper lumbar cord; *quadriplegia* points to interruption of motor tracts in the cervical cord, brainstem, or both cerebral hemispheres. Lesions of the gray matter of the spinal cord may cause an atrophic, areflexive paralysis of the legs or arms.

Paralysis of individual muscles points to a peripheral nerve lesion.

One must always remember that motor paralysis may occur in the absence of any disease in the central or peripheral nervous systems. Conditions such as myasthenia gravis, familial periodic paralysis, severe endocrine and electrolytic disturbances, and botulinus poisoning comprise this category and are considered in the section on diseases of muscle. Also, paralysis is the most common manifestation of *hysteria* or *malingering*. Usually such a diagnosis is suggested by inconsistencies of voluntary contraction (ability to perform some acts but not others that utilize the same muscles), an obvious lack of effort, lack of reflex changes, and the presence of other symptoms and signs of hysteria (see Chap. 53).

Finally, it should be noted that there may be a loss of learned patterns of movement in the absence of upper or lower motor neuron signs, ataxia, or extrapyramidal disorder. This is called *apraxia* and is described in Chap. 21.

For a more detailed discussion of this topic, see Adams and Victor: *Principles of Neurology,* 4th ed, pp 37–53.

ADDITIONAL READING

Alexander GE, Delong M: Organization of supraspinal motor systems, in Asbury AK, McKhann GM, McDonald WI (eds): *Diseases of the Nervous System*. Philadelphia, Saunders, 1986, chap 26, pp 352–369.

Asanuma H: The pyramidal tract, in Brooks VB (ed): *Handbook of Physiology, Sec 1: The Nervous System, vol 2: Motor Control*. Bethesda, MD, American Physiological Society, 1981, chap 15, pp 702–733.

Brodal A: Pathways mediating supraspinal influences on the spinal cord—The basal ganglia, in *Neurological Anatomy in Relation to Clinical Medicine*, 3rd ed. New York, Oxford University Press, 1981, chap 4, pp 180–293.

Carpenter MD, Satin J: *Human Neuroanatomy*, 8th ed. Baltimore, Williams & Wilkins, 1983.

Lance JW: The control of muscle tone, reflexes and movement: Robert Wartenburg Lecture. *Neurology* 30:1303, 1980.

Ropper AH, Fisher CM, Kleinman GM: Pyramidal infarction in the medulla: A cause of pure motor hemiplegia sparing the face. *Neurology* 29:91, 1979.

4 Abnormalities of Movement and Posture Due to Disease of the Extrapyramidal System

Here we shall consider a second group of motor abnormalities, which do not reduce muscular power but render it less effective because of rigidity, incoordination, alterations of posture, or the interposition of involuntary movements. These disorders are attributable to lesions of the basal ganglia (caudate and lenticular nuclei, subthalamic nucleus, substantia nigra, red nucleus, and pontomesencephalic reticular formation) and cerebellum.

In health, the extrapyramidal motor functions are blended with and modulated by the corticospinal and corticobulbar motor systems described in Chap. 3. Physiologic studies of primates inform us that in the performance of all planned and learned movements, the basal ganglia and cerebellum, which are partly under cerebral-cortical control, are activated before the cortico-spinal-corticobulbar systems. Also, the effects of lesions in these structures have tended to blur the distinction between the corticospinal and extrapyramidal systems. Nevertheless, such a division remains clinically useful (Table 4-1).

The extrapyramidal motor system is conventionally subdivided into two parts: (1) the basal ganglia (striatonigral system) and (2) the cerebellum.

STRIATONIGRAL DISORDERS

As indicated in Figs. 4-1 and 4-2, the premotor and supplementary motor cortices send fibers to the caudate nucleus and putamen (together referred to as the striatum), and the latter structures in turn project to the lateral and medial parts of the pallidum, the reticular (nonpigmented) part of the substantia nigra, and the thalamus. The putamen and caudate nuclei receive recurrent fibers from the pigmented cells of the substantia nigra. From the pallidum, particularly its medial segment, two bundles of efferent fibers—the ansa and fasciculus lenticularis—sweep medially and caudally to join the thalamic fasciculus, a major pathway of ascending efferent fibers from the dentate and red nuclei. Together these fasciculi project onto the ventrolateral nucleus of the thalamus, which in turn projects fibers to the precentral motor cortex (mainly area 6 and to a lesser extent area 8). A

TABLE 4-1 Clinical Differences between Corticospinal and Extrapyramidal Syndromes

	Corticospinal	Extrapyramidal
Character of the alteration of muscle tone	Clasp-knife effect (spasticity)	Plastic, equal throughout passive movement (rigidity), or intermittent (cogwheel rigidity); hypotonia in cerebellar disease
Distribution of hypertonus	Flexors of arms, extensors of legs	Flexors (predominantly) and extensors of all four limbs; flexors of trunk
Shortening and lengthening reaction	Present	Absent
Involuntary movements	Absent	Presence of tremor, chorea, athetosis, dystonia
Tendon reflexes	Increased	Normal or slightly increased
Babinski sign	Present	Absent
Paralysis of voluntary movement	Present	Absent or slight

second, more complex loop beginning in the association areas of the cerebral cortex projects to the caudate nucleus and thalamus and then back to the prefrontal cortex. In addition, there are several subsidiary loops involving the centromedian and parafascicular and mesencephalic tegmental and subthalamic nuclei.

The association cortex, via its projecting loops through the basal ganglia, is activated in the initial phases of planned movement. The ventral tier of thalamic nuclei integrate basal ganglionic and cerebellar impulses and bring them to bear on the corticospinal system.

Physiologically, the basal ganglia have been thought to function as a kind of clearing house, in which, during any intended or projected movement, one set of motor activities is facilitated and other unnecessary ones are suppressed.

Extensive lesions of the extrapyramidal motor system liberate a number of abnormalities of posture that are normally under brainstem control. The ones most clearly evidenced by disease are decerebrate rigidity and the antigravity support and righting reflexes. *In decerebrate rigidity,* in which the vestibular nuclei are separated from upper brainstem influences, all four extremities or

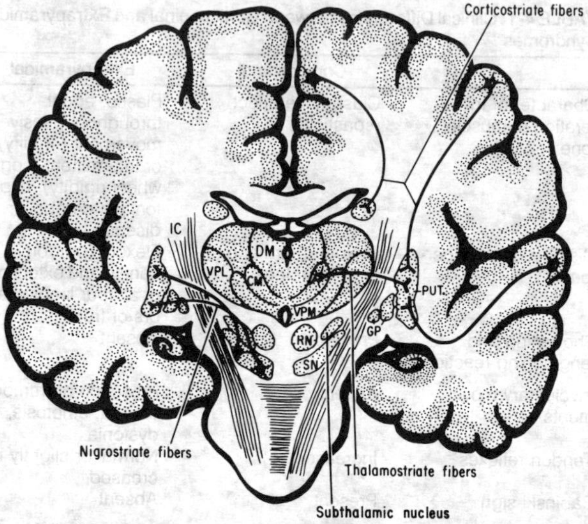

FIG. 4-1 Diagram of the striatal afferent pathways. *Corticostriate* fibers from broad cortical areas project to the putamen; fibers from the cortex on the medial surface project largely to the caudate nucleus. *Nigrostriatal* fibers arise from the pars compacta of the substantia nigra. *Thalamostriate* fibers arise from the centromedian-parafascicular complex of the thalamus. CM, centromedian nucleus; DM, dorsomedial nucleus; GP, globus pallidus; IC, internal capsule; PUT, putamen; RN, red nucleus; SN, substantia nigra; VPL, ventral posterolateral nucleus; VPM, ventral posterior medial nucleus.

the arm and leg on one side (ipsilateral to a unilateral lesion) are extended and the cervical and thoracolumbar portions of the spine are dorsiflexed; tonic neck reflexes can usually be elicited. Disorders of postural fixation and righting are demonstrated most clearly in the parkinsonian patient (see below).

Lesions that involve the corticospinal tracts predominantly result not only in paralysis of the contralateral limbs but also in the development of a fixed posture, in which the arm is maintained in flexion and the leg in extension (*decorticate posture*)

Pharmacologic studies have identified dopamine (synthesized from tyrosine and hydroxyphenylalanine to norepinephrine and epinephrine) as the nigrostriatal transmitter. The steps in the biosynthesis of the catecholamines are indicated in Table 4-2. Dopamine is elaborated by pigmented nigral cells and activates receptors on striatal cells. The other important transmitters and

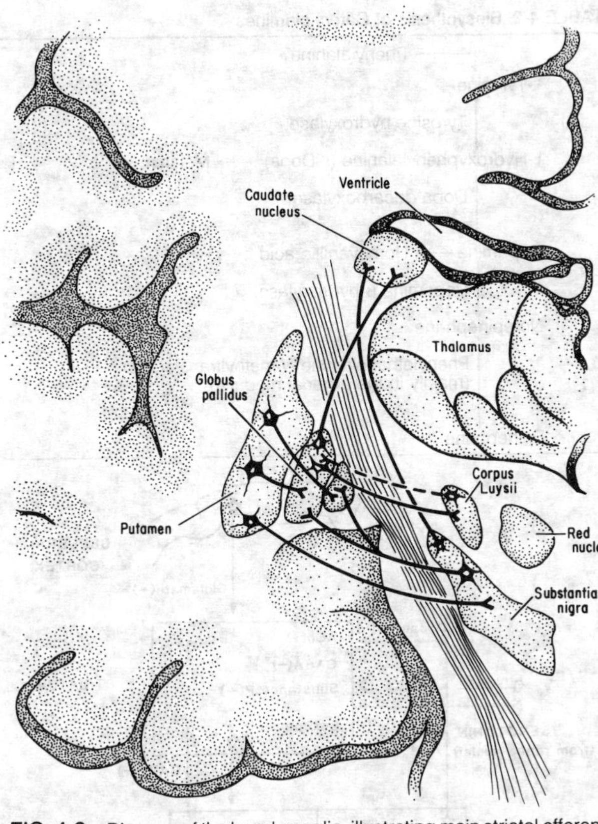

FIG. 4-2 Diagram of the basal ganglia, illustrating main striatal efferents (see text for details).

pathways involved in basal ganglionic function are illustrated in Fig. 4-3 and are described in the *Principles*.

Manifestations of Basal Ganglia Disease

In one class of extrapyramidal diseases exemplified by the Parkinson syndrome, the primary deficit is *akinesia* or *hypokinesia,* terms that refer to a disinclination of the patient to move or to use an affected part of the body. The resultant underactivity,

TABLE 4-2 Biosynthesis of Catecholamines

Phenylalanine
↓
L-Tyrosine
↓ Tyrosine hydroxylase
L-Hydroxyphenylalanine (L-Dopa) ⟶ Melanin
↓ Dopa decarboxylase
Dopamine ⟶ Homovanillic acid
↓ Dopamine β-hydroxylase
Norepinephrine
↓ Phenylethanolamine *N*-methyltransferase (mainly in the adrenal medulla)
Epinephrine

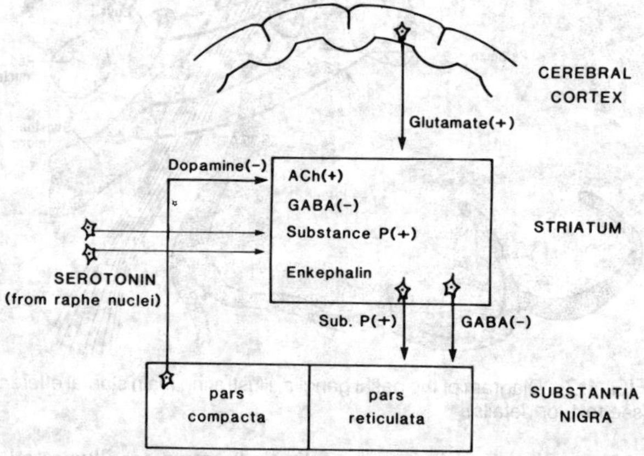

FIG. 4-3 Diagram of the chemical transmitters and pathways involved in basal ganglionic function. The symbols (+) and (−) indicate excitatory and inhibitory effects, respectively. The striatal transmitters are synthesized and released by small cells within that structure. Arrows indicate putative transmitter pathways. (*Adapted from Growdon and Fink.*)

or *poverty of movement,* extends to all of the small automatic postural adjustments which every normal person is constantly making ("the patient sits still"). Also, volitional and commanded movements are somewhat slow in being initiated (*reaction time delay*) and in being executed (*bradykinesia*). The basic defect appears to be an inadequacy of activation of the agonist (prime mover) muscles. Alternating movements are particularly hampered. Bradykinesia is regularly attended by rigidity but is not caused by it.

Rigidity is the second component of the Parkinson syndrome. The increase in tone is of plastic type, imparting an even resistance in agonists and antagonists from the start of a passive movement and throughout its range. There is no significant loss of muscle power or increase in tendon reflexes.

A rhythmic, 4- to 5-per-second, *tremor* in repose ("resting" tremor), affecting mainly the fingers, arm, and chin, is the third component and is described in Chap. 5. During passive stretching of a hypertonic muscle, slight degrees of the tremor are felt as the "cogwheel phenomenon."

These abnormalities are associated with a tendency to flexed postures—head down on chest, shoulders rounded, and arms and knees slightly flexed. Other important manifestations are a loss of righting reactions and disorders of equilibrium and postural fixation. The standing or sitting patient cannot make appropriate postural adjustments to tilting or falling. These deficits underlie the characteristic abnormality of gait, in which the patient makes a series of steps forward or backward, as though chasing his center of gravity (*festination*). Falls are frequent. Impassivity of facial expression and infrequent blinking complete the clinical picture.

The foregoing components of the Parkinson syndrome are most often manifestations of nigrostriatal lesions, but more widespread lesions involving striatum, pallidium, and substantia nigra may be associated with rigidity alone.

Involuntary movements—chorea, ballism, athetosis, and dystonia—are the other common signs of basal ganglionic disease.

Chorea refers to arrhythmic movements of a forcible, rapid, jerky type, affecting the fingers, hand, an entire limb, or some other part of the body. Grimacing and respiratory sounds are other expressions of the same disorder. Between movements the affected limbs tend to be slack. Chorea may be limited to one side of the body, i.e., hemichorea, and when the movements involve the proximal muscles of the limb and are unusually violent and flinging in nature, the disorder is referred to as *hemiballismus*. Of all the movement disorders, hemiballismus has the most consistent pathologic anatomy. The lesion in such cases is in or near the subthalamic nucleus (of Luys) of the opposite side.

Chorea is the major manifestation of Sydenham chorea and chorea gravidarum. It is also a feature of Huntington disease, but in the latter the tendency is more for the choreic movements to be confluent, i.e., choreoathetotic. Hemichorea or hemichoreoathetosis may follow recovery from hemiplegia. Excessive L-dopa in Parkinson patients results in restricted or generalized choreoathetosis, and the latter is also the most common form of tardive dyskinesia (see p. 344).

Athetosis is the term given to relatively slow, sinuous, patterned involuntary movements in which attitudes of extreme flexion and extension have a tendency to flow into one another. Between movements, the affected limbs may be spastic or rigid, depending on the anatomy of the underlying disease, but often there are abrupt lapses with hypotonia. Cocontraction of agonists and antagonists interferes with effective projected movements, and efforts to contract one agonist group may spread to involve adjacent unneeded muscles (*intention spasm*).

Athetosis may be generalized—as in Huntington disease, double athetosis (due to perinatal hypoxia), chronic hepatic encephalopathy, drug intoxication (phenothiazines, haloperidol, L-dopa), and a variety of degenerative diseases of the basal ganglia (see Chap. 41)—or it may be restricted to one group of cervical or cranial muscles—as in the oromandibular and tardive dyskinesias (p. 344). A rare paroxysmal form of choreoathetosis occurs in certain families.

Athetosis and chorea are aggravated by fatigue and emotion and attenuated by repose.

Dystonia, or torsion spasm, is manifested as an attitude or posture in one or other of the extremes of athetoid movement, with a predilection for muscles of the trunk and limb girdles and a tendency to persist. Dystonic postures may at first be reversible, or phasic, but later they may become fixed, as in the advanced stages of hemiplegia or Parkinson disease. Like choreoathetosis, dystonia occurs as a manifestation of many heredodegenerative diseases, as an acute or chronic reaction to certain drugs (phenothiazines, buterophenones), or as a restricted form of extrapyramidal disease—affecting facial, oromandibular, tongue, cervical, and hand muscles (see *Principles* for details).

Actually, choreic, athetotic, and dystonic movements so often overlap that distinctions between them are probably not fundamental. To compound the difficulty, tremor, myoclonus, and ataxia are added in some cases. Some writers on this subject avoid ambiguities of classification by calling them all dyskinesias.

Several aspects of the pathophysiology of involuntary movements have now been clarified. In dopamine-evoked athetosis, some elements of the putamen appear to be overactive. In monkeys, lesions of the subthalamic nucleus, which normally exerts a strong inhibitory influence upon the globus pallidus and ventral thalamus, produce a "choreoid dyskinesia" of the opposite arm and leg; with removal of this regulatory effect, bursts of irregular choreoid activity are recorded in the intact pallidum, where they are believed to arise. Moreover, the choreoid dyskinesia is abolished by a second lesion in the pallidum or in pallidofugal fibers or in the ventrolateral nucleus of the thalamus. It is postulated that the choreoathetotic movements of Huntington disease are also pallidal release effects from lesions in the striatum.

INCOORDINATION OF MOVEMENT (ATAXIA) DUE TO DISEASE OF THE CEREBELLUM

The structure and function of the cerebellum are somewhat better known than those of other parts of the nervous system. In the broadest terms, the organ can be subdivided into three parts (Fig. 4-4):

1. The *flocculonodular lobe,* which is phylogenetically the oldest part (hence *archicerebellum*). This part is also known as the "vestibulocerebellum," since its main afferent projections are from the vestibular nuclei; it is concerned mainly with the maintenance of equilibrium.
2. The *anterior lobe,* or *paleocerebellum,* consisting essentially of the anterior vermis and paravermian cortex. It is also called the "spinocerebellum," since its afferent projections are from proprioceptors of muscles and tendons of the limbs via the spinocerebellar tracts. The main influence of the spinocerebellum is on posture and muscle tone.
3. The *posterior lobes,* or *neocerebellum,* consist of the middle portions of the vermis and their large lateral extensions; they form the major portions of the cerebellar hemispheres. The latter receive afferent fibers from the cerebral cortex via the pontine nuclei and brachii pontis (hence "pontocerebellum") and are concerned primarily with coordination of skilled movements that are initiated at a cerebral cortical level.

The efferent connections of the cerebellar cortex, consisting essentially of the axons of Purkinje cells, terminate on the deep cerebellar nuclei. These in turn project to the cerebral cortex and certain brainstem nuclei via two main pathways: (1) the dentatorubrothalamic and dentatothalamic pathways. From the terminus of these pathways, in the ventrolateral thalamic nucleus, there is a projection to the precentral cortex; and (2) the fastigiovestibular pathways, to the vestibular and brainstem reticular nuclei. Thus, the cerebellum influences spinal motor

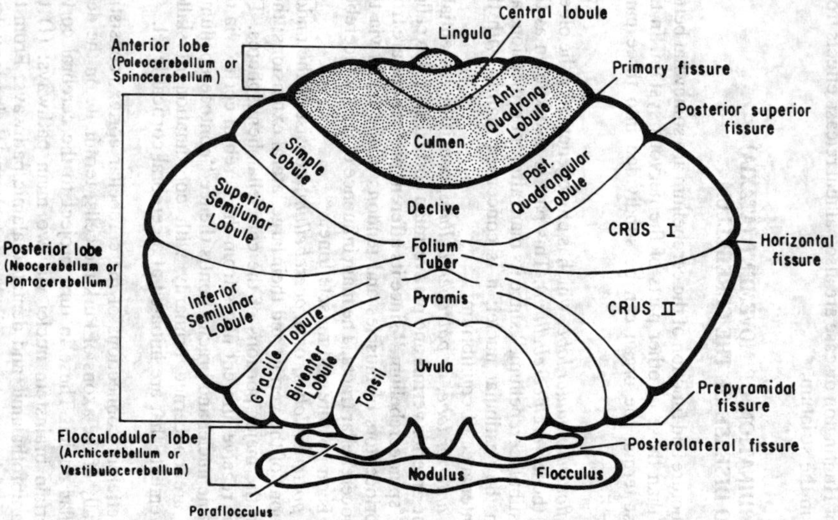

FIG. 4-4 Diagram of the cerebellum, illustrating the major fissures, lobes, and lobules and the major phylogenetic divisions (on the left).

activity indirectly, through its connections with the motor cortex and brainstem nuclei and their descending pathways.

The studies of Thach and his colleagues in primates have shown that the contribution of the cerebellum to the initiation and control of movement involves a corticopontine-cerebellar-thalamocortical circuitry, which functions in large measure before the motor cortex is activated. Interesting, then, is the fact that all planned voluntary activity is prepared by the basal ganglia and cerebellum.

Details of cerebellar anatomy and physiology will be found in the *Principles*.

Cerebellar Symptoms

Lesions of the cerebellum give rise to (1) loss of muscle tone, (2) incoordination (ataxia) of volitional movement, and (3) disorders of equilibrium and gait. Lesions of the cerebellar peduncles have essentially the same effects as the more extensive hemispheral lesions.

Hypotonia refers to the apparent decrease in resistance of muscles to palpation or to passive manipulation of the limbs and is more readily demonstrated with acute than with chronic lesions. It can be brought out by tapping the wrists of the outstretched arms, in which case the affected limb(s) will be displaced through a wider range than normal; this represents a failure of toneless muscles to fixate the arm at the shoulder. Or segments of a limb may be displaced through an abnormally wide range. Pendularity of the knee jerk betrays hypotonicity of the quadriceps and hamstring muscles.

Incoordination (ataxia) of voluntary movement (including propositional gestures) is the most prominent manifestation of cerebellar disease. It has been designated by a number of descriptive terms (dysmetria, dyssynergia, dysdiadokokinesis, etc.), but Holmes's characterization of these disturbances as *abnormalities in the rate, range, and force of movement* is less confusing and more accurate. With a unilateral lesion of the cerebellum, the movement disorder is ipsilateral.

With cerebellar lesions there may be a slight delay in the initiation of a movement, and the movement iself is slow and irregular. The velocity and force of the movement are not checked in the normal manner. These abnormalities become more prominent in acts requiring alternation of movements. Characteristically, the patient's finger (or toe) oscillates as it approaches a target or moves from side to side on the target itself. This side-to-side movement (due to a hypotonic instability of the arm at the shoulder or the leg at the hip) may assume a pseudorhythmic quality, in which case it is referred to inaccurately as an "intention tremor." The term *ataxic tremor* is more accurate. In addition, movement and attempts at sustained posture may evoke a wide-range action tremor, sometimes incorrectly called "rubral tremor."

Dysarthria that follows cerebellar lesions may take one of two forms—either a simple slowing or slurring of speech or a scanning, in which words are fragmented into syllables. The latter is uniquely cerebellar. A rhythmic tremor of the head on the trunk at a rate of 3 to 4 per second may accompany midline cerebellar lesions (*"titubation"*). A variety of abnormalities of ocular movement are commonly associated; these include saccadic dysmetria (accomplishment of voluntary gaze by a series of jerky movements), inability to hold eccentric gaze with the need to make repetitive corrective saccades (gaze-paretic nystagmus), and skew deviation (Chap. 13).

Acute lesions may cause a slight weakness and fatigability of the ataxic limbs. Incoordination of cerebellar type is distinguishable from sensory ataxia by absence of sensory deficit and relative lack of a corrective effect of vision on projected movement. Parietal lobe lesions may derange movements in much the same way as cerebellar ones.

Finally, it should be pointed out that a considerable part of a cerebellar hemisphere may suffer damage without recognizable disorder of movement.

Cerebellar disorders of equilibrium and gait are described in Chap. 6.

Table 4-3 summarizes the clinical effects of extrapyramidal and cerebellar lesions.

For a more detailed discussion of this topic, see Adams and Victor: *Principles of Neurology*, 4th ed, pp 54–77.

ADDITIONAL READING

Brooks VB: *The Neural Basis of Motor Control*. New York, Oxford University Press, 1986.

Carpenter MB, Sutin J: The corpus striatum, in *Human Neuroanatomy*, 8th ed. Baltimore, Williams and Wilkins, 1983, chap 17, pp 579–607.

DeLong MR, Alexander GE: Organization of basal ganglia, in Asbury AK, McKhann GM, McDonald WI (eds): *Diseases of the Nervous System*. Philadelphia, Saunders, 1986, chap 28, pp 379–393.

Growdon JH, Fink JS: Paralysis and movement disorder, in Wilson JD et al (eds): *Harrison's Principles of Internal Medicine*, 12th ed. New York, McGraw-Hill, 1991, pp 157–169.

Holmes G: The cerebellum of man. Hughings Jackson Lecture. *Brain* 62:1, 1939.

TABLE 4-3 Clinicopathologic Correlations of Extrapyramidal Motor Disorders

Symptoms	Principal location of morbid anatomy
Unilateral plastic rigidity with static tremor (Parkinson syndrome)	Contralateral substantia nigra plus (?) other structures
Unilateral hemiballismus and hemichorea	Contralateral subthalamic nucleus of Luys or luysialpallidal connections
Chronic chorea of Huntington type	Caudate nucleus and putamen
Athetosis and dystonia	Contralateral striatum. Pathology of dystonia musculorum deformans unknown.
Cerebellar incoordination, intention tremor, and hypotonia	Homolateral cerebellar hemisphere or middle and inferior cerebellar peduncles, brachium conjunctivum (ipsilateral if below decussation, contralateral if above)
Decerebrate rigidity, i.e., extension of arms and legs, opisthotonos	Usually bilateral in tegmentum of upper brainstem, at level of red nucleus or between red and vestibular nuclei
Palatal and facial myoclonus (rhythmic)	Ipsilateral central tegmental tract
Diffuse myoclonus	Neuronal degeneration, usually diffuse or predominating in cerebral or cerebellar cortex and dentate nuclei

Narabayashi H: Tremor mechanisms, in Schaltenbrand G, Walker AE (eds): *Stereotaxy of the Human Brain*. Stuttgart, Thieme, 1981, pp 510–514.

Thach WT Jr: The cerebellum, in Mountcastle VB (ed): *Medical Physiology*, 14th ed. St. Louis, Mosby, 1980, vol 1, pp 837–858.

Weiner WJ, Lang AE: *Movement Disorders: A Comprehensive Survey*. Mount Kisco, NY, Futura Publishing Co., 1989.

Young AB, Penney JB: Pharmacologic aspects of motor dysfunction, in Asbury AK, McKhann GM, McDonald WI (eds): *Diseases of the Nervous System*. Philadelphia, Saunders, 1986, chap 31, pp 423–434.

5 Tremor, Myoclonus, Spasms, and Tics

These disorders of movement are commonly observed in the neurologic clinic. Although they must be thought of as manifestations of disease, their clinical significance is quite variable. Moreover, their physiology is not fully understood and only rarely can their pathologic basis be established. From the student's viewpoint, once each of these phenomena has been seen, there is little difficulty in recognizing it on a second occasion and assessing its medical implications.

TREMOR

This is defined as a more or less rhythmic oscillation of a part of the body around a fixed point. It is customary to categorize tremor as being of two general types: (1) normal or physiologic and (2) pathologic.

Physiologic tremor is present in everyone and involves all muscle groups. It is of fast frequency (8 to 13 Hz) and is usually so fine as to require special instruments for its detection. Its clinical significance derives from the fact that certain metabolic varieties of tremor (e.g., hyperthyroidism) and one type of familial tremor are believed to be exaggerations of physiologic tremor ("enhanced physiologic tremor").

Pathologic tremor is what is meant when the term *tremor* is used clinically. It is of wider range and slower (4 to 7 Hz) than physiologic tremor and is mostly seen in the fingers and hands, less often in the head, tongue, or jaw, and least in the feet and legs. A number of familiar types of tremor constitute this category: parkinsonian tremor, so-called intention tremor, and certain types of essential or familial tremor.

The *parkinsonian (rest) tremor* has been mentioned in Chap. 4. It is a coarse, rhythmic, 4- to 5-Hz tremor that involves fingers, hands and arms, jaw, lips, and tongue, and rarely the feet. It is present when the limb is in an attitude of repose (resting) and is suppressed momentarily by movement. When studied physiologically, the tremor is seen to correspond with alternating bursts of activity in opposing muscle groups. Sometimes it is associated with a faster frequency action or postural tremor. Most often the resting tremor is a manifestation of the Parkinson syndrome, but it may occur as an isolated phenomenon in an elderly person without akinesia, rigidity, or mask-like facies.

Intention, or ataxic, tremor has also been referred to in Chap. 4. In contrast to the parkinsonian tremor, intention tremor is absent when the limbs are inactive and even during the first part of a voluntary movement. However, as movement continues, and particularly if precision or fine adjustment of the movement is required (e.g., touching the examiner's finger), a slow (2- to 3-Hz), irregular oscillation appears. A rhythmic oscillation of the head (titubation), trunk, or outstretched arms may be associated. The presence of this type of tremor always points to involvement of the cerebellum and its connections. Particularly severe forms of it, sometimes called rubral tremor, are seen in multiple sclerosis and Wilson disease and with vascular and other lesions that interrupt the dentatorubrothalamic pathway. This type of tremor as well as the parkinsonian tremor can be relieved by stereotactically placed lesions in the contralateral ventrolateral nucleus of the thalamus.

The adjectives *postural* and *action (kinetic)* are applied to tremors that are observed when the limbs are actively maintained in certain postures (e.g., arms outstretched with fingers apart) and they persist throughout active movement. Several types of action tremor are recognized. One appears to be an enhanced physiologic tremor, i.e., it has the same frequency as physiologic tremor but is of greater amplitude. Unlike parkinsonian tremor, this type of action tremor is characterized by bursts of alpha motoneuron activity that synchronously innervate opposing muscle groups; presumably, inequalities in the strength and timing of contraction of the opposing muscle groups account for the tremor. This type of action tremor is seen with fatigue and intense fright and anxiety, after an injection of adrenalin, during withdrawal from alcohol and other sedative drugs, in hyperthyroidism, and in one form of familial tremor.

A second type of familial tremor, inherited as an autosomal dominant trait, is of slower frequency (4 to 8 Hz). If inheritance of the tremor is not evident, it is referred to as *essential tremor,* and if it appears only late in life, it is called *senile tremor*. Most often, the tremor is limited to the upper limbs. Sometimes a side-to-side or nodding tremor of the head is added, and in advanced cases the jaw and voice may be affected. Rarely, the head tremor precedes the hand tremor by many years. Even more rarely the tremor affects the legs, most prominently during quiet standing (*orthostatic tremor*). Essential tremor is relatively common and may be so severe as to seriously impair all manual tasks.

These several types of tremor are differently responsive to

drugs. Enhanced physiologic tremor and some essential tremors are suppressed by alcohol, propranolol (20 to 80 mg tid), and mysoline (250 mg tid). The low-frequency, alternating-beat tremors are inconsistently responsive to these drugs but may be helped by Valium (5 mg tid). The tremor of Parkinson disease may be relieved by anticholinergic drugs or L-dopa, as described in relation to the treatment of that disease (p. 354). None of these medications is of predictable value in the treatment of low-frequency familial and senile tremors.

ASTERIXIS

This movement disorder consists of brief (35- to 200-ms), coarse, arrhythmic lapses of sustained posture. Asterixis can be provoked in any muscle group that is under sustained contraction but is most easily elicited by having the patient hold the arms outstretched and the hands and fingers dorsiflexed; the latter then undergo abrupt flexion movements at irregular intervals. A fine asterixis of the fingers may simulate an irregular high-frequency tremor, and only EMG can separate them. In most instances, asterixis is a manifestation of a metabolic disorder, such as impending liver coma or hypercapnia or drug intoxication (phenytoin).

CLONUS, MYOCLONUS, AND POLYMYOCLONUS

Clonus, myoclonus, and polymyoclonus are symptomatic of a large number of diverse neurologic disorders. Precise usage of these terms is essential if they are to be neurologically meaningful. The following definitions are proposed.

Clonus refers to a series of *rhythmic,* uniphasic (unidirectional) contractions and relaxations of a group of muscles. These movements involve only an agonist group of muscles, thus differing from tremors, which are diphasic (bidirectional) and involve both agonist muscles and their antagonists.

Myoclonus specifies the *arrhythmic,* shock-like contractions of a muscle or group of muscles, almost always asynchronous and asymmetric on the two sides of the body. The contractions are extremely brief in duration (50 to 100 ms), i.e., much briefer than choreic movements. Single or a few repeated contractions of this type are designated as *segmental myoclonus* or *myoclonus simplex*.

Polymyoclonus refers to *widespread* lightning-like, arrhythmic contractions of many parts of the body.

The most common type of *clonus* is that which occurs in relation to corticospinal tract lesions, when the spastic muscles are subjected to sustained stretch (p. 27). Another type of clonus, called *palatal nystagmus* or *palatal myoclonus,* is characterized by slow (1- to 2-per-second) rhythmic uniphasic movements restricted to the muscles of the palate, face, eyes, neck, and throat. This type is invariably associated with lesions that interrupt the central tegmental tract(s) in the brainstem, and the mechanism presumably is a denervation hypersensitivity of the inferior olivary nucleus and its dentate connections or some other medullary nucleus (nucleus ambiguus or nucleus reticularis). *Epilepsia partialis continua* is a special variety of clonus, in which one group of muscles is involved in a series of rhythmic monophasic contractions, continuing sometimes for months or even years on end without spreading or becoming generalized.

Thus the *myoclonias* may be restricted (*myoclonus simplex*) or generalized (*polymyoclonus*). The former may appear as a single massive contraction of the neck, shoulders, arms, and trunk in West disease, one form of infantile or childhood epilepsy (salaam seizures). One-sided myoclonic jerks characterize a particular form of childhood epilepsy—benign epilepsy with rolandic spikes (pp. 131–132).

Polymyoclonus may develop in pure or ''essential'' form as a benign nonprogressive familial disease. It may also be combined with epilepsy and dementia as in the several types of storage disease (Lafora body disease, cherry-red spot–myoclonus syndrome, lipid storage diseases). A form of polymyoclonus occurring with fast, projected movements follows recovery from hypoxic encephalopathy; it has been called *action or intention myoclonus* by Lance and Adams. In Creutzfeldt-Jakob disease, an abnormal startle response and polymyoclonus are combined with ataxia and dementia. Lithium intoxication has caused widespread myoclonus and confusion, simulating Creutzfeldt-Jakob disease.

The pathophysiology of polymyoclonus must be varied. The frequent association with cerebellar ataxia points to a cerebellar, brainstem, or thalamic localization. Specific sensory evocation—to startle, sound, visual, and proprioceptive stimuli—suggests a number of different mechanisms centered in the brainstem. One form (epilepsia partialis continua) is believed to originate in the cerebral motor cortex.

Pharmacologic responses are interesting. The massive myoclonus seizures of infancy and early childhood respond to adrenocorticotropic hormone (ACTH) and anticonvulsants. Epilepsia partialis continua is sometimes relieved by anticonvulsants. Clonazepam (8 to 12 mg/day in divided doses) is useful in the treatment of action myoclonus.

SPASMODIC TORTICOLLIS AND LINGUAL, FACIAL, AND OROMANDIBULAR SPASMS

These are involuntary spasms of a particular group of muscles. The spasms may be persistent or intermittent and tonic or irregularly clonic, resulting in a turning and retraction of the head, a forceful grimace, closure of the eyes, protrusion of the tongue, strained voice, pursing of the lips, or writer's cramp. Like all involuntary movements, they are worsened by excitement and emotional upset. The patient cannot inhibit the spasms but usually discovers that certain maneuvers modulate or obscure them. As a rule, these movement disorders appear in midadult life or later, and once started they seldom recede spontaneously; only rarely do they extend to other parts of the body. The overactive muscles undergo "work hypertrophy." No pathology has been found in the brain in the few cases coming to postmortem examination. Formerly considered by some to be psychogenic, this hypothesis was never substantiated. Current opinion is that they are restricted forms of dystonia. The following forms, which may occur singly or in combination, are recognized:

a. *Blepharospasm:* Involuntary blinking or spasms of orbicularis oculi muscles.
b. *Hemifacial spasm:* one-sided spasms of orbicularis oculi and facial muscles.
c. *Spastic dysphonia:* Strained voice due to spasm of laryngeal and respiratory muscles.
d. *Meige or Brueghel syndrome:* Forceful jaw opening associated with spasms of facial and orbicular muscles.
e. *Spasmodic torticollis:* Rotation and retraction of the head due to contraction of sternocleidomastoid, trapezius, and other neck muscles.
f. *Protrusion of the tongue.*
g. *Writer's cramp and related occupational spasms:* Contraction of hand and forearm muscles during writing or performance of other skilled motor acts.

Treatment consists of cutting or surgically denervating the offending muscle groups, to be undertaken only if medical treatment fails. The latter consists of injecting small amounts of botulinus toxin at the innervatory point in the muscle, which often relieves the spasm for several months. The administration of gradually increasing amounts of trihexyphenidyl until very large dosage is attained is helpful in some cases (see also Chap. 41).

TICS

These are quasivoluntary habit spasms; they consist of repeated twitches of a group of muscles, seemingly to relieve tension. The patient concedes that he makes the movements and that he can suppress them by force of will. The most frequent forms are blinking, sniffing, throat clearing, hitching a shoulder, or throwing the head to the side or backward.

Children 5 to 10 years old are disposed to developing tics. They last only for a few weeks if ignored. Less pressure, more rest, and a calmer environment are helpful. Some adults are inclined to exhibit tics whenever they are under pressure. If the tics are troublesome and persistent, small doses (10 to 25 mg) of chlorpromazine are helpful. Psychotherapy is of questionable value.

A syndrome of multiple tics associated with sniffing, snorting, involuntary vocalization and the compulsive utterance of obscenities is the most severe of the tic syndromes (*Gilles de la Tourette syndrome*). The condition persists for weeks, months, or years. The cause and pathologic basis are not known, but a familial clustering is found in about one-third of the cases. There are no consistent psychiatric accompaniments except for a tendency to obsessive-compulsive personality traits, but these are not present in all cases. The administration of stimulants to hyperactive boys has preceded the syndrome in some instances. In some series of cases there has been a higher than expected incidence of "soft neurologic signs" and "organic" impairment of intellect. Haloperidal (Haldol) in gradually increasing doses of 2 to 10 mg/day has been the most effective therapy. Benztropine mesylate or another anti-Parkinson drug is given simultaneously.

RHYTHMIAS (MOVEMENT STEREOTYPES)

In every institution for the mentally retarded one witnesses a remarkable variety of rhythmic rocking, head-bobbing, hand-waving, eye-rubbing, or other repetitive movements whenever the patient is idle. These are reminiscent of the headbanging of babies, but they persist throughout life, seemingly an outlet for the universal impulse to fidget and squirm or to derive gratification from rhythmic activity. Their basis is unknown and the universality of their occurrence in many different types of mental retardation argues against a fixed lesion.

STARTLE

This is a natural defensive reaction which, for reasons unknown, may in some few families be excessive and insuppressible (see *Principles of Neurology* for details).

AKATHISIA

This term denotes a state of extreme motor restlessness. The patient cannot sit still; he is constantly squirming, shifting his weight, crossing and uncrossing his legs, standing up, walking in place, and pacing the floor. Originally observed in encephalitic illnesses, it is now observed most often as a complication of neuroleptic drugs, i.e., as a symptom of tardive dyskinesia (see Chap. 40).

For a more detailed discussion of this topic, see Adams and Victor: *Principles of Neurology,* 4th ed, pp 78–92.

ADDITIONAL READING

Kennedy RH, Bartley GB, Flanagan JC, Waller RR: Treatment of blepharospasm with botulinum toxin. *Mayo Clinic Proc* 64:1085, 1989.

Lance JW, Adams RD: The syndrome of intention or action myoclonus as a sequel to hypoxic encephalopathy. *Brain* 87:111, 1963.

Lees AS, Robertson M, Trimble MR, Murray HMF: A clinical study of Gilles de la Tourette syndrome in the United Kingdom. *J Neurol Neurosurg Psychiatry* 47:1, 1984.

Lefebvre-D'Amour M, Shahani BT, Young RR: Tremor in alcoholic patients, in Desmedt JE (ed): *Physiological Tremor, Pathological Tremors, and Clonus*. Basel, Karger, 1978, pp 160–164.

Narabayashi H: Surgical approach to tremor, in Marsden CD, Fahn S (eds): *Movement Disorders*. London, Butterworth, 1982, pp 292–299.

Sheehy MP, Marsden CD: Writer's cramp—a focal dystonia. *Brain* 105:461, 1982.

6 | Disorders of Stance and Gait

Normal stance and gait require the execution of patterned alternating limb movements (central pattern generator integrity) and intact labyrinthine function, proprioception, and vision. A deficit in any one of these control mechanisms alters gait in a predictable way. A blind person or a normal one walking in the dark shortens his steps, holds the body stiffly, and tends to elevate the arms in front of the body to prevent collisions. The gait of a person with impaired labyrinthine function is somewhat cautious and unsteady and much more so on turns, slippery or uneven ground, and stairs, where he must hold onto the banister; locomotion in these circumstances is disproportionately dependent on visual cues. Loss of proprioception, if complete, makes upright stance and locomotion impossible; if partial, the base is widened, the neck and trunk are flexed slightly, and the steps are irregular and uneven in length and force.

Diseases of the nervous system also disturb stance and gait in predictable ways, and these may be of diagnostic value. But there is always a problem because the patient tends to compensate for his imbalance with certain common protective mechanisms, such as widening the base, shortening the step, and shuffling (keeping both feet on the floor at all times). These maneuvers tend to obscure the primary gait disorder.

Gait is best evaluated when the patient does not know that he is being watched, as when entering the examining room. Later tests include natural walking, running, rising quickly from a chair and stepping out, turning, walking in a circle and tandem (heel to toe), and standing with feet together and eyes open and shut.

Tabulated below are the more common disorders of gait, their distinguishing features, and usual causes.

a. *Cerebellar gait:* Wide base, unsteadiness on standing or sitting, irregularity of steps (erratic placement of feet), and lateral veering (toward side of cerebellar lesion if unilateral). On standing with feet together, a variable degree of swaying with eyes open and only slightly more swaying with the eyes closed (i.e., Romberg sign is absent).

   Common causes: multiple sclerosis, cerebellar tumors

(particularly those involving vermis), cerebellar degenerations, both hereditary and acquired ("alcoholic cerebellar degeneration"; paraneoplastic cerebellar degeneration).

b. *Sensory ataxic (tabetic) gait:* Varying difficulty in standing and walking despite retention of muscular power. Leg movements brusque, erratic in length and height of step, often with an audible stamp. Ground is watched intently for cues. Marked Romberg sign. Loss of position sense in feet and legs and usually of vibration sense as well.

   Usual causes: tabes dorsalis (now rare), Friedreich ataxia and other spinocerebellar degenerations, subacute combined degeneration of the cord (vitamin B_{12} deficiency), chronic sensory polyneuropathy, multiple sclerosis, spinal cord compression with predominant posterior column involvement.

c. *Hemiplegic and paraplegic (spastic) gaits:* In *hemiplegia,* the leg is held stiffly with failure of flexion at hip, knee, and ankle; foot is turned down and inward; hemiplegic leg advances more slowly than the normal one and may be swung outward, describing a semicircle. Outer side and toe of shoe scrape the floor. Arm may be flexed and does not swing.

   Usual causes: Most often cerebral infarction or trauma but may follow any lesion that interrupts corticospinal tract on one side.

   Paraplegic gait: In effect, a bilateral hemiplegia; legs advanced stiffly and slowly. Balance little affected if sensation is normal.

   Usual causes: cerebral diplegia due to perinatal anoxia-ischemia; chronic spinal cord disease due to multiple sclerosis, combined system diseases, chronic compression, and heredofamilial degenerations.

d. *Festinating gait:* Trunk bent forward, arms slightly flexed and do not swing, legs stiff and slightly bent at knees, steps short and shuffling. With walking, upper body advances ahead of lower part and steps become more rapid. Characteristic of Parkinson disease.

e. *Steppage or equine gait:* Steps regular and even, advancing foot hangs with toes pointing down, leg lifted high so that foot clears floor, slapping noise as foot strikes floor.

   Usual causes: if unilateral, due to compression of common peroneal nerve or to affection of anterior horn cells, as in poliomyelitis (now rare). If bilateral, due to hereditary neuropathy (Charcot-Marie-Tooth), progressive spinal muscular atrophy, and certain types of muscular dystrophy.

f. *Waddling gait:* Alternating excessive lateral movements of the trunk, imparting a roll or waddle. Due to impaired fixation of the weight-bearing hip, usually the result of weakness of gluteal muscles. Such patients have difficulty in climbing stairs and arising from a chair.

Common causes: congenital dislocation of the hips, progressive muscular dystrophy, chronic spinal muscular atrophy (Wohlfart-Kugelberg-Welander syndrome).

g. *Staggering, or drunken, gait:* Characteristic of intoxication with alcohol or other sedative drugs. Patient totters and reels and at each step threatens to lose his balance. Steps are irregular and variable and falling is prevented by facile compensatory movements. Mild degrees resemble the unsteadiness of gait that follows loss of labyrinthine function (see above).

h. *Toppling gait:* Tottering and sudden lurches, resulting in a hesitant and uncertain gait and unexpected falls, in the absence of weakness, ataxia, or loss of deep sensation. Observed in progressive supranuclear palsy (p. 355), advanced stages of Parkinson disease, and some cases of lateral medullary syndrome.

i. *Gait of normal pressure hydrocephalus:* In the absence of rigidity, tremor, or ataxia, the base is widened, gait is slowed, height of each step is diminished, and there is a tendency to shuffle. Body is held stiffly and turns en bloc.

j. *Frontal lobe disorder of gait* (frontal lobe ataxia or frontal lobe apraxia): Posture flexed, base somewhat widened, gait slow, steps small, hesitant, and shuffling (*marche à petits pas*). Initially, gait may improve with assistance and marching in step. Steps shorten progressively, with ultimate inability to make a step or to stand, sit, or turn over in bed. Final stages are associated with dementia, other frontal lobe signs such as grasping and sucking reflexes, oppositional resistance (*gegenhalten*), and rigid, flexed posture, referred to by Yakovlev as cerebral paraplegia in flexion (Fig. 6-1).

The stooped, short-stepped, cautious *gait of the elderly* person without overt neurologic disease probably represents a relatively mild degree of the frontal lobe disorder of gait.

k. *Choreoathetotic and dystonic gaits:* The various choreic, athetotic, and dystonic states, described in Chap. 4, are frequently associated with disorders of gait. The legs advance slowly and awkwardly, the result of superimposed involuntary movements and postures—plantar flexion, dorsiflexion or inversion of the foot, momentary suspension of the leg in the air, twisting of the trunk or pelvis.

l. *Gaits of the mentally retarded:* One observes a wide assortment of gait abnormalities among the mentally handicapped: ungainly stance, body and limbs in ungraceful postures, wide-based gaits with awkward lurches or stomping, unnatu-

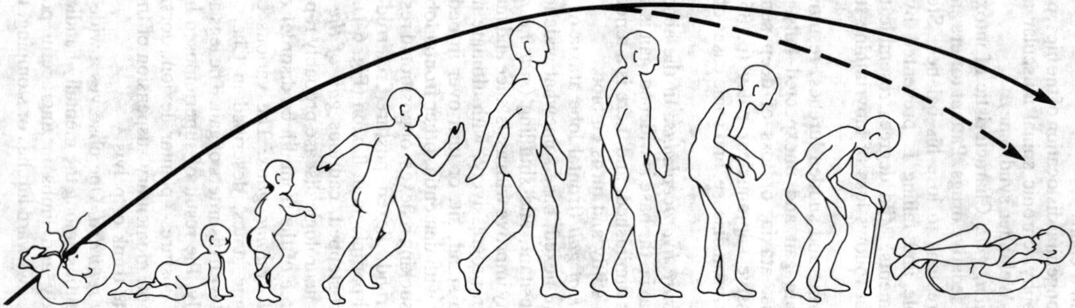

FIG. 6-1 The evolution of erect stance and gait and of paraplegia in flexion of cerebral origin, according to Yakovlev. The ripening forebrain of the infant drives the head and body up and moves the individual forward. When the "driving brain" (frontal lobe, striatum, pallidum) degenerates, the individual curls up again. Lesser degrees of this sequence may account for the nondementing gait of the elderly (upper line).

rally long or short steps. Often these gait abnormalities are associated with odd stereotyped mannerisms (rhythmias), described in Chap. 4, and failure to acquire the usual age-linked refinements of motor function.

m. *Hysterical gaits:* These do not conform to any of the gait disorders described above. The patient may not lift the leg from the floor but may drag it along or push it in front of him, as though it were on a skate. The patient may walk as though on stilts or lurch wildly in all directions or crumple to the floor (astasia-abasia), sometimes despite the capacity to move the legs in bed (see Chap. 53).

For a more detailed discussion of this topic, see Adams and Victor: *Principles of Neurology*, 4th ed, pp 93–100.

ADDITIONAL READING

Martin JP: The basal ganglia and locomotion. *Ann R Coll Surg Engl* 32:219, 1963.

Pierrot-Deseilligny E, Bergego C, Mazieres L: Reflex control of bipedal gait in man, in Desmedt JE (ed): *Motor Control Mechanism in Health and Disease*. New York, Raven Press, 1983, pp 699–716.

Sudarsky L: Geriatrics: Gait disorders in the elderly. *New Engl. J Med* 322:1441, 1990.

Sudarsky L, Simon S: Gait disorder in late-life hydrocephalus. *Arch Neurol* 44:263, 1987.

Yakovlev PI: Paraplegia in flexion of cerebral origin. *J Neuropathol Exp Neurol* 13:267, 1954.

SECTION II
PAIN AND OTHER DISORDERS OF SOMATIC SENSATION, HEADACHE, AND BACKACHE

7 Pain

The phenomena to be described in this chapter and the three chapters to follow are more recondite than disorders of motility and are made known to the physician mainly through the statements of the patient. Only to a limited extent can they be objectified by clinical examination. Nevertheless, their value as symptoms is undoubted.

Pain is at once the most frequent and worrisome symptom in medicine. Relatively few diseases are without a painful phase, and in most pain is a characteristic without which the diagnosis often remains in doubt. Because of its ubiquitous associations, the anatomy and physiology of pain assume special importance.

PAIN RECEPTORS AND PERIPHERAL AFFERENT PATHWAYS

Pain receptors are distributed throughout the body—in its integument and deep structures, including the viscera. Two types of afferent fibers have been identified: the very fine unmyelinated C fibers (0.4 to 1.1 μm in diameter) and the thinly myelinated A-delta (A-δ) fibers (1 to 5 μm in diameter). The terminal receptors of these primary pain afferents are the freely branching nerve endings. The C fibers respond mainly to mechanical and thermal stimuli; the A-δ fibers, to extremes of touch and pressure. The cell bodies of these afferent fibers lie in the dorsal root and sensory cranial ganglia. Unlike most neurons they have two axons (a peripheral one and a central one) and no dendrites. Distal axons of these cells traverse somatic segmental and splanchnic nerves; and central axons traverse the posterior roots and the glossopharyngeal, vagal, and trigeminal nerves. The *central terminations* of the cranial sensory nerves are the trigeminal and solitarius nuclei. The posterior roots of the spinal nerves terminate in certain layers or laminae (of Rexed) of the dorsal gray matter of the spinal cord (see Fig. 7-1*A* and *B*). The A-δ fibers end in lamina I (cell layer of Waldeyer), in the outermost cells of layer II (substantia gelatinosa), and in layer V. The C fibers end in lamina II. Some of the cells in these layers form ipsilateral connections with ventral and intermediolateral motor and sympathetic neurons; others decussate in the anterior spinal commissure, within one or two segments of entry, and ascend in the contralateral anterolateral fasciculus to brainstem and thalamic structures. The A-δ pain afferents release several peptide neurotransmitters, of which *substance P* is the most important in exciting secondary dorsal horn neurons. Small neurons in lamina II release an inhibitory peptide called *enkephalin,* which modulates nociceptive input to the spinal segments, brainstem, and thalamus. Opiates act by decreasing substance P and pain-evoked flexor spinal reflexes.

ASCENDING AND DESCENDING PAIN PATHWAYS

The anterolateral fasciculus of the spinal cord contains two main ascending pathways: (1) the lateral spinothalamic tract, a fast conducting pathway, which projects directly to the thalamus, mainly to the ventrobasal and posterior groups of nuclei, and then to the postcentral cortex and to the secondary sensory cortex on the upper bank of the sylvian fissure, and (2) a more slowly conducting, medially placed system, which projects via short interneuronal chains to the reticular core of the medulla and periaqueductal midbrain and then to the hypothalamus and the medial and intralaminar nuclei of the thalamus. The latter pathway, referred to as *spinoreticulothalamic* or *paleospinothalamic,* ultimately terminates diffusely in the frontal and limbic lobes. It is believed that the lateral or direct spinothalamic pathway subserves discriminative function, i.e., the identification and localization of pain sensation, whereas the more slowly conducting, polysynaptic medial pathway subserves the affective aspects of pain, i.e., the unpleasant feelings engendered by pain. The segmental arrangement of nerve fibers within major tracts is illustrated in Fig. 7-2 and the main somatosensory and reticulothalamic pathways in Figs. 7-3 and 7-4.

There are, in addition, descending pathways from brainstem structures, which have an inhibitory effect on pain. One such pathway emanating mainly from the periaqueductal region projects, via a series of brainstem cell stations, to neurons in laminae I and V of the dorsal horns. Other descending pain control systems are derived from noradrenergic and serotoninergic neu-

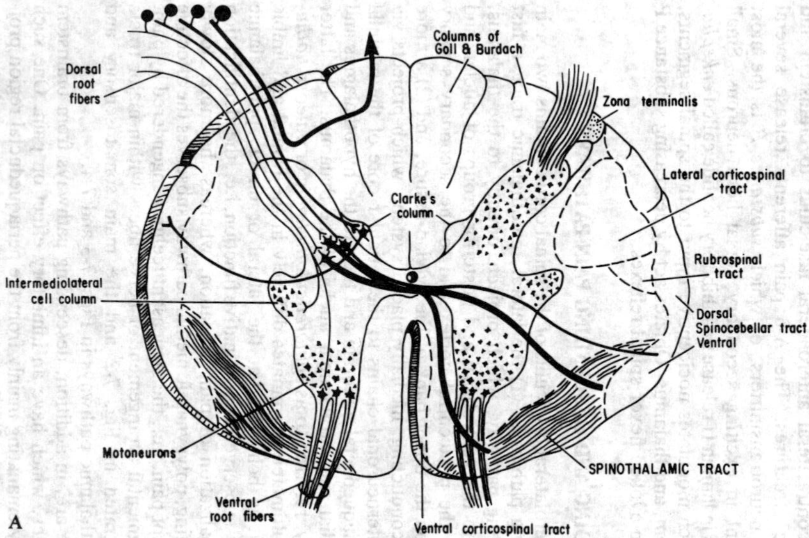

FIG. 7-1 *A.* Transverse section of spinal cord, illustrating the course of afferent fibers and major ascending pathways. Fast-conducting pain fibers are not confined to the spinothalamic tract but are scattered diffusely in the anterolateral funiculus.

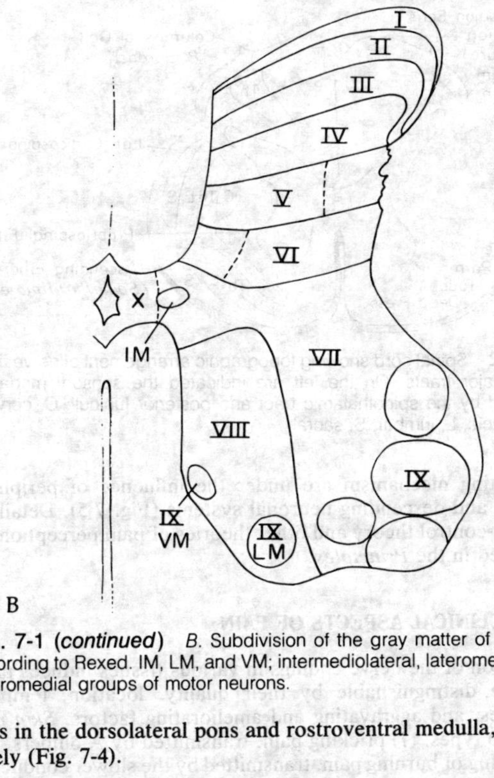

FIG. 7-1 (*continued*) *B*. Subdivision of the gray matter of the cord according to Rexed. IM, LM, and VM; intermediolateral, lateromedial, and ventromedial groups of motor neurons.

rons in the dorsolateral pons and rostroventral medulla, respectively (Fig. 7-4).

PHYSIOLOGIC ASPECTS OF PAIN

The natural stimulus for superficial pain is injury—pricking, cutting, crushing, burning, or freezing the skin. In the stomach and intestines, the effective stimuli are inflamed mucosa and distention and spasm of smooth muscle; in skeletal muscle and heart it is ischemia. In migraine, the pain is of vascular origin; in joints it is inflammation of synovial membranes. In all lesions, the receptors are excited or primed by bradykinins, histamine, prostaglandins, serotonins, and potassium ions.

A complex physiology in the dorsal horn of the spinal cord has been postulated to control or modulate incoming pain impulses. Small neurons believed capable of providing an inhibi-

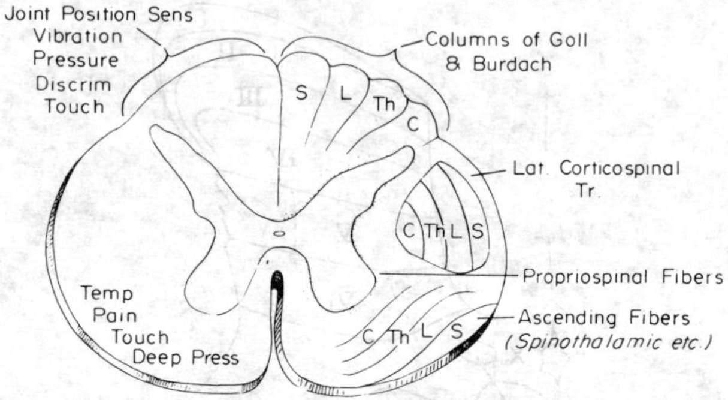

FIG. 7-2 Spinal cord showing topographic arrangement of nerve fibers within major tracts. On the left are indicated the sensory modalities mediated by the spinothalamic tract and posterior funiculi: C, cervical; Th, thoracic; L, lumbar; S, sacral.

tory gating mechanism are under the influence of peripheral afferent and descending neuronal systems (Fig. 7-5). Details of the gate-control theory and other theories of pain perception are discussed in the *Principles*.

SOME CLINICAL ASPECTS OF PAIN

Activation of the nerve endings in various tissues induces pains that are distinguishable by their quality, location, temporal attributes, and aggravating and ameliorating factors. *Skin pain* is of two types: (1) pricking pain, transmitted by A-δ fibers, and (2) stinging or burning pain, transmitted by the slower conducting C fibers. *Deep pain* is aching in quality, occasionally knife-like or burning (as in "heartburn"), and poorly localized. Nevertheless, its location bears a fixed relationship to skeletal or visceral spinal segments to which it is conducted. Usually pain from deep structures is projected to the skin, presumably because there are so many more superficial afferents than visceral ones in each segment; this process is called *referred pain*. If a receptive pool of neurons in the spinal cord is made hyperactive by a disease (e.g., of gall bladder), the status of the neurons in adjacent segments may be altered, and pain from another organ, such as the heart, may then be shifted caudally from its usual location (*aberrant reference*).

Hyperalgesia refers to an increased sensitivity and a lowered threshold to painful stimuli, as occurs with inflammation or a

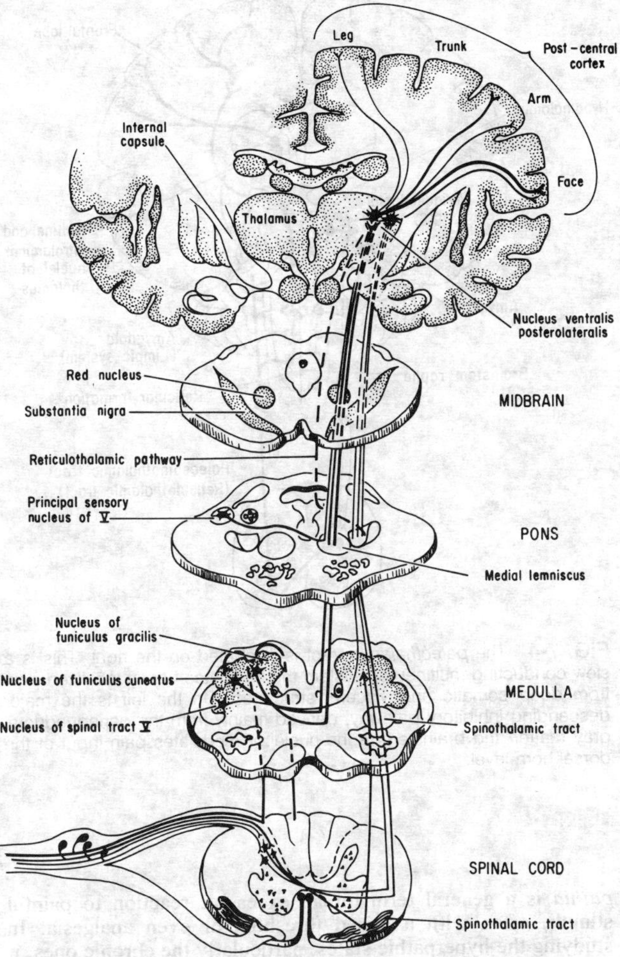

FIG. 7-3 Diagram of the main somatosensory pathways.

superficial burn of the skin. With hyperalgesia there may also be *allodynia,* in which pain is produced by stimuli that do not normally induce pain (touch, pressure, warmth, etc.). *Hyper-*

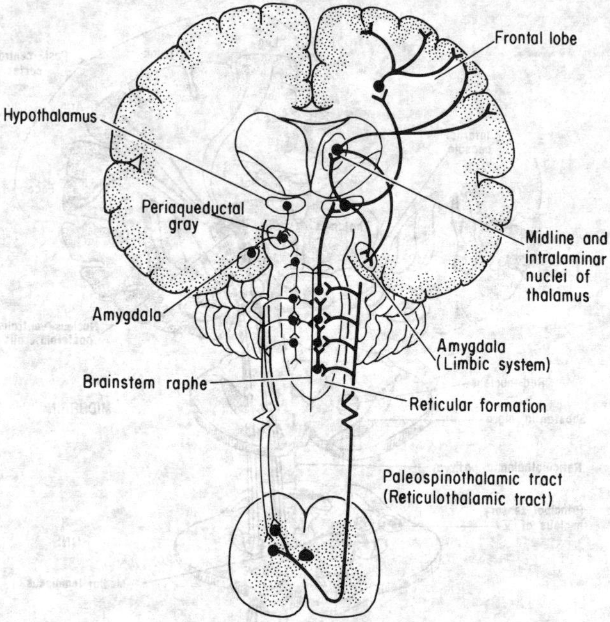

FIG. 7-4 The *paleothalamic* tract is illustrated on the right. This is a slow-conducting multineuron system that mediates poorly localized pain from deep somatic and visceral structures. On the left is the major descending inhibitory pathway, derived mainly from the periaqueductal gray matter and brainstem raphe nuclei. It modulates pain input at the dorsal horn level.

pathia is a general term for an excessive reaction to painful stimuli, often with a raised threshold or even analgesia. In studying the hyperpathic states, particularly the chronic ones, it becomes apparent that unlike touch, thermal sense, etc., pain is not only a sensory experience but also an affective one. The sensory part may be abolished by a nerve or spinal cord or thalamic lesion, but the patient may be left with the affective component.

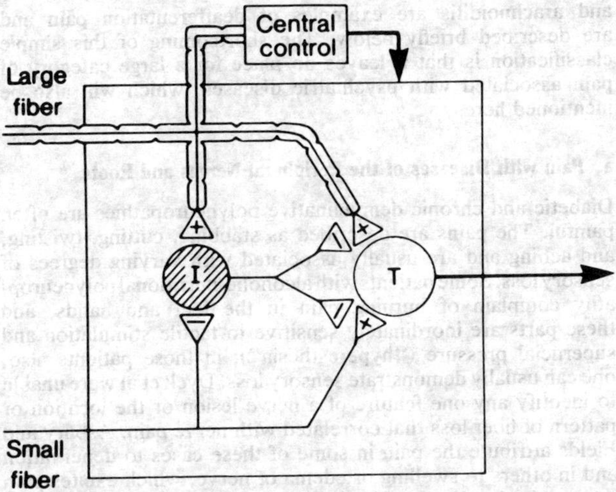

FIG. 7-5 The gate control hypothesis of Melzack and Wall: a stimulus presented to the skin activates both large- and small-diameter fibers. If the stimulus is light, large-fiber input predominates, the inhibitory interneuron (I) is excited, and the transmission cell does not fire. If the stimulus is intense, small-fiber input predominates, the inhibitory interneuron is shut off, and the transmission cell (T) is activated, resulting in pain. (*Adapted from Fields and Levine.*)

PAIN SYNDROMES

With a few important exceptions (acute headache and acute pain of spinal origin) neurologists are called upon to deal with pain that is chronic or recurrent. The latter types of pain have been subdivided by Gybels and Sweet into two categories: One, designated as *somatic pain*, is thought to be based on prolonged or intermittent activation of nociceptors, the same ones that are responsible for the perception of acute pain; the other, referred to as *central* or *deafferentation* pain, results from a variety of injuries to the nervous system. The latter type depends not upon activation of peripheral receptors but upon a change in what Gybels and Sweet call the central "signal elaborating system." Headache and cervical and lumbosacral spine pains are the main examples of the first category and are considered in Chaps. 9 and 10, respectively. Painful neuropathies, avulsion of the brachial plexus, spinal cord trauma, postzoster neuralgia, thalamic pain, and arachnoiditis are examples of deafferentation pain and are described briefly below. The shortcoming of this simple classification is that it leaves no place for a large category of pain associated with psychiatric diseases, which will also be mentioned here.

a. Pain with Diseases of the Peripheral Nerves and Roots

Diabetic and chronic demyelinative polyneuropathies are often painful. The pains are described as stabbing, cutting, twisting, and aching and are usually associated with varying degrees of sensory loss. Some patients with alcoholic-nutritional polyneuropathy complain of burning pain in the feet and hands, and these parts are inordinately sensitive to tactile stimulation and superficial pressure ("hyperesthesia"); in these patients also, one can usually demonstrate sensory loss. Dyck et al were unable to identify any one feature of a nerve lesion or the location or pattern of fiber loss that correlated with nerve pain. Asbury and Fields attribute the pain in some of these cases to denervation and in others to swelling or edema of nerve, which excites pain endings in the sheaths of the nerves themselves.

Some lesions of nerve are more likely to be painful than others. Avulsion of the brachial plexus almost always gives rise to chronic pain. Partial injury of a single nerve in the arm or leg may result in a severe burning type of pain, which, once started, may persist for years (*causalgia*). The leading explanation of causalgic pain is that an artificial synapse has been created at the point of nerve injury, permitting the activation of afferent somatic sensory fibers by sympathetic efferent ones (ephaptic transmission). But a hypersensitivity of nocifensive C receptors has also been demonstrated by Cline et al.

Herpes zoster, especially in the elderly, is often the forerunner of a chronic painful state (Chap. 31). The lesions lie in the spinal ganglia and roots but severing the nerve roots affords no relief, pointing to a central spinal mechanism. An altered state (disinhibition) of secondary spinal neurons due to denervation is the usual postulated mechanism, but there are so many descending modulating and feedback systems that a number of alternate explanations are equally plausible.

Tabes dorsalis, with its lancinating pains and gastric crises, is another (now rare) painful radicular disorder, the spinal ganglia being intact.

Probably the most frequent pain syndrome encountered by neurologists is the one due to compressive and irritative lesions of the lumbosacral roots and related to *ruptured discs*, repeated laminectomies and myelography, and focal arachnoiditis.

Whether the mechanism is peripheral or central has not been determined.

b. Spinal Cord Pain

Arm, shoulder, and neck pains are distressing symptoms in approximately 30 percent of patients with syringomyelia. Decompression of the syrinx and the frequently associated Chiari malformation usually provides no relief. Cordotomy for chronic pain in the lower extremity may give rise to intractable pain at the segmental level of the operative site, presumably due to injury of the posterior horn of spinal gray matter. Transection of the spinal cord as a result of trauma, infarction, or myelitis may be a cause of intractable pain, even if all sensory tracts are interrupted. The source of the pain appears to be the sensory neurons in the gray matter in the upper stump of the cord; intrathecal morphine delivered by a catheter or excision of the upper stump may relieve the pain. Complete section of the posterior trigeminal root, a procedure that leaves the patient with pain in the analgesic areas in 10 to 15 percent of cases, is another example of *analgesia dolorosa*.

c. Thalamic Pain

This syndrome, almost always the result of infarction, is discussed in the next chapter and in Chap. 32, on cerebrovascular disease.

d. Pain with Psychiatric Disease

Chronic pain may be the predominant complaint of patients with endogenous depression; and most patients with persistent pain are depressed. Differentiating these states is often difficult, and sometimes one must resort to a therapeutic trial of antidepressant medication or even electroconvulsive therapy. If these measures ablate the pain, the depression is probably primary. On the other hand, depression that recedes as pain is brought under medical control is probably secondary.

Intractable pain may also be a leading symptom of hysteria. Failure to recognize this association may have dire consequences for the patient, who may become addicted to narcotics or be subjected to repeated unnecessary surgical procedures (see Chap. 53).

Hysteria in men (compensation neurosis or malingering) is characterized by complaints of persistent headache, neck pain (whiplash injuries), and low-back pain. Drug addicts may simulate the symptoms of intractable migraine or renal or biliary colic. In these cases, the complaint of pain becomes the means of obtaining drugs or monetary compensation. Long delay in the settlement of litigation serves only to entrench the symptoms and prolong the disability. An objective appraisal of the injury, an unambiguous statement of the psychiatric diagnosis, and encouragement to settle the legal claims as quickly as possible are the most effective means of dealing with these complaints.

Chronic Pain of Indeterminate Cause

This is the most difficult group, the pain that remains after all medical, neurologic, and psychiatric causes have been excluded by careful and repeated examinations. The majority of patients in this group are addicted to opioids, and the need for the drug prompts the regular recurrence of pain. Many are also depressed, and compensation for real or imagined injuries may play a part. Hospitalization of the patient and breaking the drug habit are the first steps in management since the ambulatory treatment of addiction almost never succeeds and pain cannot be assessed in the addicted individual. Settling legal issues, treating the symptoms of depression, training the patient to tolerate his pain, and encouraging him to engage in challenging and satisfying activities are the other methods utilized by centers for the management of difficult pain problems.

The use of opiates and other analgesics in the treatment of intractable pain is considered in Chap. 40. When there is no medical, neurologic, or psychiatric basis for the pain, it is better to be guided by the above-mentioned principles than to prescribe opiates or subject the patient to ablative neurosurgery.

For a more detailed discussion of this topic, see Adams and Victor: *Principles of Neurology,* 4th ed, pp 103–117.

ADDITIONAL READING

Asbury AK, Fields HL: Pain due to peripheral nerve damage: An hypothesis. *Neurology* 34:1587, 1984.

Cline MA, Ochoa J, Torebjork HE: Chronic hyperalgesia and skin warming caused by sensitized C nociceptors. *Brain* 112:621, 1989.

Dyck PJ, Lambert EH, O'Brien PC: Pain in peripheral neuropathy related to rate and kind of fiber degeneration. *Neurology* 26:466, 1976.

Fields HL: *Pain*. New York, McGraw-Hill, 1987.

Fields HL, Levine JD: Pain: A clinical approach based on physiological principles, in Isselbacher KJ et al (eds): *Update II. Harrison's Principles of Internal Medicine*. New York, McGraw-Hill, 1982, pp 205–220.

Gybels JM, Sweet WH: *Neurosurgical Treatment of Chronic Pain: Physiologic and Pathologic Mechanism of Human Pain*. New York, Karger, 1989.

Light AR, Perl ER: Peripheral sensory systems, in Dyck PJ et al (eds): *Peripheral Neuropathy,* 2nd ed. Philadelphia, Saunders, 1984, vol I, chap 9, pp 210–230.

Mountcastle VB: Central nervous mechanisms in sensation, in Mountcastle VB (ed): *Medical Physiology,* 14th ed. St. Louis, Mosby, 1980, vol I, part 5, chaps 11–19, pp 327–605.

Nathan PW: The gate-control theory of pain. A critical review. *Brain* 99:123, 1976.

Sinclair D: *Mechanism of Cutaneous Sensation.* Oxford, Oxford University Press, 1981.

Wall PD: The role of substantia gelatinosa as a gate control, in Bonica JJ (ed): *Pain.* New York, Raven Press, 1980, pp 205–231.

8 General Somatic Sensation

Included under this title are all forms of sensation arising in the skin, muscles, and joints. One form of somatic sensation—pain—has been accorded a chapter of its own because of its clinical importance. Other forms of somatic sensation include touch, pressure, warmth, and cold (which, because of the location of their receptors, are called *cutaneous* or *exteroceptive*). The senses of position, movement, and deep pressure (both painful and painless), which arise from deeper somatic structures, are called *proprioceptive*.

PERIPHERAL SENSORY MECHANISMS

Originally it was thought that each modality of sensation is subserved by a morphologically unique end organ, which transduces a particular type of stimulus (specificity theory of von Frey). More recent physiologic evidence distinguishes only two functional groups of receptors: encapsulated endings and nonencapsulated, freely branching cutaneous endings. Each of these end organs is then classed as a mechanoreceptor, a thermoreceptor, or a nociceptor, depending upon its preferential (but not specific) sensitivity to mechanical, thermal, or noxious stimuli, respectively. Moreover, it has been found that the *quality* of sensation depends not on the type of ending but on the type of nerve fiber to which it is attached, i.e., *the afferent channel*. By contrast, *intensity* of sensation is related to the frequency of stimulation. Fibers conveying thermal sensation are unmyelinated or thinly myelinated and slow conducting, like pain fibers. Touch, pressure, and proprioceptive afferents are large, myelinated, and fast conducting. Cutaneous afferent fibers form the superficial sensory nerves, their only efferent fibers being autonomic. The proprioceptive afferents are part of the deep, predominantly muscular nerves. Some deep afferents enter the splanchnic system.

Each afferent channel consists of a cell body located in the dorsal root ganglion and two extensions: (1) a peripheral nerve fiber (axon) with its multiple terminal endings and (2) a central axon connected to the spinal cord or, if a cranial sensory nerve, to sensory nuclei in the brainstem. The ensemble of the nerve cell body and its axons is called the *primary sensory unit*. The cutaneous area innervated by one unit varies in different parts of the body, and any one area of skin is innervated by more than one unit.

When a disease involves the most peripheral parts of the nervous system, it nearly always impairs more than one modality of sensation, probably because many fibers of different sizes are implicated. However, motor function may be spared entirely. Since proprioceptive afferents travel with muscular nerves, they are often involved together. As a rule, lesions of proximal parts of nerves involve both sensory and motor fibers. A disease affecting small myelinated and unmyelinated fibers, as would be expected, impairs pain and temperature function as well as the function of the postganglionic autonomic fibers, to which they are apposed.

When a peripheral nerve to a given area of skin is severed, all forms of sensation are lost, as is piloerection and sweating. But within days the periphery of the area is invaded by collaterals from adjacent intact pain and thermal sensory units. Tactile units, however, seem to have little capacity for such collateralization. As a result, the zone of tactile loss is larger than that for pain and temperature. In the marginal zone of restored sensation, painful stimuli are unpleasant and diffuse and cannot be localized accurately. Observations such as these gave rise to the concept, now considered invalid, of two sensory systems, protopathic and epicritic (for details, see *Principles*).

SENSORY PATHWAYS

Each sensory spinal (dorsal) root contains all the fibers from skin, muscles, connective tissue, ligaments, tendons, joints, bones, and viscera that lie within the distribution of a single body segment, or somite. The distribution of the dorsal roots on the surface of the body is illustrated in Figs. 8-1 and 8-2.

It is in the dorsal roots, at their points of entrance into the spinal cord, that sensory fibers are first rearranged according to function. Large, heavily myelinated fibers enter the cord just medial to the dorsal horn and divide into descending and ascending branches. Within a few segments of their entrance into the cord, the *descending fibers* synapse with nerve cells in the posterior and anterior horns, including large anterior horn cells; these subserve segmental reflexes. Other dorsal root fibers, after synapsing in the dorsal horns, form the spinocerebellar pathways. *Ascending fibers* run uninterrupted in the ipsilateral posterior columns of Goll and Burdach (also called gracilis and

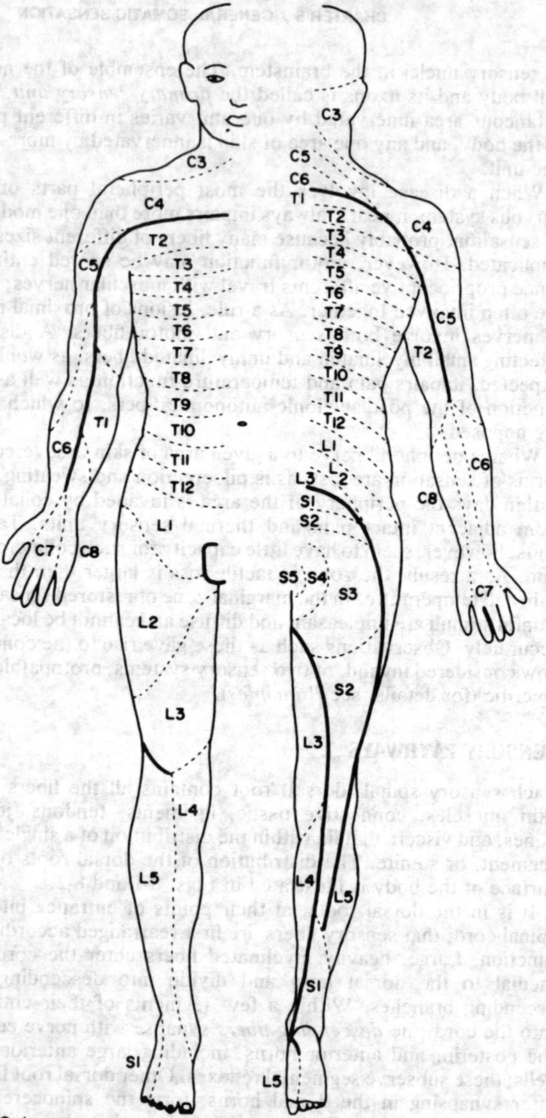

FIG. 8-1 Distribution of the sensory spinal roots on the surface of the body, front and back. (*From D Sinclair, Mechanisms of Cutaneous Sensation, Oxford, Oxford University Press, 1981.*)

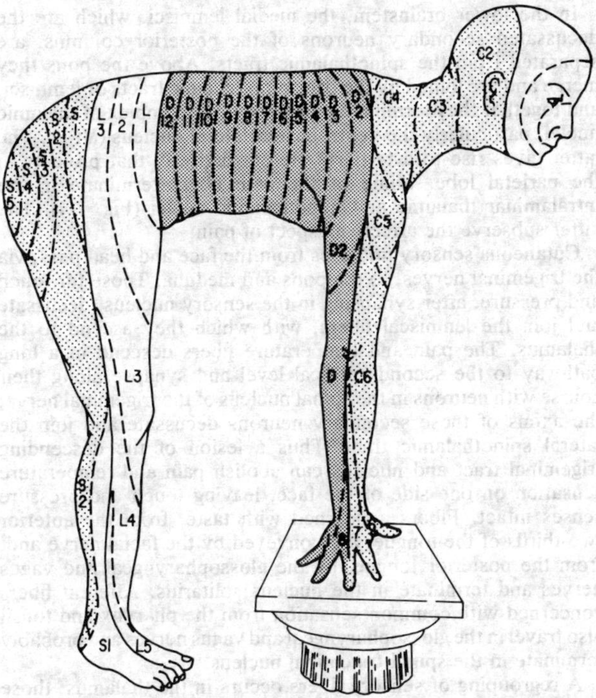

FIG. 8-2 Distribution of the sensory spinal roots on the surface of the body, seen from the side.

cuneatus) to the lower medulla, where they synapse in the nuclei of Goll and Burdach and the accessory cuneate nuclei. These nuclei are the source of the medial lemnisci (see Fig. 7-3). Posterior column fibers convey sensations of touch, pressure, vibration, direction of movement, position of joints, and stereoesthetic sense (whereby one is able to judge the size, shape, and texture of an object by touch).

A second group of thinly myelinated or unmyelinated dorsal root fibers enter the cord on the lateral aspect of the dorsal horn. Within a segment or two of their entry, they synapse with dorsal horn cells; the latter give rise to secondary sensory fibers, most of which decussate and ascend in the anterolateral fasciculus as the lateral and anterior spinothalamic tracts, as illustrated in Fig. 7-3.

In the lower brainstem, the medial lemnisci, which are the decussated secondary neurons of the posterior columns, are separated from the spinothalamic tracts. Above the pons they merge and are joined by the trigeminothalamic tracts or lemnisci, and together they terminate in the posterior complex of thalamic nuclei, particularly the ventroposterolateral nucleus (VPL). The latter gives rise to a tertiary afferent pathway that projects to the parietal lobe. Some of the pain fibers terminate in the intralaminar thalamic and hypothalamic nuclei (Fig. 7-4). The latter subserve the affective aspect of pain.

Cutaneous sensory impulses from the face and head pass, via the trigeminal nerves, to the pons and medulla. Those for touch and pressure, after synapsing in the sensory nucleus, decussate and join the lemniscal fibers, with which they ascend to the thalamus. The pain and temperature fibers descend in a long pathway to the second cervical level and synapse along their course with neurons in the spinal nucleus of the trigeminal nerve; the axons of these secondary neurons decussate and join the lateral spinothalamic tract. Thus a lesion of the descending trigeminal tract and nucleus can abolish pain and temperature sensation on one side of the face, leaving touch and pressure senses intact. Fibers concerned with taste, from the anterior two-thirds of the tongue, are conveyed by the facial nerve and, from the posterior tongue, by the glossopharyngeal and vagus nerves and terminate in the nucleus solitarius. Afferent fibers concerned with common sensation from the pharynx and tonsil also travel in the glossopharyngeal and vagus nerves and probably terminate in the spinal trigeminal nucleus.

A regrouping of sensory fibers occurs in the thalamus; those subserving discriminative sensation ascend to the postcentral (primary) and suprasylvian (secondary) sensory cortices. The projecting thalamic nuclei also receive fibers from the sensory cortices. Conscious awareness of sensory stimuli is believed to occur at the thalamic level, for always some sensation remains after complete ablation of the cerebral cortex. The cortical contribution is to provide the ability to localize stimuli and make other sensory discriminations and to interpret stimuli in terms of previous sensory experience of both cutaneous and visual types.

SENSORY SYNDROMES

The location and pattern of sensory findings are of value in topographic diagnosis and thereby, as stated in Chap. 2, in etiologic diagnosis. The type and location of the sensory changes depend strictly on the anatomy of the lesion. The spinal cord is essentially a segmental structure, each segment innervating its own area of skin and muscles; thus, one need only consult a map, such as the ones illustrated in Figs. 8-1 and 8-2, to determine the location of a radicular or segmental spinal cord lesion. Similarly, each peripheral nerve has a more or less constant cutaneous and muscular distribution. Again, it is easier to consult a map, as in Fig. 8-3, than to commit to memory the details of innervation of every part of the body.

Lesions of Single Peripheral Nerves and Roots

With respect to peripheral nerve lesions, the clinical findings will vary depending on whether the involved nerve is predominantly muscular, cutaneous, or mixed. With interruption of a *cutaneous nerve,* the area of sensory loss is always less than its anatomic distribution because of overlapping innervation from adjacent nerves. Also, for reasons given above, loss of tactile sensation is usually a more accurate measure of a cutaneous nerve lesion than is loss of pain and temperature. Sensory nerve fibers of different sizes and degrees of myelination are susceptible to certain pathologic agents and resistant to others. For example, compression may ablate the function of large touch and pressure fibers and spare the small pain, thermal, and autonomic fibers; ischemia and procaine have the opposite effects.

Interruption of a *muscular nerve* will cause a total paralysis or only a partial paralysis, because certain large muscles are innervated by more than one nerve.

A lesion of a single sensory root (e.g., compression by a prolapsed disc) may impair cutaneous sensation in a segmental distribution but never produces a complete loss of sensation, for the reason that adjacent roots always overlap in their cutaneous distribution. In plexus and peripheral nerve lesions, all trace of segmental arrangement is lost because plexuses and nerves are made up of fibers derived from several roots. Sensory changes that characterize the involvement of multiple nerves (polyneuropathy) are described in Chap. 44. Sensory syndromes due to involvement of multiple sensory roots (e.g., tabetic neurosyphilis, some cases of diabetes mellitus) are difficult to distinguish from a posterior column syndrome (see below).

Spinal Sensory Syndromes

The lesions giving rise to these syndromes are shown diagramatically in Fig. 8-4.

A *complete transverse lesion* of the spinal cord abolishes all motor and sensory functions below the level of the lesion. In a narrow band at the upper level of the analgesic zone, where loss

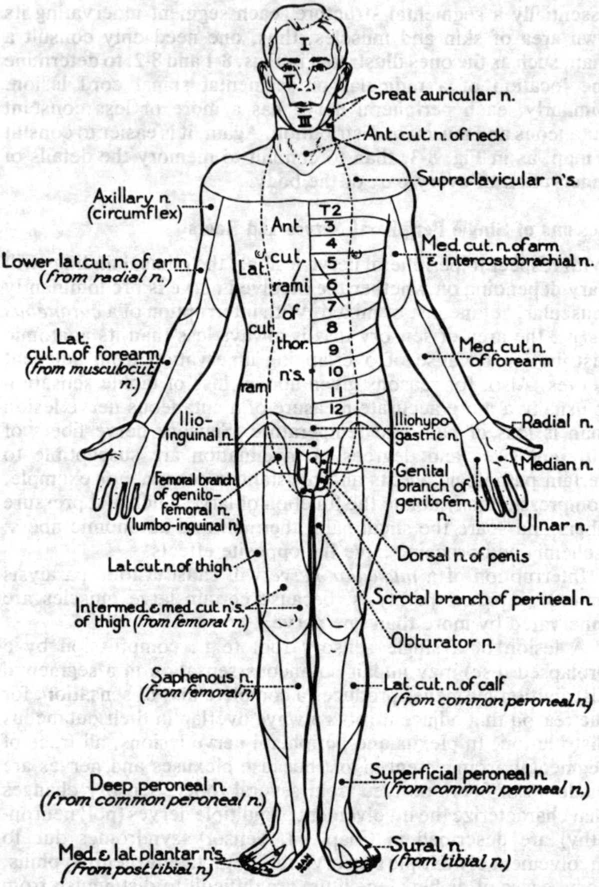

FIG. 8-3 The cutaneous fields of peripheral nerves. (*From W Haymaker, B Woodhall, Peripheral Nerve Injuries, 2nd ed, Philadelphia, Saunders, 1953.*)

of sensation is only partial, pressing or rubbing the skin lightly may be painful.

A lesion of one side of the cord results in a contralateral loss of perception of pain and thermal sense, beginning one to two dermatomes below the level of the lesion, and a loss of vibratory,

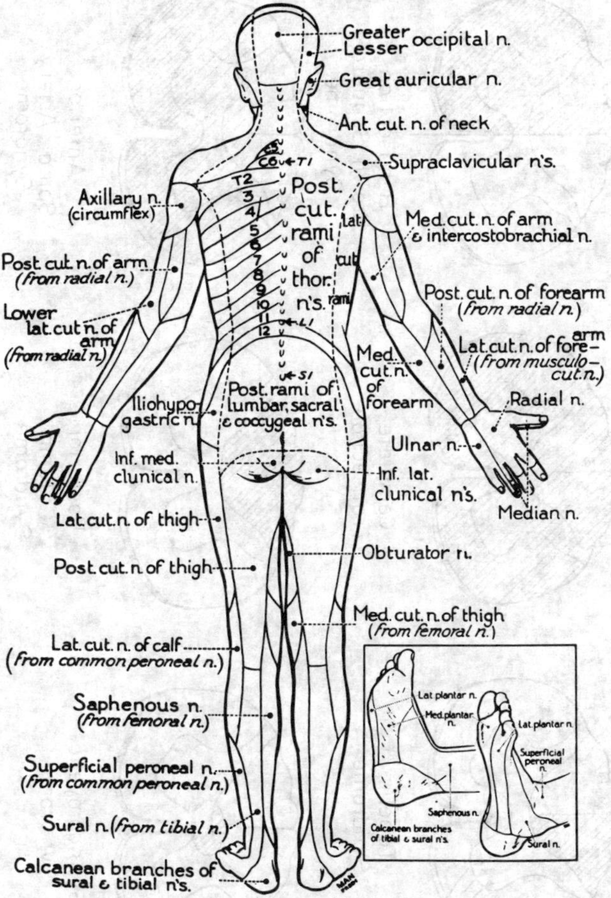

FIG. 8-3 (*continued*)

postural, and discriminatory sensation ipsilaterally. Tactile sense is affected little if at all because it utilizes bilateral pathways. There is also an upper motor neuron paralysis on the side of the lesion. This combination of sensorimotor loss is known as the *Brown-Séquard syndrome*.

Lesions that damage only the *anterior half of the cord* (anterior

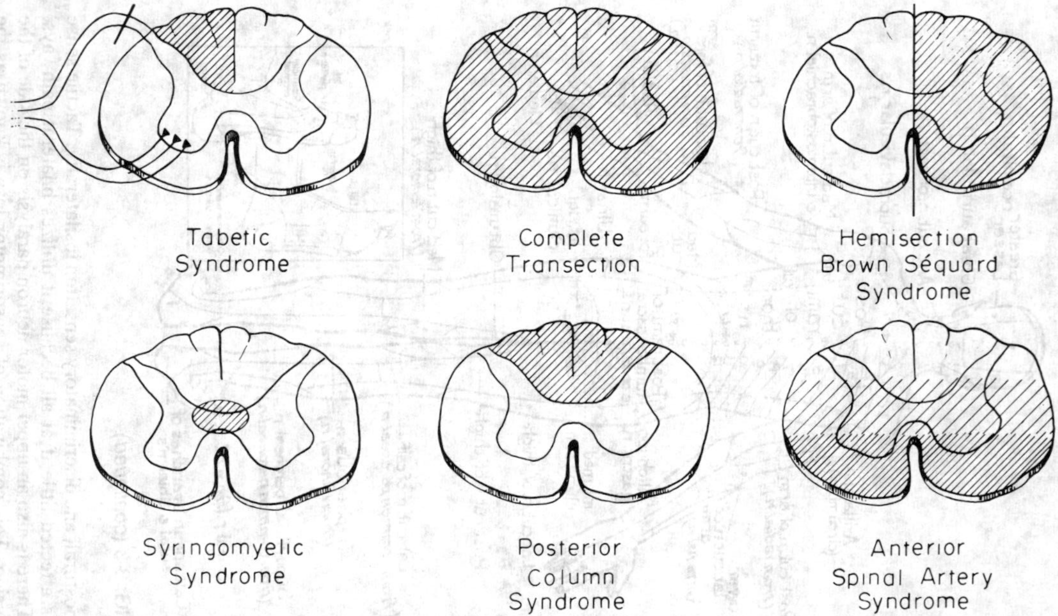

FIG. 8-4 Some of the sites of lesions that produce characteristic spinal cord syndromes (shaded areas indicate lesions).

spinal artery syndrome) cause a bilateral loss of pain and temperature sense, with sparing of posterior column sensation. Contrariwise, *lesions limited to the posterior columns* cause a loss of position and vibratory sense and all types of sensory discrimination, a Romberg sign, a characteristic ataxic or "tabetic" gait (Chap. 6), and an ataxia of the arms and astereognosis in the hands (with high cervical lesions); tactile sensation is little affected, and the response to painful and thermal stimuli and to tickling may actually be increased (Nathan et al).

Partial lesions of the spinal cord, as would be expected, are expressed by limited sensory deficits. Section of an anterior quadrant (*spinothalamic cordotomy*) abolishes pain and temperature but not tactile sensation on the opposite side. The loss may recede after some months, when multisynaptic afferent pain neurons in the gray matter of the cord become more active.

Compressive lesions of the cord and intramedullary lesions have variable effects on sensation, depending upon their precise location. The sensory fibers in the posterior and lateral columns are laminated. As new fibers enter the posterior columns at successively ascending levels, fibers from the lower segments are displaced medially and posteriorly. An opposite lamination pertains in the spinothalamic tract; at each ascending segment, crossing fibers for pain and temperature are added to the inner side of the tract so that the longest fibers from the sacral segments come to lie most superficially (Fig. 7-2). Thus a cord lesion may cause either an ascending or a descending deficit, depending on the direction in which it expands. With lateral compression of the cord, sensory loss begins in the legs and then ascends; an expanding central lesion would involve spinothalamic tract function in the reverse direction.

Involvement of the posterior horn may cause an ipsilateral radicular sensory loss and pain over one or more segments. Lesions that involve the anterior commissure and extend over many segments cause a segmental loss of pain and temperature on one or both sides, with sparing of tactile sensation. This type of dissociated sensory loss is characteristic of *syringomyelia* (Chap. 34). Certain lesions of the posterior columns appear to affect some fibers more than others. It is not unusual to find a loss of vibratory sense with preservation of position sense; occasionally the opposite occurs.

Sensory Loss with Lesions of the Brainstem, Thalamus, and Parietal Lobe

In the lower brainstem, e.g., lateral tegmentum of the medulla, a lesion may involve the descending fibers and nucleus of the trigeminal nerve and the contiguous lateral spinothalamic tract. The result is an ipsilateral loss of pain and temperature sensation over the face and a contralateral loss over the neck, arm, trunk, and leg. The medial lemniscus, which lies more medially, is usually not affected. However, in the upper pons and midbrain, where these tracts merge, a lesion may impair all forms of sensation contralaterally, including tactile sensation.

Lesions of the *ventrolateral thalamus* (usually vascular) may also abolish all forms of sensation contralaterally. As improvement occurs and the sensory deficit lessens, there may be spontaneous ("thalamic") pain on the affected side and all stimuli, including affective ones, give rise to pain and discomfort of a diffuse, persistent type. The pain may be present even when the threshold for perception of pain and thermal stimuli is raised *(analgesia dolorosa)*. A similar state is known to accompany lesions of the parietal white matter.

The effects of parietal cortical lesions on the discriminatory qualities of sensation have already been mentioned. Other effects of parietal lesions on sensation and the function of the parietal lobe as a sensory integrating mechanism are discussed in Chap. 21.

TESTING OF SENSORY FUNCTION

This is the most difficult part of the neurologic examination, demanding, as it does, the close attention and objective attitude of an alert and cooperative patient. Moreover, test procedures are relatively insensitive and their evaluation is difficult, since they are subjective, i.e., they depend on the patient's interpretation of sensory experiences.

Tactile sensation is conventionally tested with a wisp of cotton. The patient, with eyes closed, is asked to indicate each contact. The light application of the examiner's or the patient's roving fingertips is a useful method of mapping an area of tactile loss. *Pain* sensation is usually tested by pinpricks delivered about one per second and not over the same spot, the patient being asked to distinguish between blunt and sharp. Areas or levels of pain loss are best delineated by proceeding from a region of impaired sensation toward the normal, and the changes are confirmed by dragging a pin lightly over the parts in question. The proper evaluation of thermal sense requires that large test objects be used, preferably Erlenmeyer flasks containing hot and cold water, and the patient is asked to state whether one flask feels warmer or colder than another. The temperature of the water can be measured by thermometers that extend through the flask stopper, and the severity of thermal loss can be roughly quantitated by determining the differences in temperature that the patient is able to distinguish.

Vibration sense is tested by placing a tuning fork with a low rate and long duration of vibration (128 dv) over the bony prominences and comparing the point tested with a more normal part of the patient or a corresponding part of the examiner. The perception of passive *movement* and *position sense* are tested most efficiently in the fingers and toes, since the defects are reflected maximally in these parts. The digit is grasped firmly at the sides and moved quickly, and the patient is instructed to report each movement as being "up" or "down" from the previous position.

Supplementation of these tests by refined quantitative methods is required for research purposes.

Discriminative or *"cortical" sensory functions* are assessed by testing the patient's ability to distinguish two points from one (two-point discrimination), to localize cutaneous tactile or painful stimuli, to recognize numbers or letters written on the hands (graphesthesia), and to recognize the shape and size of objects placed in the hand (the primary sense data being intact).

Details of sensory testing and their implications will be found in the *Principles*.

For a more detailed discussion of this topic, see Adams and Victor: *Principles of Neurology*, 4th ed, pp 118–133.

ADDITIONAL READING

Brodal A: The somatic afferent pathways, in *Neurological Anatomy*, 3rd ed. New York, Oxford University Press, 1981, pp 46-147.

Carmon A: Disturbances of tactile sensitivity in patients with unilateral cerebral lesions. *Cortex* 7:83, 1971.

Light AR, Perl ER: Peripheral sensory systems, in Dyck P et al (eds): *Peripheral Neuropathy*, 2nd ed. Philadelphia, Saunders, 1984, vol I, chap 9, pp 210-230.

Lindblom U, Ochoa J: Somatosensory function and dysfunction, in Asbury AK, McKhann GM, McDonald W (eds): *Diseases of the Nervous System*. Philadelphia, Saunders, 1986, pp 283-298.

Nathan PW, Smith MC, Cook AW: Sensory effects in man of lesions in the posterior columns and of some other afferent pathways. *Brain* 109:1003, 1986.

9 Headache and Other Craniofacial Pains

Headache is essentially a symptom without a sign. With a few notable exceptions (auscultation of a bruit, palpation of thickened arteries) physical examination of the head during or between headaches yields little useful information.

The frequency and multiplicity of causes of headache bring it to the notice of physicians in many specialties. Although usually benign and lacking assignable cause, it is often enough the expression of significant intracranial disease to require consultation with a neurologist or neurosurgeon.

By consensus, headache refers to pain in the cranium. Pains in the face, jaws, throat, and neck are set apart, for they turn attention to a different set of diagnostic possibilities. They will be considered briefly in the latter part of this chapter and elsewhere in the book.

Headache may have its source in a large number of cranial structures, all of which are innervated by unmyelinated C fibers and thinly myelinated A-δ fibers contained in the trigeminal, glossopharyngeal, and vagus nerves and first two to three cervical roots. These pain-sensitive structures include the eye, ear, paranasal sinuses, large extra- and intracranial arteries, dural sinuses, periosteum of the skull, skin, cranial muscles, and upper cervical spine. The pathophysiologic mechanisms whereby pain is evoked in each of these structures varies.

As in all painful states, it is helpful in patients with headache to make careful inquiry as to the quality of the headache, its intensity, location, temporal profile, associated symptoms, and clinical course, and the conditions that evoke, intensify, and relieve the pain. Films of the skull and sinuses, CT scans and MRI, EEG, and CSF examination are useful ancillary procedures but are required in only a minority of cases. The art of medicine is to know when to use them.

A large proportion of the general public is subject to headache from time to time. It is usually ascribed to nervousness or tension, and relief is obtained with aspirin or acetaminophen. One can only speculate as to the cause of the common everyday headache. Everyone has experienced the frontal-nasal discomfort of upper respiratory infections, the clues to which are nasal blockage and discharge. Only sphenoid sinusitis, which may refer pain to the vertex, and persistence of headache after the infection or allergic rhinitis has passed occasion diagnostic problems. Hyperopia and astigmatism may be associated with pain in the forehead, especially in young people with "eye strain," but the latter diagnosis is made far more often than it exists. Myopia seldom causes headache. Special importance attaches to the association of ocular pain with glaucoma and iridocyclitis and with temporal arteritis which, if not recognized, may result in a loss of sight (see further on). Arthritis of the upper cervical spine may be a source of occipitocervical pain, usually worse after a period of inactivity; its reference to the forehead is puzzling, however. Febrile states of all types may be manifest by headache, raising always the specter of meningitis.

These generalizations are familiar to every physician and seldom raise problems in diagnosis. Not so are certain instances of intracranial and extracranial disease and migraine, which because of their subtle variations may be diagnostically difficult.

In the clinical approach to the patient, it is important to determine whether the headache is a new development, unlike any headache that the patient had experienced before, or merely the recurrence of a frequently experienced headache. Different also is the approach to a patient whose headaches in recent days, weeks, or months have become more frequent, severe, or continuous. In these circumstances, CT scans, MRI, or other investigative measures may be required to reassure the patient (and the physician) that a brain tumor or other intracranial lesion has not been overlooked.

The common types of headache and their clinical features are listed in Table 9-1. Additional features of these and less common forms of headache are described below.

HEADACHE OF ABRUPT ONSET OR RAPID DEVELOPMENT

The common causes are ruptured saccular aneurysm, primary or hypertensive intracerebral hemorrhage, ruptured arteriovenous malformation (AVM), and bacterial meningitis. These disorders represent medical emergencies, and the headache in each case is notable for its severity. The hypertensive hemorrhage nearly always progresses to stupor or coma with major neurologic deficit. Subarachnoid hemorrhage from an aneurysm or AVM may leave the patient conscious with few or no focal or lateralizing signs; nausea, vomiting, and stiff neck are frequent, however (Chap. 32). Headache associated with fever and signs of meningeal irritation, seizures, drowsiness, and confusion are indicative of a bacterial or viral meningitis (Chaps. 30 and 31). Diagnostic

TABLE 9-1 Common Types of Headache

Type	Site	Age and sex	Clinical characteristics
Common migraine	Frontotemporal Uni- or bilateral	Children, young to middle-aged adults, more common in women	Throbbing, worse behind one eye or ear; becomes dull ache and generalized; sensitive scalp
"Neurologic" migraine	Same as above	Same as above	Same as above Family history frequent
Cluster (histamine headache, migrainous neuralgia)	In or around one eye and temple	Adolescent and adult males (80–90%)	Intense, nonthrobbing pain, unilateral
Tension headaches	Generalized	Mainly adults, both sexes, more in women	Pressure (nonthrobbing), tightness, aching
Meningeal irritation (meningitis, subarachnoid hemorrhage)	Generalized, or bioccipital or bifrontal	Any age, both sexes	Intense, steady deep pain, may be worse in neck
Brain tumor	Unilateral or generalized	Any age, both sexes	Variable intensity; may awaken patient; steady pain
Temporal arteritis	Unilateral or bilateral, usually temporal	Over 50 years, either sex	Throbbing, then persistent aching and burning, scalp arteries thickened and tender

Diurnal pattern	Life profile	Provoking factors	Associated features	Treatment
Upon awakening or later in day; lasts hours to 1–2 days	Irregular intervals, weeks to months; tends to decrease in middle age and during pregnancy	Bright light, noise, tension, alcohol; relieved by darkness and sleep	Nausea and often vomiting	Ergotamine and phenergan at onset; propranolol or amitriptyline for prevention
Same as above	Same as above	Same as above	Scintillating lights, blindness, and scotomas; unilateral numbness, weakness, dysphasia, vertigo	Same as above
Usually nocturnal, one or more hours after falling asleep; occasionally diurnal	Nightly or daily for several weeks to months; recurrence after many months or years	Alcohol in some	Lacrimation, stuffed nostril, rhinorrhea, injected conjunctivum	Ergotamine before anticipated attack; amitriptyline; corticosteroids and lithium in recalcitrant cases
Continuous, variable intensity, for days, weeks, or months	One or more periods of months to years	Fatigue and nervous strain; fear of brain tumor	Depression, worry, anxiety	Antianxiety and antidepressant drugs
Rapid evolution—minutes to hours	Single episode	None	Neck stiff on forward bending; Kernig and Brudzinski signs	For meningitis or bleeding (see text)
Lasts minutes to hours; increasing severity	Once in a lifetime: weeks to months	None; sometimes position	Papilledema, vomiting, impaired mentation, seizures, focal signs	Corticosteroids, mannitol, treatment of tumor
Intermittent, then continuous	Persists for weeks to a few months	None	Loss of vision; polymyalgia rheumatica; fever, weight loss, increased sedimentation rate	Corticosteroids

difficulty is posed by febrile states with meningismus (stiff neck but normal CSF). Not infrequently a patient presents to an emergency ward with a violent headache for which no cause is found; CT scans, MRI, and CSF are normal. It may be a first attack of migraine or some other headache that will become recurrent. In such patients close follow-up is essential.

CHRONIC RECURRENT HEADACHE

Migraine

This is the most frequent type. Two forms are identifiable clinically: (1) classic or neurologic migraine and (2) common migraine. Both forms occur with great frequency. Classic migraine affects an estimated 1 to 2 percent of the general population and common migraine, in which diagnosis is less certain, as much as 10 percent.

Criteria that identify *classic migraine* are episodes (lasting hours or a day or longer) of throbbing and usually hemicranial pain of varying degrees of severity preceded by visual disturbances (sparkles, bright zig-zag lines, spreading scotomata) and less often by hemisensory disturbances, hemiparesis, or aphasia, usually on the side opposite the pain. These prodromata last 5 to 15 min and usually disappear before the headache begins. At its maximal intensity, the headache is associated with nausea and often with vomiting. Rest in bed and shunning of light and noise are desired if the pain is severe. The scalp may be tender in the region of the headache and jarring of the head is painful. Sleep tends to alleviate the pain. Additional criteria are a family history of "sick headaches" and response of the headache to ergot preparations.

Common migraine is similar but occurs without neurologic prodromata. Generalized headache is somewhat more common than with classic migraine. Occasionally classic migraine and, even more rarely, common migraine are followed by a lasting neurologic deficit—most often a homonymous hemianopia or hemisensory deficit, rarely hemiparesis, aphasia, or oculomotor palsy (*complicated migraine*). A special form of migraine is thought to occur in the territory of the *basilar artery*; the visual phenomena may occupy all of both visual fields and are accompanied by brainstem signs, sometimes with stupor. The headache that follows is usually occipital.

The onset of both types of migraine is usually in adolescence, but they may begin in childhood or in early or mid-adult life. Attacks usually occur once every month or two, sometimes more frequently, and rarely the patient lapses into a state of virtually continuous migraine ("decompensated migraine" or "status migrainosus''). In childhood, the male-to-female ratio is about equal; later the incidence is twice as high in females. It disappears during pregnancy in 80 percent of cases, and it is prudent to discontinue medication during pregnancy. Birth control hormones tend to aggravate migraine and increase the risk of permanent sequelae. The premenstrual type of headache is thought to be nonmigrainous. In late adult life, migraine may disappear or be reduced to only the neurologic prelude, without the attendant headache.

Neither the etiology nor the pathogenesis of migraine is fully understood. Most authorities contend that it is a hereditary disorder; classic migraine occurs in several family members of the same and successive generations in 60 to 80 percent of cases. The figures for common migraine are less convincing. No one personality type has proved to be disproportionately vulnerable. In none of the so-called psychosomatic diseases or neuroses is the incidence of migraine higher than in the population at large. The worsening of migraine that occurs during periods of intense nervousness, anxiety, and depression is usually due to the superimposition of tension headache.

The conventional view of the pathogenesis of classic migraine, dating from the early observations of Wolff and colleagues, has been that vascular spasm accounts for the neurologic symptoms and vasodilatation for the headache and tenderness. The pulsatile character of the headache and its relief by carotid compression, the occasional occurrence of ischemic infarction, and the reduced blood flow (only in classic migraine, not in common migraine), all incriminate a vascular factor. More recent hypotheses place greater emphasis on the role of sensitized nerve endings in the blood vessels, which release substance P, the latter causing vasoconstriction and regional reduction in blood flow. Yet another hypothesis favors an initial disturbance in the hypothalamus and limbic cortex. None of these hypotheses explains the periodicity of migraine.

Tension Headache

This is the most frequent type encountered in general practice, constituting about two-thirds of all headache cases and affecting, at one time or another, about 25 percent of the general population. The main features are outlined in Table 9-1. The headache, though bilateral and usually diffuse, may predominate in any part of the cranium. Aching, fullness, tightness, or pressure are the common descriptive terms. Persistence of the headache, with only mild fluctuations, for weeks, months, or even years is characteristic. Sleep is rarely disturbed, however. Accompanying symptoms are those of anxiety and depression, though in some patients these features are not prominent. In these respects, the headaches of the posttraumatic instability syndrome are similar (Chap. 33). Not infrequently, tension headache may be superimposed on typical attacks of migraine.

Sustained, excessive muscle contraction has been the postulated mechanism of the pain, but it probably explains only a small proportion of the cases (see *Principles* for details).

Cluster Headache (Migrainous Neuralgia, Horton's Histamine Cephalgia)

This type occurs nightly, less often daily, for a period of many weeks to months (a cluster) and then disappears as mysteriously as it came. It occurs predominantly in young adult males (male-female ratio of 5:1). The pain is intense and nonpulsatile in and around one eye and is accompanied by tearing, conjunctival congestion, rhinorrhea, and sweating and flushing of the forehead and cheek. It lasts for 20 to 30 min and subsides rapidly. A common pattern is abrupt onset within an hour or two after falling asleep; it is of such intensity as to awaken the patient and set him to pacing. At the peak of severity it may occur several times a day. The entire cluster may recur several times, usually on the same side. In some patients, a cluster is provoked by consumption of alcohol. A chronic form, recurring daily for many years without respite, is known.

Other Varieties of Headache

Postlumbar puncture headache Characteristic is the occurrence of headache and pain in the neck and upper back a few minutes after sitting up or standing and relief on lying down. A rent in the spinal dura permits CSF to seep into the epidural tissues for hours or days after the lumbar puncture. The low CSF pressure, which is further reduced in the upright position, leads to caudal displacement of the brain and traction on dural attachments and sinuses. Once the leakage stops and the pressure is restored, the postural headache ceases.

Spontaneous, low-pressure headaches lasting several days may follow a sneeze or strain that has caused rupture of the arachnoid surrounding a nerve root.

Headache of brain tumor Headache is a significant symptom in approximately two-thirds of patients with intracranial tumor. With supratentorial tumors, the pain is usually anterior to the interauricular circumference of the skull, and with posterior fossa tumors, it is postauricular. Early on, the location of the headache correlates with the site of the tumor. Usually, the headache is deep-seated and nonthrobbing, and lasts a few minutes to hours. Nocturnal and early morning occurrence of the headache are characteristic features but are not specific. The headaches increase in frequency and severity as the tumor grows. With elevated intracranial pressure, the headache tends to be bilateral and fronto-occipital. Unanticipated vomiting may accompany tumor headaches.

Cranial arteritis This is an inflammatory disease of extracranial arteries, sometimes occurring in conjunction with polymyalgia rheumatica. The patient is nearly always elderly and has some systemic symptoms, an elevated sedimentation rate, and palpably thickened, tender, temporal arteries on one side of the head (other nonpalpable arteries may be affected). Diagnosis is confirmed by biopsy of an artery. If untreated, the disease lasts for many months to a year or longer, the great danger being an abrupt onset of visual loss (often permanent) or an ophthalmoplegia from occlusion of an ophthalmic artery.

Headaches related to *cough, exertion,* and *sexual activity* are not uncommon but present no special difficulties in diagnosis or management.

TREATMENT

The control of an attack of *migraine* is most effective if the drug to be used is given at the very onset of an attack. If mild, 650 mg (two tablets) of aspirin or an equivalent amount of other nonnarcotic analgesic, repeated as necessary, may be sufficient. Metoclopromide (10 mg), taken concomitantly, promotes gastric absorption and reduces nausea. For severe attacks, ergotamine tartrate is the most effective medication. This can be taken sublingually (1 to 2 mg), by subcutaneous injection (0.25 to 0.5 mg), in combination with caffeine (Cafergot) orally or by suppository, or by inhalation (Medihaler). Each of these ergot preparations may be repeated in 30 to 60 min, but only once or twice.

Dihydroergotamine (DHE), 1 mg intramuscularly or subcutaneously, has less side effects (nausea, aching in the legs) than ergotamine tartrate. Also DHE is more effective in terminating an established headache and status migrainosus.

For the *prevention of migraine,* oral propranolol (Inderal, 20 to 80 mg tid) is the most effective drug, reducing the frequency and severity of headache in about 75 percent of patients. Clonidine (0.05 mg tid), indomethacin (150 to 200 mg/day), cyproheptadine (Periactin, 4 to 16 mg/day), or a course of methysergide (Sansert, 2 to 6 mg/day), amitryptiline (25 mg tid),

TABLE 9-2 Types of Facial Pain

Type	Site	Clinical characteristics	Aggravating-relieving factors	Associated diseases	Treatment
Trigeminal neuralgia (tic douloureux)	Second and third divisions of trigeminal nerve, unilateral	Men/women = 1:3; over 50 years; paroxysms (10–30 s) of stabbing, burning pain; persistent for weeks or longer; trigger points; no sensory or motor paralysis	Touching trigger points, chewing, smiling, talking, blowing nose, yawning	Idiopathic; in young adults, multiple sclerosis; vascular anomaly; tumor of fifth cranial nerve	Carbamazepine; phenytoin; alcohol injection, coagulation, or surgical decompression of nerve
Atypical facial neuralgia	Unilateral or bilateral; cheek or angle of cheek and nose; deep in nose	Predominantly female 30–50 years; continuous intolerable pain; mainly maxillary areas	None	Depressive and anxiety states; hysteria; idiopathic	Antidepressant and antianxiety medication
Postzoster neuralgia	Unilateral; usually ophthalmic division of fifth nerve	History of zoster; aching, burning pain; jabs of pain; paresthesiae, slight sensory loss Dermal scars	Contact, movement	Herpes zoster	Carbamazepine, antidepressants, and sedatives

Costen syndrome	Unilateral, behind or front of ear, temple, face	Severe aching pain, intensified by chewing; tenderness over temporomandibular joints; malocclusion, missing molars	Chewing, pressure over temporo-mandibular joints	Loss of teeth, rheumatoid arthritis	Correction of bite; surgery in some
Tolosa-Hunt syndrome	Unilateral, mainly retro-orbital	Intense sharp, aching pain, associated with opthalmoplegias and sensory loss over forehead; pupil usually spared	None	Lesion of cavernous sinus or superior orbital fissure	Surgery: corticosteroids for granulomatous lesions
Raeder paratrigeminal syndrome	Unilateral, frontotemporal and maxilla	Intense sharp or aching pain, ptosis, miosis, preserved sweating	None	Tumors, granulomatous lesions, injuries in parasellar region	Depends on type of lesion
Carotidynia, lower half headache sphenopalatine neuralgia, etc.	Unilateral face, ear, jaws, teeth, upper neck	Both sexes, constant dull ache 2–4 h	Compression of common carotid at or below bifurcation reproduces pain in some	Occasionally with cranial arteritis, carotid tumor, migraine and cluster headache	Ergotamine acutely; methysergide for prevention

phenelzine (Nardil, 30 to 60 mg/day), and phenytoin (in children) have been helpful in individual cases. Prednisone (45 mg/day for 3 to 4 weeks) or a calcium channel blocker (verapamil, nifedipine) can be tried in refractory cases. Each of these drugs has significant side effects, and one resorts to them only if the headaches are severe and disabling and cannot be controlled by the early use of ergotamine tartrate or DHE.

Cluster headaches can be treated with single doses of ergotamine at bedtime (for nocturnal attacks) or once or twice during the day, in anticipation of a headache. Once the diagnosis has been established, most physicians go directly to a course of prednisone, beginning with 75 mg daily and reducing the dose at 3-day intervals, unless the headaches reappear. In chronic cases, lithium carbonate (600 to 900 mg daily, with blood levels of 0.7 to 1.2 meq/L) may be successful, according to recent reports. Indomethacin may be effective in some chronic cases.

Antidepressive and anxiolytic medication—amitryptiline, norpramine, imipramine, or one of the MAO inhibitors—or benzodiazepines are the standard treatment for *tension headaches* with symptoms of anxiety and depression. Patients in whom sustained excessive muscle contraction is prominent may benefit from massage and lidocaine (xylocaine) injection of tender points in the temporal or neck muscle.

OTHER CRANIOFACIAL PAINS

There are many types, for the most part rare. Only trigeminal neuralgia occurs with any degree of frequency, and it will be discussed with disorders of the cranial nerves (Chap. 45). The other types are summarized in Table 9-2.

For a more detailed discussion of this topic, see Adams and Victor: *Principles of Neurology*, 4th ed, pp 134–154.

ADDITIONAL READING

Broderick JP, Swanson JW: Migraine-related strokes. *Arch Neurol* 44:868, 1987.

Drummond PD, Lance JW: Extracranial vascular changes and the source of pain in migraine headache. *Ann Neurol* 13:32, 1983.

Fisher CM: Late-life migraine accompaniments—further experience. *Stroke* 17:1033, 1986.

Kittrelle JP, Grouse DS, Seybold ME: Cluster headache. *Arch Neurol* 42:496, 1985.

Lance JW: *The Mechanism and Management of Headache,* 4th ed. London, Butterworth, 1982.

Moskowitz MA: The neurobiology of vascular head pain. *Ann Neurol* 16:157, 1984.

Oleson J: The ischemic hypothesis of migraine. *Arch Neurol* 44:321, 1987.
Raskin NH: *Headache*, 2nd ed. New York, Churchill Livingstone, 1988.
Wolff HG: in Dalessio DJ (ed): *Wolff's Headache and Other Head Pain*, 5th ed. New York, Oxford University Press, 1987, pp 59–60.
Ziegler DK, Hurwitz A, Hassanein RS, et al: Migraine prophylaxis. A comparison of propranolol and amitriptyline. *Arch Neurol* 44:486, 1987.

10 Pain in the Back, Neck, and Extremities

In the study of painful disorders of these parts, the principal role of the neurologist is to help decide whether a disease of the spine has implicated the spinal cord and the spinal roots and nerves. (The neurology of spinal cord and root compression is discussed in Chap. 34.) But the neurologist also participates in searching for the underlying disease and determining the mechanism of the pain. The latter objectives demand a knowledge of many diseases outside the field of neurology.

PAIN IN THE LOWER BACK AND LEGS

The periosteum of the lumbosacral vertebrae, the ligaments that bind them together, their articulations, and the muscles that provide spinal motility and postural support all contain pain receptors. Pain can be produced by direct injury to these structures or by the attendant protective reflex contraction of muscles; or pain can be referred to the low back from diseased extravertebral structures (lower abdominal and genitourinary). Certain spinal diseases, particularly ruptured intervertebral discs, spondylotic stenosis, and spondylolisthesis, and intraspinal trauma and tumors may implicate spinal roots and nerves. Pain from disease of the spine and that from involvement of sensory roots may then be combined. Segmental truncal pain from protective paravertebral muscle spasm and pain referred to parts remote from the lesion add to the difficulties of localization and diagnosis.

Types of Low-Back Pain

a. *Pain due to involvement of lumbosacral structures* is a steady, aching (at times sharp) pain that is poorly localized but felt nevertheless in the general vicinity of the affected part. If severe, it is accompanied by involuntary spasm of the corresponding paravertebral muscles. Certain movements and the assumption of certain postures are thereby prevented. Pressure and percussion over the involved segment(s) may elicit tenderness.
b. *Pain of reflex muscle spasm* is a pressing, aching pain

in palpably taut muscles. Tender points, small knots of contracted muscles, may be palpable.

c. *Referred pain* is of two types: One is projected from the spine to extravertebral structures, e.g., buttock and hamstring muscles, and the other from viscera (ovary, uterus, prostate, colon) to the low back. Referred pain is usually diffuse and aching but at times is more superficial and burning. The intensity of the referred pain corresponds roughly to that of the primary disease.

d. *Radicular or root pain* is more intense than referred pain and is characterized by a proximal-distal radiation in the territory of the root. It is sharp, knife-like, and intensified by movement, cough, or strain and is usually superimposed on a background of aching pain.

Examination of the Back

Much information can be obtained from simple *inspection* of the back, buttocks, and lower extremities in various positions. When standing, the presence of an excessive curvature (of the normal dorsal kyphosis or lumbar lordosis), a gibbus (from spine fracture), a step deformity (from lumbar spondylolisthesis), a pelvic tilt (from a lateral prolapsed disc), a sagging gluteal fold (from an S1 root lesion) are all helpful diagnostic signs.

The patient is then observed walking, sitting, and lying down. All the natural motions may be impeded. Forward bending with knees extended may be limited by pain and spasm, the lumbar spine may be straight and immobile, and tautness of the sacrospinalis muscles may be visible. With degenerative spine disease, straightening up from a flexed position may be slow and uncomfortable. In unilateral sciatica there is often a list to the painful side (sometimes to the opposite side), and the affected leg may be held slightly flexed at the hip and knee. However, hyperextension of the lumbar spine is usually not restricted or painful, either with prolapsed disc or lumbosacral strain. It is restricted with vertebral fracture or inflammatory disease of the articular facets or other structures. One also looks for muscle atrophy on the side of the pain.

Of the tests performed by the examiner, straight-leg raising is the most useful. In cases of prolapsed disc, with the patient supine, lifting the leg with the knee fully extended is limited by pain and hamstring muscle spasm (Lasègue sign). Straight-leg raising may also be limited on the opposite side and evokes pain in the affected leg. Abduction and rotation of the hip are painful in diseases of the hip joint.

A search for tender areas is the last step. The finding of such

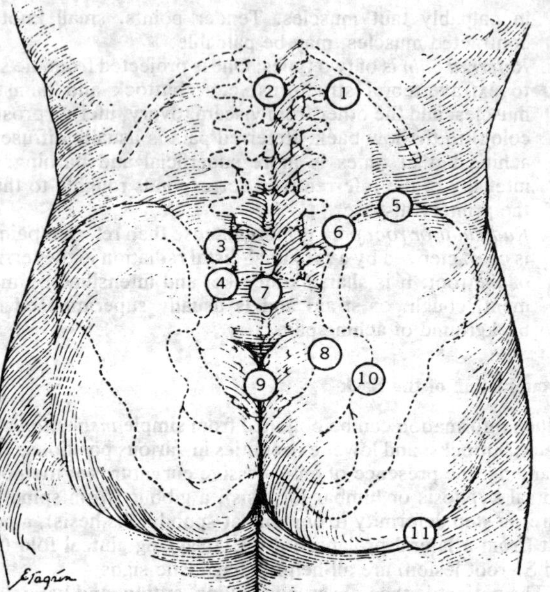

FIG. 10-1 (1) Costovertebral angle. (2) Spinous process and interspinous ligament. (3) Region of articular facet (fifth lumbar to first sacral). (4) Dorsum of sacrum. (5) Region of iliac crest. (6) Iliolumbar angle. (7) Spinous processes of fifth lumbar to first sacral vertebrae (tenderness = faulty posture or occasionally spina bifida occulta). (8) Region between posterior superior and posterior inferior spines. Sacroiliac ligaments (tenderness = sacroiliac sprain, often tender with fifth lumbar to first sacral disc). (9) Sacrococcygeal junction (tenderness = sacrococcygeal injury, i.e., sprain or fracture). (10) Region of sacrosciatic notch (tenderness = fourth to fifth lumbar disc rupture and sacroiliac sprain). (11) Sciatic nerve trunk (tenderness = ruptured lumbar disc or sciatic nerve lesion).

areas, as indicated in Fig. 10-1, is suggestive of disease in the designated structures.

Ancillary Procedures

The selection of laboratory tests depends on the nature of the back problem and the level of one's suspicion of the presence of disease. Helpful measurements include complete blood count, sedimentation rate, serum immunoelectrophoresis, Ca, P, acid and alkaline phosphatase, and rheumatoid factor. Tuberculin skin test and brucella antibody test should be carried out if there is a suspicion of inflammatory disease. Plain films of the spine, bone scans, CT scans with or without enhancement or myelography, MRI, and in cases of discogenic disease, electromyography and nerve conduction studies are important ancillary procedures. Myelography is customarily reserved for patients in whom there is a strong suspicion of ruptured disc, tumor, or stenosis and a likelihood of surgery.

Common Conditions Causing Low-Back Pain

The age of the patient makes certain diagnostic possibilities more or less likely. Postural abnormalities (scoliosis, kyphosis), congenital malformations (e.g., spondylolisthesis), and osteochondritis (Scheuermann disease) are the most frequent causes of chronic back pain in childhood and adolescence. Lumbosacral sprains, rheumatoid spondylitis, ankylosing spondylitis, discogenic disease, and trauma are the predominant types of back pain in early and middle adult years. Stenosing spondylosis, osteoporosis with vertebral collapse, and metastatic tumor tend to occur in older individuals.

Lumbosacral strain or sprain At any age, but mostly in physically vigorous individuals, this disorder may cause intense low-back pain and muscle spasm. Plain films of the lumbosacral region are usually negative. Unless there are paresthesias, weakness unrelated to pain, or reflex changes, there is no way of deciding whether this condition is due to a prolapsed disc or to a ligamentous or muscular lesion. Bed rest, the application of cold and heat, and sufficient analgesic medication relieves the pain in a few days. Hospitalization is only a matter of convenience. A history of one or several such episodes is elicited frequently in patients who are later found to have a ruptured disc.

Spondylolisthesis This disorder, in which a vertebral body, along with its pedicles and articulatory processes, slips forward on the vertebra below (usually L5 on S1, less often L4 on L5), reveals itself in late childhood and adolescence. Low-back pain, limitation of motion, a palpable "step" of the spinous process forward from the one below, and an exaggerated lumbar lordosis are the usual manifestations. In severe cases, the lower lumbar roots may be compressed, with slight weakness or sensory changes in the legs, diminished ankle reflexes, and disturbances of bladder function. The symptoms are increased by standing and walking, like those of lumbar stenosis (see below). Treatment is surgical.

Ruptured intervertebral disc Trauma (usually a flexion injury) or fraying of the annulus fibrosus and posterior longitudinal ligaments allows the soft nucleus pulposus to extrude posterolaterally into the spinal canal and compress a spinal root. The injury need not be severe because of underlying degenerative changes; a sudden twist or lifting from a flexed position of the trunk may be sufficient. The sites of rupture are usually at L5-S1 and L4-L5 and are progressively less frequent at the upper lumbar and lower thoracic levels. The other common sites are C6-C7 and C5-C6.

Usually pain and paresthesias are more conspicuous than weakness. With unilateral root compression weakness is mild, and despite overlapping effects, one finds S1 lesions to weaken ankle flexors; L5, extensors of ankle and big toe; L4, ankle everters; L3, knee extensors; L2, thigh adductors; and L1, hip flexors.

Protrusion of the L4-L5 disc, by compressing the L5 root, causes sciatica along the lateral surface of the thigh and calf and dorsal surface of the foot and first three toes. With an L5-S1 disc (compression of first sacral root), the pain is in the posterior thigh and calf, lateral border of the foot, and fourth and fifth toes; the ankle jerk is reduced or absent. Straight-leg raising stretches L5 and S1 roots, hence the Lasègue sign. With an L3-L4 disc the pain extends to the anterior thigh and the knee jerk is diminished. Large central disc rupture may cause bilateral symptoms with severe weakness of the legs and paralysis of bladder and bowel (cauda equina syndrome). The mechanism of root compression by protruded discs is illustrated in Fig. 10-2.

Bed rest relieves the pain of root compression, unless there is a large free fragment. If bed rest fails, MRI or a lumbar myelogram with or without CT scan confirms the diagnosis and serves as a guide to hemilaminectomy and excision. Large central protrusion with signs of cauda equina compression demands immediate myelography and surgical removal. If diagnostic procedures disclose a protruded disc but there is no sciatica, a protracted period of conservative therapy (rest during periods of pain, analgesics, exercises to strengthen abdominal and back muscles, corset) should be tried before resorting to laminectomy.

Only about 1 percent of patients with low-back pain have unmistakable signs of root compression unrelieved by conservative measures and requiring surgical decompression. Of those operated upon, as many as 10 percent in some series need further surgery and as many as 25 percent are left with troublesome back pain ("failed back syndrome"; see *Principles* for details).

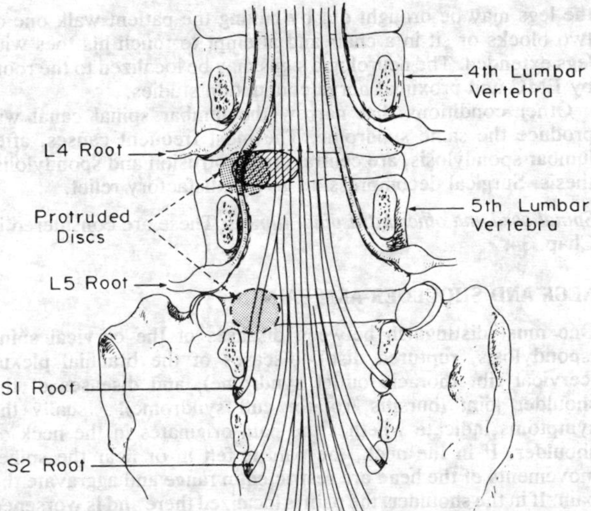

FIG. 10-2 Mechanisms of compression of the fifth lumbar and first sacral roots. A lateral disc protrusion at the L4-L5 level usually involves the fifth lumbar root and spares the fourth; a protrusion at L5-S1 involves the first sacral root and spares the fifth lumbar root. Note that a more medially placed disc protrusion at the L4-L5 level may involve the fifth lumbar root as well as the first (or second and third) sacral root.

Degenerative arthritis Wear and tear and repeated subclinical trauma are blamed for degenerative changes in the most mobile parts of the spine (low cervical and lumbar). This leads to osteophyte formation, both anteriorly and posteriorly into the spinal canal, infolding of the posterior longitudinal ligament, bulging of discs, subchondral sclerosis, and thickening of the ligamentum flavum (*lumbar spondylosis*). There is pain in the affected region, associated with stiffness and limitation of motion. Treatment follows conservative lines if no stenotic compression of roots is present.

Superimposition of the osteoarthritic changes on a narrower-than-normal canal may cause compression of lumbosacral roots; this is referred to as *lumbar spinal stenosis*. Patients have pain in the low back and legs. The pain increases on standing and walking and may resemble the intermittent claudication associated with vascular disease. Weakness and numbness of the feet are added in some cases. Sitting and flexing the trunk reduces or abolishes the symptoms. Weakness and reflex loss in the legs may be brought out by having the patient walk one or two blocks or sit in a chair and attempt to touch his toes with legs extended. The neurologic signs may be localized to the roots by EMG and proximal nerve conduction studies.

Other conditions that narrow the lumbar spinal canal will produce the same syndrome. The most frequent causes, after lumbar spondylosis, are central disc protrusion and spondylolisthesis. Surgical decompression gives satisfactory relief.

Spinal cord and other intraspinal tumors These are considered in Chap. 34.

NECK AND SHOULDER-ARM PAIN

One must distinguish between diseases of the cervical spine (spondylosis, ruptured disc), diseases of the brachial plexus (cervical rib, thoracic outlet syndrome), and diseases of the shoulder joint (bursitis, rotator cuff syndrome). Usually the symptoms indicate whether the pain originates in the neck or shoulder. If in the neck, the pain is felt in or near the spine; movements of the head are restricted in range and aggravate the pain. If in the shoulder, the pain is localized there and is worsened by lifting, abducting, or rotating the upper arm. More deceptive is the relatively rare thoracic outlet syndrome, in which the pain is mainly in the shoulder and upper arm or inner parts of the hand and forearm.

Cervical Disc Protrusion

This may result from injury, especially with hyperextension of the neck (as in diving, chiropractic manipulation), or it may develop without explanation. A lateral protrusion at C5-C6 compresses the sixth cervical root. There is pain along the ridge of the trapezius and tip of the shoulder, with radiation to the anterior part of the upper arm, radial forearm, and often to the thumb, and there are paresthesias and mild sensory impairment in the same regions. The biceps and supinator reflexes are diminished, and there may be slight weakness in flexion of the forearm.

Protrusion of the disc between C6 and C7, compressing the C7 root, causes pain in the shoulder blade, with radiation into the pectoral region, axilla, posterolateral aspect of the upper arm, dorsal forearm, and index and middle fingers; paresthesias and sensory loss correspond to the distribution of the pain. There may be weakness in extension of the forearm and a diminished or absent triceps reflex.

Rupture of a disc may occur at other cervical levels, but that at C6-C7 accounts for 70 percent of cases and that at C5-C6 for 20 percent.

Treatment follows along the same lines as were indicated for lumbar disc disease. In the case of cervical root compression, immobilization of the neck with a soft collar or by traction with a halter is often helpful.

Degenerative Diseases of the Cervical Spine

Osteoarthritis, the most common member of this group, affects men more often than women. Not well understood is its tendency to worsen abruptly and to induce symptoms of radicular disease. This suggests trauma or an inflammatory joint change, but evidence for either is usually lacking. The usual symptoms are cervical aching pain radiating into the occiput, shoulder, and upper arms and restriction of movement of the head. With advanced disease and the formation of bony ridges (ossification of protruded disc material), the spinal cord may be compressed (*cervical spondylosis*), resulting in spastic weakness and loss of position and vibratory sense in the legs. Osteophytic spur formation in an around the vertebral foramina may cause symptoms and signs of root compression. In patients with congenital narrowing of the cervical spinal canal (less than 10 to 11 mm in anteroposterior diameter), relatively mild trauma or osteoarthritic changes may result in cord and root compression. Temporizing, using analgesic medications, and immobilization of the neck (soft collar, traction) may relieve the symptoms. Failure to do so may require surgical measures (see discussion of cervical spondylosis, Chap. 34).

Rheumatoid arthritis of the cervical spine may, in its advanced form, give rise to a number of acute and chronic spinal cord syndromes. The most serious is acute spinal cord compression due to vertebral subluxation, particularly atlanto-axial subluxation.

Thoracic outlet syndrome (cervical rib syndrome, anterior scalene syndrome) is a rare condition seen most often in the adult woman with drooping shoulders and poor muscle tone. The lower trunk of the brachial plexus, the subclavian vein, and subclavian artery, together or in various combinations, are compressed in the lateral cervical region by a cervical rib, fascial bands, or possibly the anterior and medial scalene muscles. Shoulder and arm pain, slight weakness and atrophy of muscles in an ulnar distribution, dusky discoloration of the hand and forearm, venous distension, and ischemic changes in hand and arm are the usual clinical manifestation (see *Principles* for clinical details and treatment).

Pain Due to Diseases of Extremities

Here one must ditinguish pain due to rheumatoid and hypertrophic arthritis, atherosclerosis of iliac and femoral arteries, polymyalgia rheumatica, and reflex sympathetic dystrophy. Only the latter is of neurologic interest, and it will be described with diseases of the peripheral nervous system (Chap. 44).

For a more detailed discussion of this topic, see Adams and Victor: *Principles of Neurology,* 4th ed, pp 155–180.

ADDITIONAL READING

Alexander E Jr, Kelly DL, Davis CH Jr, et al: Intact arch spondylolisthesis. A review of 50 cases and description of surgical treatment. *J Neurosurg* 63:840, 1985.

Borenstein DG, Wiesel SW: *Low Back Pain. Medical Diagnosis and Comprehensive Management.* Philadelphia, Saunders, 1989.

Empting L: Chronic low back pain and failed back syndrome, in Johnson RT (ed): *Current Therapy in Neurologic Disease–3.* Philadelphia, BC Decker, 1990, pp 61–64.

Gilliatt RW: Thoracic outlet syndromes, in Dyck PJ et al (eds): *Peripheral Neuropathy,* 2nd ed. Philadelphia, Saunders, 1984, pp 1409–1424.

Imparato AM, Riles TS: Peripheral arterial disease, in Schwartz SI et al (eds): *Principles of Surgery,* 5th ed. New York, McGraw-Hill, 1989, pp 933–1010.

Powell MC, Szyprty P, Wilson M, et al: Prevalence of lumbar disc degeneration observed by magnetic resonance in symptomless women. *Lancet* 2:1366, 1986.

Shannon N, Paul EA: L4/5, L5/S1 disc protrusions: Analysis of 323 cases operated on over 12 years. *J Neurol Neurosurg Psychiatry* 42:804, 1979.

Weinstein PR, Ehni G, Wilson CB: *Lumbar Spondylosis, Diagnosis, Management and Surgical Treatment.* Chicago, Year Book, 1977.

SECTION III
DISORDERS OF THE SPECIAL SENSES

11 | Disorders of Smell and Taste

The senses of smell and taste are unique in that they are responsive only to chemical stimuli. Clinically, these senses are subtly combined. Many gustatory experiences are largely olfactory, and patients are often deceived into thinking that they have lost their sense of taste when actually the loss is one of olfaction.

While sources of pleasure—we delight in certain aromas and savor our food—the senses of smell and taste seldom contribute in any fundamental way to health and survival (an exception might be the capacity to smell smoke). Nevertheless, disorders of these senses are frequent sources of complaint, and they may point to the presence of intracranial or systemic disease.

OLFACTORY SENSE

Clinical Disorders of Smell

Anosmia Loss of the sense of smell is a frequent symptom, but only if bilateral is it appreciated by the patient. Olfaction is tested by blocking one nostril and then the other and asking the patient to sniff nonirritating olfactory stimuli, such as coffee, tobacco, and vanilla. If the subject can detect and describe (but not necessarily identify) these odors, the olfactory nerves are intact. Commercial scratch-and-sniff test kits are available.

Numerous nasal disorders may cause anosmia or hyposmia by damaging the ciliated receptor cells in the nasal mucosa: chronic rhinitis of infective or allergic type, heavy smoking, influenza, and atrophic rhinitis (leprosy, local radiation). Receptor cells may be congenitally absent, as in albinos.

Concussive head injury and particularly fractures of the ethmoid bone cause anosmia by interrupting the delicate central processes of the olfactory receptor cells as they pass through the cribriform plate to the olfactory bulbs. The anosmia may be unilateral or bilateral and is often permanent. Subarachnoid hemorrhage, chronic meningitis, and cranial surgery, in which the frontal lobes and olfactory bulbs are retracted from the ethmoid bone, may have the same effect.

The olfactory bulb and tract (second olfactory neuron) may be involved by a meningioma of the olfactory groove, in which case the optic nerve is often implicated as well. The association of unilateral anosmia and optic atrophy with a contralateral papilledema is known as the Foster Kennedy syndrome. Rarely, a large aneurysm causes the same syndrome. Children with anterior meningoencephaloceles and hydrocephalus are usually anosmic, and some of them exhibit CSF rhinorrhea as well.

A large proportion of patients with multiple sclerosis and Parkinson disease are hyposmic or anosmic, and odor recognition may be reduced in patients with Huntington chorea and Alzheimer disease. An impaired capacity to discriminate between odors, the primary perceptual aspects of olfaction being intact, is a characteristic feature of the alcoholic form of Korsakoff psychosis. Presumably these disorders are due to involvement of the higher order olfactory systems in medial-temporal and thalamic regions.

Parosmia or dysosmia This refers to a perversion of the sense of smell; it occurs with partial injuries of the olfactory bulbs or local nasopharyngeal infections, such as ozena or empyema of the nasal sinuses. Parosmia of extreme degree, in which every article of food has an intolerably disagreeable odor (and taste), is sometimes a manifestation of a depressive illness. Parosmia of minor degree, in which unpleasant odors persist for several hours and are reawakened by other olfactory stimuli (phantosmia) is not abnormal.

Olfactory hallucinations These are always of central origin. They are observed most often as the brief initial manifestation (lasting only seconds) of seizures that originate in the mesial-temporal cortex (“uncinate seizures”). Gustatory hallucinations are sometimes conjoined. Olfactory hallucinations accompanied by delusions signify a psychiatric disease, most frequently endogenous depression or schizophrenia. Rarely, hallucinations that occur during the alcohol withdrawal period are olfactory in type. Olfactory hallucinations may also occur in patients with senile dementia, but in such cases one needs always to consider the presence of an associated late-life depression.

GUSTATORY SENSE

There are four primary taste sensations: salt, sweet, bitter, and sour. The receptors are exquisitely sensitive taste buds distributed mainly over the surface of the tongue and to a lesser extent over the palate, pharynx, and larynx. Each receptor is preferentially but not solely sensitive to one type of stimulus, which in the case of taste is a chemical substance in solution. From the anterior two-thirds of the tongue, taste fibers run first in the lingual nerve and then in the chorda tympani, which is a branch of the facial nerve. From the posterior third of the tongue and soft palate, the taste fibers run in the glossopharyngeal nerve, and from the pharynx and larynx, they run in the vagus nerve. All of the primary taste fibers converge on the nucleus solitarius (the "gustatory nucleus"). The second sensory neuron for taste projects to the ventroposteromedial nucleus of the thalamus, probably bilaterally, and also to the hypothalamus and other basal forebrain limbic structures. The end station for taste fibers is probably in the tongue-face area of the postrolandic sensory cortex, since gustatory hallucinations have been produced by electrical stimulation of this region.

Taste is tested by withdrawing the tongue with a gauze sponge and placing a few crystals of salt or sugar on discrete parts of the tongue. The tongue is then wiped clean and the subject reports what he had tasted. If the taste loss is bilateral, mouth washes with dilute solutions of sugar, salt, citric cid, and caffeine are used. Special instruments are available for measuring the thresholds for taste and olfactory perception, but they are impractical for bedside testing.

Clinical Disorders of Taste

The causes of taste impairment are remarkably diverse. Heavy smoking, particularly pipe smoking, is probably the most common cause. Since taste stimuli, like olfactory ones, are effective only in a fluid medium, disorders that cause extreme dryness of the tongue (Sjögren syndrome, pandysautonomia, radiation therapy) will lead to a loss or reduction in taste sensation (ageusia or hypogeusia).

The influenza-like illnesses that impair the sense of smell (see above) also damage the taste buds and diminish or pervert the sense of taste (dysgeusia). Other conditions that may have the same effects are scleroderma, hepatitis, viral encephalitis, myxedema, adrenal insufficiency, and a deficiency of vitamins B_{12} and A. A wide variety of drugs may cause persistent distortions of taste, the most common ones being penicillamine (used in Wilson disease and rheumatoid arthritis), the antineoplastic drugs procarbazine and vincristine, and griseofulvin, amitriptyline, antithyroid drugs, chlorambucil, and cholestyramine.

Henkin et al have described a special form of hypogeusia in which the taste and aroma of food is unpleasant to the point of being revolting. Patients with this disorder have reportedly responded to small oral doses of zinc sulfate.

Taste is frequently lost over the anterior one-half of the tongue in Bell's palsy (see Chap. 45). Invasion of the lingual nerve or chorda tympani by tumor will have a similar effect. Brief gustatory hallucinations may precede a temporal lobe seizure, indicating that taste sensibility is represented in the cerebral cortex, probably in area 43 of the parietal operculum and in the adjacent parainsular cortex.

For a more detailed discussion of this topic, see Adams and Victor: *Principles of Neurology,* 4th ed, pp 183–189.

ADDITIONAL READING

Brodal A: *Neurological Anatomy in Relation to Clinical Medicine,* 3rd ed. Fair Lawn, NJ, Oxford University Press, 1981, pp 640–654.

Douek E: *The Sense of Smell and Its Abnormalities*. London, Churchill Livingstone, 1973.

Hauser-Hauw C, Bancaud J: Gustatory hallucinations in epileptic seizures. *Brain* 110:339, 1987.

Henkin RI, Larson AL, Powell RD: Hypogeusia, dysgeusia, hyposmia, and dysosmia following influenza-like infection. *Ann Otol* 84:672, 1975.

Pryse-Phillips W: Disturbances in the sense of smell in psychiatric patients. *Proc Roy Soc Med* 68:26, 1975.

Schiffman SS: Taste and smell in disease. *N Engl J Med* 308:1275; 1337, 1983.

12 | Common Disturbances of Vision

The diverse composition of the eye, containing, as it does, epithelial, vascular, connective, muscular, pigmentary, and nervous tissue elements, renders it vulnerable to a wide variety of diseases. For this reason it concerns specialists in several branches of medicine other than ophthalmology.

To the neurologist, the eyes are the most important of all sense organs. A large part of human motility and reactions to the environment are under visual control. Thus, nature has placed motor centers next to the visual ones. It has even been suggested that the peculiar neural arrangement wherein one-half of the body is represented in the opposite half of the brain is due to the biconvex lens of the eye, which projects all visual input from the right half of our world to the left hemisphere.

Since the eye is the sole organ of vision, impairment of vision is the main symptom of eye disease. Positive phenomena such as phosphenes and visual illusions and hallucinations are relatively unimportant. Other eye symptoms are irritation, photophobia, pain, diplopia and strabismus, and drooping of the eyelids.

The eyes are examined with two objectives: one is to search in the eye and its adnexa for changes that might clarify the diagnosis of some systemic disease; the other, to find the cause of reduced vision. In Table 12-1 are listed the more common nonneurologic abnormalitites of the eye and the local and systemic diseases of which they are a part. Some of them also impair vision.

APPROACH TO THE PROBLEM OF VISUAL LOSS

Examination for visual loss First one measures *visual acuity* by means of a Snellen chart or, at the bedside, by a "near card," on which the letters have been reduced proportionately, to be read at a distance of 14 in. If the patient reads only the top line of the Snellen chart at 20 ft rather than 200 ft, the acuity is stated as 20/200 or 6/60, in meters. Normal vision is 20/20 or 6/6. If the patient has a refractive error, his glasses should be worn during the test.

If visual impairment cannot be corrected to 20/20 with lenses

TABLE 12-1 Ocular (Nonretinal) Manifestations of Local and Systemic Diseases

Ocular abnormality	Diseases
Conjunctivitis and uveitis with ulceration and fibrosis of cornea	Herpes simplex and zoster, mucocutaneous-ocular syndromes (Stevens-Johnson, Reiter, Behcet), lymphoma, sarcoid
Vascularization of conjunctiva	Ataxia-telangiectasia, orbital-vascular malformations
Keratitis	Congenital syphilis, tuberculosis, ocular pemphigus, malignant exophthalmos
Corneal depositions	
Calcium salts (band keratopathy)	Vitamin D intoxication, sarcoid, hyperparathyroidism, multiple myeloma, rheumatoid arthritis
Cystine crystals	Cystinosis
Chloroquine crystals	Treatment with chloroquine
Clouding with polysaccharides	Mucopolysaccharidoses
Cholesterol	Arcus senilis
Kaiser-Fleischer ring (copper)	Wilson disease
Cataract	Diabetes mellitus, galactosemia, myotonic dystrophy, prolonged corticosteroid therapy, radiation therapy, aging
Vitreous hemorrhage	Trauma, ruptured aneurysm or AVM, diabetic proliferative retinopathy
Vitreous deposits	
Calcium (asteroid hyalosis)	Aging
Amyloid	Systemic amyloidosis
"Floaters"	Usually benign; sometimes retinal detachment

(either for myopia or heteropia), there must be some reason other than an uncorrected refractive error for the diminished visual acuity. It may be an interference with light transmission through the refractive media (cornea, lens, or vitreous). One can inspect each of these structures by depth focusing with an ophthalmoscope. If each of these structures and the retina appear to be normal, then the fault must lie in the optic nerves, chiasm, tracts, lateral geniculate bodies, geniculocalcarine tracts, or occipital lobes (see *Principles* for detailed anatomy of these structures).

Next one examines the *visual fields*. At the bedside this is done by having the patient cover one eye and aligning the other with the corresponding eye of the examiner. By bringing a target (a moving finger or a white disc mounted on a stick) into the

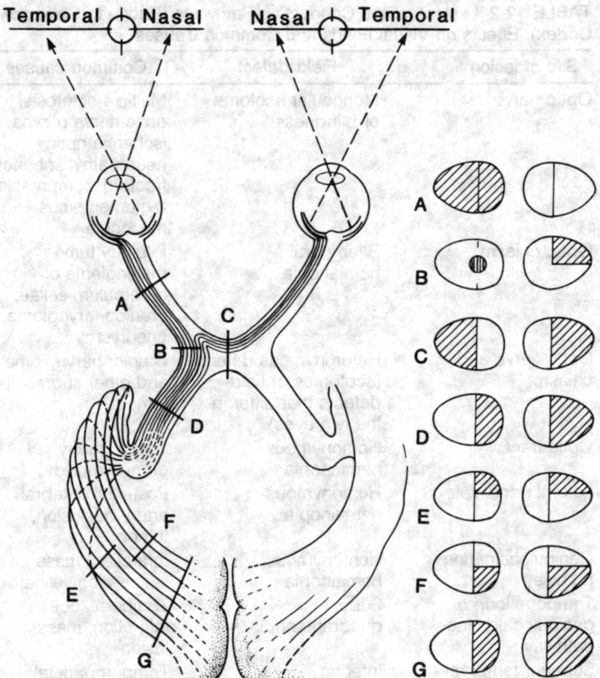

FIG. 12-1 Diagram showing the effects on the fields of vision produced by lesions at various points along the optic pathway: *A*, complete blindness in left eye; *B*, the usual effect is a left junction scotoma in association with a right upper quadrantanopia. The latter results from interruption of right retinal nasal fibers that project into the base of the left optic nerve (Wilbrand's knee). A left nasal hemianopia could occur from a lesion at this point but is exceedingly rare; *C*, bitemporal hemianopia; *D*, right homonymous hemianopia; *E* and *F*, right upper and lower quadrant hemianopia; and *G*, right homonymous hemianopia.

visual field, from the periphery toward the center and equidistant between patient and examiner, the visual fields of patient and examiner can be compared. Perimetry and tangent screen testing are more accurate. The patterns of visual field loss from lesions in different parts of the visual pathway are illustrated in Fig. 12-1. The common causes of these visual field defects are summarized in Table 12-2.

The third step in the examination is a careful *ophthalmoscopic*

TABLE 12-2 Lesions of the Conducting Pathways (Retina to Calcarine Cortex). Effects on Visual Fields and Common Causes

Site of lesion	Field defect	Common causes
Optic nerve	Monocular scotoma or blindness	Multiple sclerosis; optic nerve glioma, ischemic optic neuropathy; sphenoid fracture, compression by tumor; sinus mucocele
Optic chiasm	Bitemporal hemianopia	Pituitary tumor; meningioma of tuberculum sellae; craniopharyngioma; aneurysms
Optic nerve and chiasm	Heteronymous defect (scotomas or field defects that differ in the two eyes)	Craniopharyngioma and other suprasellar tumors
Optic tract	Homonymous hemianopia	Tumor; rarely demyelinative
Lateral geniculate	Homonymous hemianopia	Posterior cerebral artery occlusion; tumor
Geniculocalcarine pathway	Homonymous hemianopia	Infarction, mass lesion, demyelinative
Temporal loop of geniculocalcarine pathway	Superior quadrantanopia	Temporal lobe infarction; mass lesion
Superior temporal lobe	Inferior quadrantanopia or noncongruent homonymous hemianopia	Temporoparietal infarction; mass lesion
Occipital lobe and calcarine cortex	Homonymous hemianopia, congruent	Posterior cerebral artery occlusion
	Central homonymous hemianopic scotomata	Infarction of one occipital pole
	Homonymous altitudinal hemianopia (loss of vision in corresponding upper or lower visual fields)	Infarction above and below calcarine sulcus
	Bilateral cortical blindness	Bilateral infarction. May be central if only occipital poles are affected.

inspection of the retina through a pupil dilated with a short-acting mydriatic (10% phenylephrine). Common shortcomings in the ophthalmoscopic examination are a failure to examine the macular area (which lies 3 to 4 mm lateral to the optic disc and accounts for 95 percent of visual acuity), to search the periphery of the retina, and to appreciate the variations in the appearance of the normal disc. Ophthalmoscopy permits identification of most of the diseases that involve the retina and the optic nerve head.

Ancillary examinations A number of special tests are useful in the investigation of neuro-ophthalmic disorders. The *electroretinogram (ERG)* measures the electrical field generated by the retinal elements. It is impaired in diseases affecting the retinal receptors but is normal with optic nerve lesions. This test is particularly helpful in certain retinal degenerations, which cause only minimal changes in the retina and pigment epithelium and are not easily detected by ophthalmoscopy.

Pattern shift visual evoked potentials detect conduction delays caused by subtle (subclinical) lesions at various points in the visual pathways (Chap. 2).

Other useful procedures are CT scanning, MRI, ultrasound examination of the orbit, and fluorescein retinography.

COMMON CAUSES OF VISUAL LOSS

Acute retinal lesions Sudden painless loss of vision always suggests an ischemic lesion of the retina or optic nerve due to occlusive disease of the central retinal artery or vein or posterior ciliary arteries. Macular and vitreous hemorrhages and retinal detachment are less common causes. Thrombotic or embolic occlusion of the central retinal artery renders the retina ischemic. With occlusion of the central retinal vein, there is engorgement of the retinal veins and diffuse retinal hemorrhages. With ischemic optic neuropathy there may initially be few ophthalmoscopic changes; later the optic disc becomes pale. Mainly these acute vascular accidents occur on a background of hypertensive atherosclerotic disease.

More chronic vascular changes, taking the form of straightening of the retinal arterioles, arteriolar-venular compression, and segmental narrowing of arterioles, are indicative of hypertension. In malignant hypertension, there are, in addition, a number of extravascular lesions—papilledema, hemorrhages, and exudates. These retinal changes are referred to as *hypertensive retinopathy,* and the advanced changes are characteristic of hypertensive encephalopathy.

TABLE 12-3 Common Clinical Types of Visual Loss

Clinical problem	Etiology
A. Acute (minutes to hours) blindness in one eye	Vitreous hemorrhage; ischemic optic neuropathy; temporal arteritis; occlusion of central retinal artery or vein; glaucoma (usually painful); acute iridocyclitis; retrobulbar neuritis
B. Acute bilateral blindness	
1. Retinal lesions	Episode of hypotension; malignant hypertension; eclampsia; retinal burns (sunlight); methyl alcohol
2. Optic nerves	Retrobulbar neuritis
C. Chronic bilateral partial field defects	
1. Bilateral scotomas	Optic (retrobulbar) neuritis; nutritional amblyopia; ischemic optic neuropathy; hereditary optic atrophy
2. Heteronymous field defects	Lesions of chiasm and nerve(s): suprasellar tumors, arachnoiditis
3. Bitemporal hemianopia	Pituitary adenoma, meningioma, aneurysm, some craniopharyngiomas
4. Homonymous hemianopia Upper quadrantanopia (anterior and lower temporal lobe) Lower quadrantanopia (temporoparietal)	May be acute or chronic effects of tumor, abscess, hemorrhage, or infarction
5. Homonymous altitudinal hemianopia (above or below horizontal diameter)	Basilar or bilateral posterior cerebral artery occlusion

Syphilis, toxoplasmosis, histoplasmosis, tuberculosis, and sarcoidosis may cause destructive inflammatory foci in the retina.

Degenerative diseases of the retina The most common is *retinitis pigmentosa (RP)*. This is a hereditary disease in which the outer receptor layer of the retina degenerates, allowing melanin of the pigment epithelium to collect in the thinned retina. The melanin deposits resemble bone corpuscles. The disease begins in adolescence and progresses slowly over years. The peripheral parts of the retina are first and more severely affected, constricting the visual fields and impairing twilight vision predominantly. RP may occur alone or in conjunction with degeneration of other parts of the nervous system—corticospinal tracts, cerebellum, ocular muscles, and myocardium (Kearns-Sayre syndrome), Refsum disease, Bassen-Kornzweig disease, Batten-Mayou lipid storage disease, and endocrine-hypothalamic disease (Laurence-Moon-Biedl syndrome).

Papilledema Papilledema, or "choked disc," is a reflection of raised intracranial pressure. Here the disc margins are elevated and the retinal veins are congested and no longer pulsate. There may be peripapillary hemorrhages, but the macular and peripheral retina are normal. Cerebral tumors, abscesses, intracranial hemorrhage, and hydrocephalus are the usual causes. Visual acuity usually remains normal, but the blind spots enlarge and the visual fields become constricted. With high pressure of long standing, rapid visual failure may occur. Swelling of the optic nerve fibers and stasis of axoplasmic flow are thought to underlie the development of papilledema.

Inflammatory and demyelinative lesions, if located at the optic nerve head, may cause swelling of the disc and even peripapillary hemorrhages ("*papillitis*"), but always there is simultaneous visual impairment. With lesions located further back in the optic nerve the retina and optic disc may appear normal, although later temporal pallor of the disc is seen. Diagnosis of the latter lesions is made from the characteristic visual field abnormalities (Fig. 12-1) and the findings on special ophthalmologic tests. This form of optic (retrobulbar) neuropathy is nearly always due to a demyelinative process and is discussed in Chap. 35.

These and other common clinical types of visual loss and their causes are summarized in Table 12-3.

For a more detailed discussion of this topic, see Adams and Victor: *Principles of Neurology,* 4th ed, pp 190–205.

ADDITIONAL READING

Chester EM: *The Ocular Fundus in Systemic Disease*. Chicago, Year Book Medical Publishers, 1973.

Hayreh SS: Anterior ischemic optic neuropathy. *Arch Neurol* 38:675, 1981.

McDonald WI: Diseases of the optic nerve, in Asbury AK, McKhann GM, McDonald WI (eds): *Diseases of the Nervous System*. Philadelphia, Saunders, 1986, chap. 37, pp. 496–506.

Pearlman AL: Visual system, in Pearlman AL, Collins RC (eds): *Neurobiology of Disease*. New York, Oxford University Press, 1990, chap 7, pp 124–149.

Tso MOM, Hayreh SS: Optic disc edema in raised intracranial pressure III: A pathologic study of experimental papilledema. *Arch Ophthalmol* 95:1448, 1977; IV: Axoplasmic transport in experimental papilledema. Ibid 95:1458, 1977.

13 Disorders of Ocular Movement and Pupillary Function

The extraocular muscles, by their coordinated action, permit a visual stimulus to fall precisely on the two foveas and maintain foveal fixation when the stimulus or the subject is moving. For the latter functions, the labyrinths are essential. The precision with which the two eyes are coordinated in foveation is the most impressive sensory guidance mechanism in human neurophysiology. It makes possible two forms of ocular movement: one in which the eyes turn simultaneously in the same direction, called *conjugate or versional movements,* and the other in which the eyes move in opposite directions (convergence or divergence), called *disconjugate or vergence movements*. The vestibular system influences versional but not vergence movements.

Diseases of the nervous system result in three types of disordered ocular movement: (1) a misalignment of the eyes due to weakness or paralysis of individual ocular muscles, so that a stimulus no longer falls exactly on the foveas of the two eyes (there is then a characteristic diplopia and strabismus); (2) a failure of conjugate movement or gaze, in which the two eyes do not move synchronously in one direction (up or down or to the right or left; in gaze palsies there is no diplopia or strabismus); and (3) a mixture of ocular muscle and gaze palsies.

THE TESTING OF EYE MOVEMENTS

To determine if the axes of the two eyes are parallel, one observes the eyes as the patient looks straight ahead and fixates on a distant target. If one eye deviates inward (esotropia) or outward (exotropia), covering the normal eye will result in refixation of the deviant eye onto the target, indicating an imbalance of ocular muscle tone (congenital or nonparalytic strabismus) rather than an ocular muscle palsy. Another way of detecting an ocular imbalance is for the examiner to hold a light between his eyes and to observe the reflected image on the patient's pupils; in the eccentric eye, the light does not fall on the center of the pupil. At the same time one also observes the width of the two palpebral fissures and relative prominence of the two eyes.

Next one examines versional or conjugate movements, which are of two types. In one, the movements are initiated by will or by command ("look to the right or left") or reflexly, as when a sudden visual or auditory stimulus causes a turning of the eyes (and usually the head) toward it. These movements are referred to as *saccadic* and are normally very rapid (about 200 ms) and accurate. With certain diseases, such as Wilson disease and Huntington chorea, there may occur a marked slowness of saccadic movements. The movements may be fragmented into a series of saccades and fail to reach the target (*hypometria*) or there may be an overshooting of the eyes (*hypermetria*) with coarse corrective saccades. The latter disorders are indicative of defective cerebellar control of the pontine paramedian reticular formation (PPRF) and abducens nucleus (see Fig. 13-1). Yet another abnormality is a failure to initiate voluntary saccades, which is characteristic of ocular apraxia of childhood (Cogan syndrome) and ataxia-telangiectasia (see further on).

Versional movements of the second type are relatively slow and largely involuntary and are tested by asking the patient to follow a moving target, first to one side and then the other and up and down ("pursuit" or "smooth tracking" movements). A slowly rotating striped drum evokes pursuit movements; the eyes follow the stripes and then make a quick corrective saccade to refocus the eyes centrally. The repeated rapid movements of refixation are called *optokinetic nystagmus*. With parieto-occipital lesions, with or without hemianopia, the slow movement of the eyes to the side of the lesion are diminishd or abolished. (*Note:* Cerebral control of visual pursuit movements is ipsilateral.) Pursuit movements, like the fast saccadic ones, may be slowed, fragmented, or dysmetric.

When the patient fixates on a visual target and his head is passively turned, *vestibulo-ocular movements* are elicited. The movement normally is smooth and proportionate to the speed of head turning. The stimulated semicircular canals project information to the contralateral abducens nucleus, which simultaneously innervates the ipsilateral lateral rectus muscle and, via the medial longitudinal fasciculus, the opposite medial rectus muscle. Receptors in neck muscles are integrated with the vestibular end organs to produce coordinated head and eye movements. *Caloric testing* utilizes the same mechanisms; stimulation of the semicircular canals by irrigation with cold water causes conjugate deviation of the eyes toward the stimulus. Warm water has the opposite effect.

Other useful tests are observation of eye movements on forced flexion of the head (*doll's-head maneuver*) and forced closure of

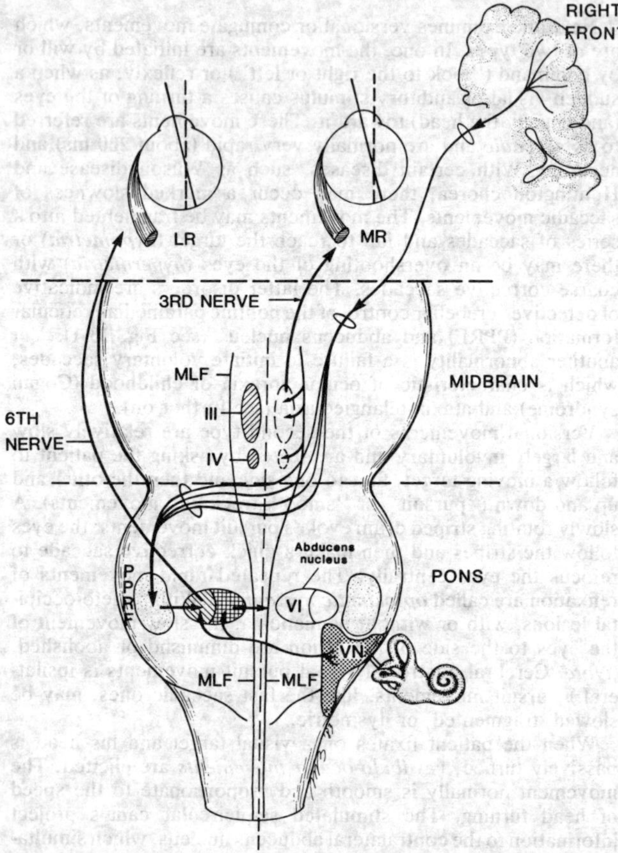

FIG. 13-1 The supranuclear pathways subserving *voluntary* conjugate horizontal gaze to the left. Pathway originates in the right frontal cortex, descends in the internal capsule, decussates at the level of the rostral pons and descends to synapse in the left pontine paramedian reticular formation (PPRF). Cortical (parieto-occipital) control of *pursuit movements* is ipsilateral. Further connections with the ipsilateral sixth nerve nucleus and contralateral medial longitudinal fasciculus are also indicated. Cranial nerve nuclei III and IV are labeled on left; nucleus of VI and vestibular nuclei (VN) are labeled on right. LR, lateral rectus; MR, medial rectus; MLF, medial longitudinal fasciculus.

the eyelids (*Bell phenomenon*). Retention of reflex upward deviation in these maneuvers and failure of voluntary elevation indicate that nuclear and peripheral mechanisms are intact and that the defect is supranuclear.

Vergence or disconjugate eye movements are tested by having the patient focus on a stimulus as it moves toward him. The eyes turn inward; concomitantly the pupils constrict and the ciliary muscles relax to thicken the lens (near or accommodative triad). If convergence (or divergence) is inadequate, diplopia results.

Finally, the size of the pupils and the pupillary reactions to light and near stimuli are recorded.

DISORDERS OF CONJUGATE MOVEMENT (GAZE)

Frontal lobe lesion, acute: Weakness or paralysis of contralateral gaze; eyes deviate to side of lesion; temporary (few days); retention of pursuit and vestibulo-ocular movements.

Bilateral frontal lesions (erroneously called apraxia of gaze): Loss of fast voluntary movements to either side, with retention of visual pursuit and vestibulo-ocular movements.

Parieto-occipital lesion: Loss of pursuit movements to side of lesion; retained voluntary, commanded, and vestibulo-ocular movements; loss of slow phase of optokinetic nystagmus to side of lesion and of fast phase contralaterally.

Midbrain periaqueductal lesion: Paralysis of vertical gaze, more often of upgaze than downgaze (Parinaud syndrome); loss of horizontal gaze with large lesions; convergence and retraction nystagmus may occur on attempted upward gaze.

Pontine lesion: Ipsilateral palsy of horizontal gaze; eyes deviate away from lesion.

Progressive supranuclear palsy: Loss of vertical and later horizontal eye movements; lid retraction.

Parkinson disease: Saccadic eye movements are hypometric; pursuit movements are cogwheel (fragmented).

Ocular apraxia: Eyes move horizontally in direction opposite to head movement in fast willed and commanded movements and are absent on pursuit; vertical movements intact; no optokinetic or vestibulo-ocular movements; seen as a congenital condition (Cogan syndrome) and in ataxia-telangiectasia.

NUCLEAR AND INFRANUCLEAR DISORDERS

Oculomotor (third nerve) palsy: Paralysis or weakness of superior, medial, and inferior rectus muscles, levator palpebrae, and usually of pupillary light and near reactions. With complete lesions, there is ptosis of eyelid, deviation of the eye outward and slightly downward (due to unopposed actions of abducens and superior oblique), and dilatation of pupil. With incomplete lesions, strabismus is less and pattern of diplopia on ocular movement conforms to that in Fig. 13-2. Compressive lesions of oculomotor nerve usually dilate the pupil; ischemic lesions (e.g., in diabetes) usually do not.

Abducens (sixth nerve) palsy: Paralysis of lateral rectus with medial deviation of eye. If partial, there is uncrossed diplopia (image of abducting eye is projected lateral to image of adducting eye) on looking to the side of the lesion (Fig. 13-2). If lesion is central, it is often combined with a palsy of horizontal gaze or internuclear ophthalmoplegia (see below).

Trochlear (fourth nerve) palsy: Extorsion and weakness of downward movement, most marked (diplopia) on looking downward and inward.

Causes of third, fourth, and sixth nerve palsies: Common central causes are infarction (basilar artery and basilar branches), tumor (pontine glioma), hemorrhage, demyelinative disease, and Wernicke encephalopathy (abducens weakness is bilateral). Peripheral causes are infarction of nerve (particularly with diabetes mellitus), basilar skull fractures, tumor (meningeal carcinomatosis), aneurysms or thrombosis of cavernous sinus (often with involvement of ophthalmic division of fifth nerve), ruptured saccular aneurysm (third nerve), giant compressive aneurysms, arteritis, and increased intracranial pressure (bilateral sixth).

FIG. 13-2 Diplopia fields with individual muscle paralysis. The dark glass is in front of the right eye, and the fields are projected as the patient sees the images. *A.* Paralysis of right external rectus. Characteristic: right eye does not move to the right. Field: horizontal homonymous diplopia increasing on looking to the right. *B.* Paralysis of right internal rectus. Characteristic: right eye does not move to the left. Field: horizontal crossed diplopia increasing on looking to the left. *C.* Paralysis of right inferior rectus. Characteristic: right eye does not move downward when eyes are turned to the right. Field: vertical diplopia (image of right eye lowermost) increasing on looking to the right and down. *D.* Paralysis of right superior rectus. Characteristic: right eye does not move upward when eyes are turned to the right. Field: vertical diplopia (image of right eye uppermost) increasing on looking to the right and up. *E.* Paralysis of right superior oblique. Characteristic: right eye does not move downward when eyes are turned to the left. Field: vertical diplopia (image of right eye lowermost) increasing on looking to left and down. *F.* Paralysis of right inferior oblique. Characteristic: right eye does not move upward when eyes are turned to the left. Field: vertical diplopia (image of right eye uppermost) increasing on looking to left and up. (*Adapted from DG Cogan, Neurology of the Ocular Muscles, 2nd ed, Springfield, IL, Charles C Thomas, 1956.*)

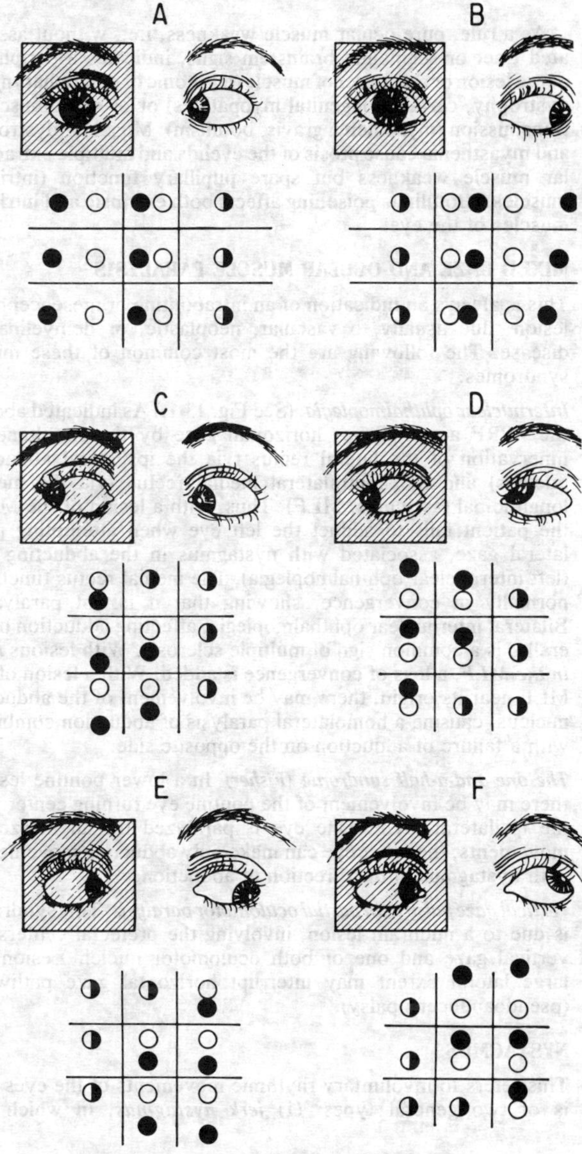

FIG. 13-2

As a rule, pure ocular muscle weakness, i.e., without associated tract or segmental brainstem signs, indicates a peripheral nerve lesion or a disorder of muscle (myotonic or oculopharyngeal dystrophy, certain congenital myopathies) or of neuromuscular transmission (myasthenia gravis, botulism). Muscular dystrophy and myasthenia cause ptosis of the eyelids and multiple extraocular muscle weakness but spare pupillary function (intrinsic muscles). Botulinus poisoning affects both extrinsic and intrinsic muscles of the eye.

MIXED GAZE AND OCULAR MUSCLE PARALYSIS

This is always an indication of an intrapontine or mesencephalic lesion, due usually to vascular, neoplastic, or demyelinative disease. The following are the most common of these mixed syndromes.

Internuclear ophthalmoplegia (See Fig. 13-1.) As indicated above, the PPRF accomplishes horizontal gaze by the simultaneous innervation of the lateral rectus (via the ipsilateral abducens nucleus) and the contralateral medial rectus (via the medial longitudinal fasciculus, MLF). Thus, with a lesion of the MLF, the patient fails to adduct the left eye when attempting right lateral gaze, associated with nystagmus in the abducting eye (left internuclear ophthalmoplegia). The medial rectus functions normally in convergence, showing that it is not paralyzed. Bilateral internuclear ophthalmoplegia, affecting adduction bilaterally, is a common sign of multiple sclerosis. With lesions *high in the MLF*, a loss of convergence is added. With a lesion of the MLF near its origin, there may be involvement of the abducens nucleus, causing a homolateral paralysis of abduction combined with a failure of adduction on the opposite side.

The one-and-a-half syndrome (Fisher) In a lower pontine lesion, there may be involvement of the pontine eye turning center plus the ipsilateral MLF. One eye is paralyzed for all horizontal movements; the other eye can make only abducting movements, with nystagmus in the direction of abduction.

Vertical gaze palsy with partial oculomotor paralysis This syndrome is due to a midbrain lesion, involving the pretectal centers for vertical gaze and one or both oculomotor nuclei. Lesions of large lateral extent may interrupt horizontal gaze pathways (pseudoabducens palsy).

NYSTAGMUS

This refers to involuntary rhythmic movements of the eyes and is of two general types: (1) *jerk nystagmus,* in which the movements alternate between a slow phase and a rapid, corrective phase (by custom, the nystagmus is named according to the direction of the fast phase), and (2) *pendular nystagmus,* in which the oscillations are equal in the two directions, although on lateral gaze two distinct phases may become evident, with the fast phase to the side of gaze. A very fine, rhythmic nystagmus, appearing at the end point of gaze, is physiologic and is abolished by allowing the eyes to move 10° to 15° toward the midline.

The several varieties of pendular and jerk nystagmus, their identifying features, and causative diseases are summarized in Table 13-1.

OTHER DISORDERS OF OCULAR MOVEMENT

Ocular bobbing consists of fast downward (or upward) movements of both eyes followed by a slow return to the central position; or the initial movements may be slow followed by a rapid return. It is usually observed in comatose patients with extensive pontine lesions but may occasionally accompany obstructive hydrocephalus and metabolic encephalopathy.

Ocular myoclonus is a fast (1- to 2-Hz) jerking of the eyes to one side. Usually it is identified by the finding of similar rhythmic movements of the palate, face, neck, or thoracic muscles. The lesion (vascular or tumor) involves the central tegmental tracts between the red nuclei and the medulla.

Opsoclonus refers to rapid multidirectional conjugate movements of the eyes ("dancing eyes"). *Ocular flutter* is a closely related disorder in which bursts of very rapid horizontal oscillations occur around the point of fixation. These disorders occur as a paraneoplastic syndrome with carcinoma; neuroblastoma and viral encephalitis of childhood are other causes.

Sustained spasms of convergence may occur with lesions of the upper midbrain tegmentum. As an isolated phenomenon, it is usually a hysterical symptom.

ABNORMALITIES OF THE PUPILS

The size of the pupil is controlled by the degree of retinal illumination and the state of the optic nerves and tracts, superior colliculi, oculomotor nuclei (Edinger-Westphal) and nerves, ciliary ganglia, and irides. In addition, a sympathetic hypothalamic-cervical cord pathway, with exit mainly at T2, sends preganglionic fibers through the superior cervical ganglion and postganglionic fibers along the internal carotid artery to pupillodilator muscles (see Chap. 25). The pathways involved in the pupillary light reflex are illustrated in Fig. 13-3.

Parasympathetic stimulation constricts the pupil and sympa-

TABLE 13-1 Types of Nystagmus

Type of nystagmus	Identifying features	Causes
Pendular	Always binocular; oscillations in one plane	Albinism and other congenital diseases of retina and refractive media; congenital nystagmus with normal vision
Spasmus nutans	Occurs in infancy with head-nodding and wry neck	Cause unknown; prognosis good
Jerk nystagmus		
Optokinetic	Involuntary slow pursuit followed by fast corrective saccade (refixation)	Lost with parietal lesion and with acute frontal lesion (transient)
Labyrinthine-vestibular	Mixed horizontal and torsional nystagmus associated with vertigo, nausea and vomiting, staggering, often tinnitus and deafness; greater amplitude to side away from lesion	Menière disease; acute labyrinthitis; vestibular neuronitis; 8th N tumor; lateral medullary infarct
Fastigiovestibular	Greatest amplitude toward side of lesion; little or no vertigo or nausea and vomiting	Multiple sclerosis, brainstem infarction and tumor; hereditary ataxias (*continued on p. 119*)

thetic stimulation dilates it, i.e., parasympathetic and sympathetic paralyses have the opposite effects. Usually, lesions that interrupt the parasympathetic innervation of the pupil also interfere with accommodation. This is true of botulinus and diphtheria infections, the Landry-Guillain-Barré syndrome, and the periaqueductal (Parinaud) syndrome. But in certain oculomotor neuropathies, pupillary constriction to light is lost while that on convergence is retained. The functional integrity of the sympathetic and parasympathetic innervation of the pupils can be determined pharmacologically. The small pupil that is due to sympathetic denervation (Horner syndrome) fails to dilate in response to 4 to 10% cocaine. If the lesion is in the postganglionic neuron, the pupil still does not react to hydroxyamphetamine (1%); however, if the lesion is central or preganglionic, the pupil will dilate with the latter drug. A tonic (Adie) pupil constricts to a tiny pupil with 0.1% pilocarpine (denervation supersensitivity).

TABLE 13-1 Types of Nystagmus (*continued*)

Type of nystagmus	Identifying features	Causes
Gaze paretic	Inability to sustain horizontal gaze with drifting of eyes to midline	Cerebellar lesion
Drug induced	Usually horizontal, may be vertical and asymmetrical	Intoxication with alcohol, phenytoin, barbiturates
Upbeat	Precise anatomy uncertain	Multiple sclerosis, infarction, tumors, Wernicke disease
Downbeat	Lesions in medullary-cervical region	Chiari malformation, syringobulbia, basilar invagination, Wernicke disease
Special types		
Monocular in abducting eye	Incompletely developed internuclear ophthalmoplegia	Multiple sclerosis, vascular lesions, Wernicke disease
Retraction and convergence	Slow abduction followed by quick adduction and retraction of both eyes; midbrain lesions with paralysis of upward gaze	Infarcts, tumors (pinealoma)
See-saw	Torsional-vertical oscillation; intorting eye moves up, extorting eye down, then reverse	Sellar or parasellar masses

A large pupil that is due to a mydriatic (anticholinergic) drug does not constrict, even to 1.0% pilocarpine.

A blind eye abolishes the reflex constriction to direct light (*afferent defect*) and also the reflex constriction that normally occurs in the opposite eye (*consensual reflex*). However, the pupil of the blind eye is still capable of consensual constriction from a light stimulus to the normal eye. Damage to the retina or optic nerve may weaken the direct light reflex, and after a brief constriction, the pupil dilates (Gunn pupil sign). Inequality of the pupils (*anisocoria*), unaccompanied by other pupillary abnormalities, is present in many normal individuals.

Other pupillary syndromes of importance are outlined in Table 13-2.

For a more detailed discussion of this topic, see Adams and Victor: *Principles of Neurology*, 4th ed, pp 206–225.

TABLE 13-2 Major Pupillary Syndromes

Type	Main features	Causes
Horner syndrome	Ptosis upper eyelid (paresis of Müller's muscle, miosis, apparent enophthalmos (narrowed palpebral fissure); ipsilateral anhydrosis and warmth of face	Lesions involving sympathetic pathway in brainstem and cervical cord (no anhydrosis) or in upper thorax, neck, internal carotid, cavernous sinus, or orbit
Adie syndrome (pupillotonia)	Blurred vision, anisocoria, more common in women, knee and ankle jerks often absent; pupil slowly dilates only to strong maximal stimulation, dilatation sustained	Idiopathic degeneration of ciliary ganglia and postganglionic parasympathetic fibers
Argyll Robertson pupil	Pupils small, irregular, unequal; do not react to light, but near response is intact; no response to mydriatics; iris atrophy; vision intact	Neurosyphilis, especially tabes; occasionally diabetes
Other light-near dissociation syndromes	Pupils do not react to light; react on accommodation; pupils normal size; vision intact	Neurosyphilis; diabetes; high midbrain lesions (pinealoma, multiple sclerosis)
Dilated pupil	Unreactive to light and accommodation	Part of oculomotor palsy, always with some degree of extraocular muscle weakness; if a solitary finding, usually due to a mydriatic drug

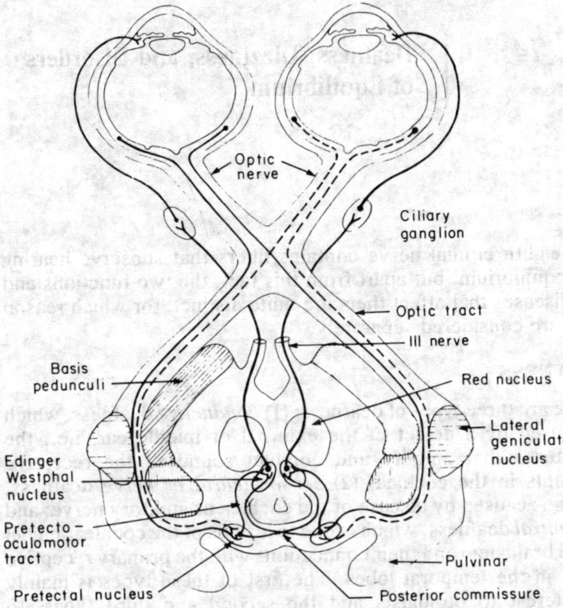

FIG. 13-3 Diagram of the pupillary light reflex. (*Adapted from FB Walsh, WF Hoyt, Clinical Neuro-Ophthalmology, 3rd ed, Baltimore, Williams & Wilkins, 1969.*)

ADDITIONAL READING

Caplan LR: "Top of the basilar" syndrome. *Neurology* 30:72, 1980.

Corbett JJ, Thompson HS: Pupillary function and dysfunction, in Asbury AK, McKhann GM, McDonald WI (eds): *Diseases of the Nervous System*. Philadelphia, Saunders, 1986, chap 46, pp 606–617.

Daroff RB: Ocular oscillations. *Ann Otol Rhinol Laryngol* 86:102, 1977.

Glaser JS (ed): *Neuro-ophthalmology*, 2nd ed. Philadelphia, Lippincott, 1990.

Keane JR: Acute bilateral ophthalmoplegia: 60 cases. *Neurology* 36:279, 1986.

Leigh RJ, Zee DS: *The Neurology of Eye Movements*, 2nd ed. Philadelphia, FA Davis Co, 1991.

Rush JA, Younge BR: Paralysis of cranial nerves III, IV, and VI. Cause and prognosis in 1000 cases. *Arch Ophthalmol* 99:76, 1981.

Spector RW, Troost BT: The ocular motor system. *Ann Neurol* 9:517, 1981.

14 Deafness, Dizziness, and Disorders of Equilibrium

The eighth cranial nerve contains fibers that subserve hearing and equilibrium, but apart from this fact, the two functions and the diseases that affect them are quite distinct, for which reason they are considered separately.

DEAFNESS

There are three types of deafness: (1) *conductive* deafness, which is caused by a defect of the external or middle ear, i.e., the structures that amplify and conduct sound to the receptive elements in the cochlea; (2) *sensorineural or nerve* deafness, which is caused by disease of the cochlea or auditory nerve; and (3) *central* deafness, which is due to lesions of the cochlear nuclei in the brainstem and their connections with the primary receptive areas in the temporal lobes. The first of these types is mainly of interest to otologists and the second and third types, to neurologists, although specialists in both fields must be able to differentiate all types of deafness.

Tests of Hearing

The patient's report of hearing loss is usually reliable, and the examiner can confirm this by testing the patient's ability to hear whispered voice in each ear. A number of simple tuning fork tests are helpful in separating conductive from neurosensory deafness. When a tuning fork, vibrating at 512 Hz (middle C) is applied to the middle of the forehead, the sound is normally heard in both ears. In nerve deafness, the sound is localized in the normal ear and in conductive deafness, in the affected ear (*Weber test*). In the *Rinne test,* the vibrating fork is applied to the mastoid bone, and as soon as the sound ceases, the fork is held at the auditory meatus. Normally, air conduction (AC) is greater than bone conduction (BC). In middle ear deafness BC > AC (negative Rinne); in nerve deafness, the reverse is true (positive Rinne), although both AC and BC may be quantitatively reduced.

Sensorineural deafness, if partial, affects high tones more than low tones; the opposite occurs in conduction deafness. This is determined most accurately by the use of an electric audiometer and the construction of an audiogram, which is an essential procedure in any investigation of hearing loss.

Special Audiologic Procedures

Often it is difficult to distinguish between lesions that affect the organ of Corti (the cochlear receptor) and those of the auditory nerve (retrocochlear lesions). It is important to make this distinction because retrocochlear lesions, one of the most common of which is an acoustic neuroma, are often surgically treatable. In addition to the audiogram, a number of special laboratory tests are helpful. These are loudness recruitment and threshold "tone decay" (the most helpful), speech discrimination, short-increment sensitivity index, Békésy audiometry, and brainstem auditory evoked responses (see *Principles* for details). MRI provides clear images of the brainstem and internal auditory meati and can identify tiny intracanalicular tumors.

Tinnitus

This refers to sounds emanating from the ear: ringing, buzzing, humming, whistling, hissing, clicking, or pulse-like sensations. Tinnitus is of two general types: *tonal,* which can be heard only by the patient (subjective), and a far less frequent type, *nontonal,* which can sometimes be heard by the examiner as well as by the patient (hence objective).

Tonal tinnitus, transient and of short duration, is experienced by most normal adults in very quiet surroundings (physiologic tinnitus); under ordinary conditions it is masked by the ambient noise level. Usually a persistent complaint of tinnitus signifies a disturbance of the tympanic membrane, ossicles, inner ear, or cochlear nerve. As a generalization, a ringing or high-pitched musical sound is associated with an impairment of cochlear or neural function. Tinnitus due to middle ear disease (e.g., otosclerosis) tends to be more constant, of variable intensity, and of lower pitch.

Nontonal tinnitus consists of noises that are conducted to the ear from various structures of the head and neck: clicks from the eustachian tube, a bruit transmitted from neck vessels or from an intracranial arteriovenous malformation, or the rhythmic (1- to 2-per-second) beat of palatal myoclonus.

Table 14-1 lists the common causes of deafness and tinnitus.

DIZZINESS AND VERTIGO

Dizziness is among the most common of all neurologic complaints, and an essential step in dealing with it is to determine

TABLE 14-1 Common Causes of Deafness and Tinnitus

Type	Site of lesion	Treatment
	Conduction	
Chronic otitis, mastoiditis	Middle ear, mastoid air cells	Control of infection
Otosclerosis	Ossicles	Surgery
Disorders of external ear or eustachian canal	—	Symptomatic
	Cochlear	
Degenerative deafness (>35 types)	End organ (cochlea) often with retinal, systemic, or neurologic abnormalities	See *Principles*
Infections	Cochlea, nerve (?)	For measles, mumps, herpes zoster, otitis media, etc.
Presbycusis	Cochlea and spiral ganglion	
Drugs (kanamycin, streptomycin, gentamycin)	Organ of Corti	Preventive
Explosions, intense noise	Organ of Corti	—
Ménière disease	Organ of Corti	See text, under vertigo
	Auditory nerve	
Tumor, trauma	Usually both portions of eighth nerve	Surgery in some cases
Postmeningitis		
	Cental	
Unilateral	Cochlear nuclei	—
Bilateral	Temporal lobes (infarction, tumor)	Surgery in some cases of tumor

how the patient is using the word. Most often it refers to a feeling of light-headedness or giddiness brought on by an anxiety state with hyperventilation. The patient, given a choice of terms, usually likens it to a swaying sensation rather than a feeling of rotation or other movement characteristic of vertigo. If uncertainty exists, 3 min of deep breathing will usually reproduce the feeling of swaying and light-headedness, thus precluding the need to search for labyrinthine or vestibular disorders.

Other clinical settings in which one encounters pseudovertiginous symptoms are severe anemia, chronic obstructive pulmonary disease, orthostatic hypotension, in patients chronically ill and recently bedfast, and in some elderly but otherwise asymptomatic persons. Rising quickly from a sitting or recumbent position may be followed by a swaying type of dizziness and "spots before the eyes"; the symptoms abate after several seconds, during which time the patient must stand still and steady himself.

True vertigo usually comes in attacks, which, if severe, are accompanied by nausea and vomiting, sometimes with pallor and perspiration, difficulty in walking, and the need to sit or lie down. In its most common form the patient reports a whirling or turning sensation, either of objects in the environment or of himself. Less frequently other feelings of movement are described, such as tilting or leaning or being impelled to one side. Nystagmus, horizontal and rotary in type, is usually present during an attack. Certain motions of the body may be provocative. The site of disease is almost always in some part of the labyrinthine-vestibular apparatus, i.e., in the semicircular canals, vestibular nerve, or vestibular nuclei of the brainstem. Rarely, there is a lesion of the vestibulocerebellum (flocculonodular lobe) or cerebrum (e.g., a seizure arising in the temporoparietal region).

The common causes of an acute attack of vertigo are benign positional vertigo, Ménière disease, and vestibular neuronitis.

Benign positional vertigo is the most frequent. It is characterized by brief (a minute or less) attacks of vertigo and nystagmus with certain critical positions of the head, such as lying down or turning over in bed or tilting the head backward. Symptoms may recur periodically for several days or months. *Hearing is unaffected*. Diagnosis is confirmed by moving the patient from the sitting position to recumbency with the head tilted 30° over the end of the table and 30° to one side. This maneuver produces a brief attack of vertigo and nystagmus; return to the sitting position changes the direction of the vertigo and nystagmus. After three or more trials, the attacks can no longer be elicited.

In Ménière disease, the attacks of vertigo are characteristically abrupt, several minutes to an hour in duration, and of such severity that the patient must lie still, with the faulty ear uppermost. Rotational or caloric-induced nystagmus is impaired or lost on the involved side. Tinnitus and deafness are usually associated and may worsen during an attack.

Vestibular neuronitis is distinguished by the occurrence of a single protracted attack of vertigo, which persists in severe form for several days and, to a lesser degree, for several weeks. There is no response to caloric stimulation on one side, and *tinnitus and deafness are absent*. Rare recurrent and bilateral forms have been described. The cause of this disorder and exact site of the lesion have not been established. An inflammatory lesion of the vestibular portion of the eighth nerve is presumed.

TABLE 14-2 Vertiginous Syndromes with Lesions of Different Parts of the Vestibular System

	Other neurologic findings	Disorders of equilibrium	Type of nystagmus*	Hearing	Laboratory exam
Labyrinthine, *unilateral* (trauma, Ménière disease, vestibular neuronitis, labyrinthitis, benign positional)	None	Ipsilateral past pointing and lateral propulsion to side of lesion	Horizontal or rotary to side opposite lesion, paroxysmal, positional	Normal, or conduction or neurosensory deafness with recruitment	Vestibular paresis by caloric testing, directional preponderance
Labyrinthine, *bilateral* (aminoglycoside intoxication; idiopathic vestibulopathy)	None	Slightly wide base and tottering to both sides	Bilateral fine horizontal or rotary	Normal, or sensorineural deafness	Vestibular paresis by caloric testing, bilateral
Vestibular nerve and ganglia (vestibular neuropathy, herpes zoster)	Auditory eighth, seventh, and sometimes other cranial nerve abnormalities	Ipsilateral past pointing and lateral propulsion to side of lesion	Vestibular, positional	Usually sensorineural deafness, without recruitment; speech discrimination diminished	Radiography and CT may be normal or abnormal; vestibular paresis on caloric testing; directional preponderance

Cerebellopontine angle (acoustic neuroma, glomus and other tumors)	Ipsilateral fifth, seventh, ninth, tenth cranial neuropathies; cerebellar ataxia; increased intracranial pressure (late)	Ataxia and falling ipsilaterally	Gaze-paretic, positional, coarser to side of lesion	Sensorineural deafness without recruitment	CT and MRI abnormal; vestibular paresis on caloric testing; directional preponderance. Increased CSF protein
Brainstem and cerebellum (infarcts, tumors, viral infections)	Multiple cranial neuropathies, brainstem tract signs, cerebellar ataxia	Ataxia present with eyes open	Coarse horizontal and vertical, gaze-paretic	Usually normal	Hyperactive labyrinths or directional preponderance on caloric testing; CT and MRI abnormal in some cases
Higher (cerebral) connections	Aphasia, visual field, hemimotor, hemisensory, and other cerebral abnormalities, seizures	No change	Usually absent	Normal	No change in caloric responses; CT and EEG may be abnormal

*See Chap. 13 for description of types of nystagmus.

Treatment During an acute attack of Ménière disease, the patient recognizes the need to remain immobile in a position that minimizes the vertigo. Fortunately, the severe vertigo is usually of brief duration; if protracted, the administration of one of several antihistaminic drugs is helpful: dimenhydrinate (Dramamine), cyclizine (Marezine), meclizine (Bonine, Antivert), or promethazine (Phenergan) in doses of 25 to 50 mg every 4 h. Trimethobenzamine (Tigan) in 200-mg suppositories every 6 h is useful in controlling the nausea and vomiting. If the attacks are frequent and disabling, permanent relief can be obtained by surgical destruction of the labyrinth (if the disease is strictly unilateral and hearing loss is nearly complete); or the vestibular portion of the eighth nerve can be sectioned or decompressed (by separating the nerve from an aberrant vessel).

Benign positional vertigo requires no special therapy. The aforementioned antihistaminics are useful in patients with vestibular neuronitis.

These and other common vertiginous syndromes, their sites of origin, and their main clinical features are summarized in Table 14-2.

For a more detailed discussion of this topic, see Adams and Victor: *Principles of Neurology*, 4th ed, pp 226–246.

ADDITIONAL READING

Baloh RW: *Dizziness, Hearing Loss, and Tinnitus: The Essentials of Neurotology*. Philadelphia, Davis, 1984.

Baloh RW, Honrubia V, Jacobson K: Benign positional vertigo: Clinical and oculographic features in 240 cases. *Neurology* 37:371, 1987.

Baloh RW, Jacobson K, Honrubia V: Idiopathic bilateral vestibulopathy. *Neurology* 39:272, 1989.

Brodal A: The cranial nerves, in *Neurological Anatomy,* 3rd ed. New York, Oxford University Press, 1981, pp 448–577.

Cascino G, Adams RD: Brainstem auditory hallucinosis. *Neurology* 36:1042, 1986.

Konigsmark BW: Hereditary progressive cochleovestibular atrophies, in Vinken PJ, Bruyn GW (eds): *Handbook of Clinical Neurology,* vol 22. Amsterdam, North-Holland, 1975, chap 22, pp 481–497.

Konigsmark BW: Hereditary diseases of the nervous system with hearing loss, in Vinken PJ, Bruyn GW (eds): *Handbook of Clinical Neurology,* vol 22. Amsterdam, North-Holland, 1975, chap 23, pp 499–526.

Shuknecht HF, Kitamura K: Vestibular neuronitis. *Ann Otol Rhinol Laryngol* 90:1, 1981.

SECTION IV
EPILEPSY AND DISORDERS OF CONSCIOUSNESS

15 Epilepsy and Other Seizure Disorders

Epilepsy is one of the most frequent of all neurologic disorders. Often it is the only manifestation of a disease state that is otherwise inapparent but persists for a lifetime and requires regular medical care. In many other cases, seizures complicate intercurrent medical and neurologic illnesses or brain injuries.

The term *epilepsy* refers to recurrent seizures that were recognized by Hughlings Jackson more than a century ago as being due to the intermittent, sudden, excessive discharge of cerebral cortical neurons. The term *convulsion* applies to any given seizure in which motor manifestations predominate. *Seizure* is the more appropriate term, since many attacks are purely sensory or akinetic and also because the term can be qualified, e.g., psychic seizure and convulsive seizure.

Seizures take many forms, varying according to cause, location of the lesion, EEG correlates, and the level of maturity of the nervous system at the time of their occurrence. Many classifications have been elaborated on the basis of these and other features. For all practical purposes, however, only two major categories need be recognized:

1. *Primary, generalized seizures,* i.e., bilaterally symmetrical, without local onset. These are of two main types: one known first to the French and now to everyone as *grand mal* and the other, consisting of a brief lapse of consciousness, as *petit mal* or *absence* seizures.
2. *Partial seizures,* i.e., seizures beginning locally. These are also of two main types: *simple,* in which consciousness is not impaired, and *complex,* with impairment of consciousness. These seizures vary with the site of the discharging focus and may become generalized. Partial seizures are also called *focal*

or *secondary* seizures, emphasizing the facts that they usually have an identifiable structural cause and that there is a need to ascertain the localization and nature of the epileptogenic lesion. By contrast, the nature of primary generalized seizures is unknown; no pathologic basis has been estáblished and usually there is no apparent cause (hence "idiopathic").

In all forms of epilepsy, the EEG is the most effective way of identifying a seizure discharge and MRI and CT scanning provide the best means of demonstrating the epileptogenic lesion.

PRIMARY GENERALIZED SEIZURES

Grand Mal

Sometimes without warning and sometimes after a brief (seconds) unnatural visceral sensation, the patient abruptly loses consciousness and emits a cry as the entire musculature is engaged in a violent contraction. The patient falls to the ground, the jaws snap shut, often biting the tongue; breathing is arrested, and if the bladder is full, it is emptied. The tonic contraction is sustained for about 20 s, and the patient becomes cyanotic. Then the tonic contraction breaks into a series of clonic contractions, which last for a minute or less as a rule. Less often the sequence differs, a clonic phase preceding the tonic phase (clonic-tonic-clonic seizure). At the end of the final clonic phase, breathing resumes and the patient lies comatose, flaccid, and breathing quietly. After a few minutes, consciousness is regained, but the patient is confused and drowsy. Afterward he complains of a headache, a sore, bitten tongue, aching of overexercised muscles, and the aftereffects of a hurtful fall. Rarely, vertebras are crushed and serious craniocerebral injury is incurred.

If one seizure after another occurs before full recovery from the preceding one, and more particularly before consciousness is regained, the condition is known as *tonic-clonic or convulsive status epilepticus*.

Petit Mal (Absence)

This consists of a brief lapse of consciousness, which comes without warning, lasts for 2 to 10 s, and is followed by immediate and full resumption of consciousness. Often there is blinking of the eyelids or rhythmic (3-per-second) movement of the arms or fingers. The patient remains sitting or standing and afterward may be unaware that anything has happened. Hyperventilation may induce an attack.

Petit mal is a disease of childhood, with onset between 4 and 12 years of age. The attacks tend to become less frequent (but rarely disappear) in adolescence, at which time a major seizure may appear for the first time. The EEG shows a characteristic generalized 3-per-second spike and wave abnormality.

Petit Mal Variants

In these varieties of epilepsy, loss of consciousness is less complete and myoclonus more prominent than in typical absence. The spike-and-wave EEG discharge may occur at a frequency of 2 to 2.5 per second, or there may be a 2- to 6-Hz multiwave and spike complex.

A special form, called the Lennox-Gastaut syndrome, consists of atonic (astatic) postural lapses succeeded by various combinations of minor tonic-clonic and postural seizures, intellectual impairment (not part of typical petit mal), and a distinctive slow (1- to 2.5-per-second) spike-wave EEG pattern. Often this syndrome is preceded by massive myoclonus, continuous multifocal spikes and delta waves of large amplitude ("hypsarrhythmia"), and an arrest in development—a triad known as the West syndrome. The seizures of the Lennox-Gastaut syndrome are frequently associated with extensive lesions of the brain, thus differing from the other primary generalized epilepsies. These seizures may persist into adult life and are often recalcitrant to all forms of treatment.

PARTIAL, OR FOCAL, SEIZURES

Seizures that make up this category, in distinction to primary generalized ones, usually have readily identifiable structural causes. The recognition of the clinical type of focal seizure, particularly at its outset, is of prime importance, because it enables one to localize the discharging lesion. These correlates are listed in Table 15-1.

Both simple and complex patterns occur. *Simple, or elementary, partial seizures* are unaccompanied by a loss of consciousness if the motor, sensory, or psychic symptoms remain confined to one side. Focal motor seizures, attributable to a lesion of the opposite frontal lobe, are characterized by forceful turning of the eyes and head to the side opposite the discharging focus, often with tonic contraction and then clonic movements of the limbs on that side. The *jacksonian motor seizure,* in which there is, within seconds, an orderly spread ("march") of clonic movements from the muscles first affected to other muscles on the same side, is quite uncommon and has the same localizing significance as focal motor seizures of the usual type.

Rolandic epilepsy and *epilepsia partialis continua* are special types of focal motor epilepsy. The former begins between 5 and

TABLE 15-1 Common Seizure Patterns

Clinical type	Localization
Somatic motor	
Jacksonian (focal motor)	Prerolandic gyrus
Masticatory	Amygdaloid nuclei
Simple contraversive	Frontal
Head and eye turning associated with arm movement	Supplementary motor cortex
Somatic and special sensory (auras)	
Somatosensory	Contralateral postrolandic
Unformed images, lights, patterns	Occipital
Auditory	Heschl gyri
Vertiginous	Superior temporal
Olfactory	Mesial temporal
Gustatory	Parietal and/or rolandic operculum
Visceral: autonomic	Insular-orbital-frontal cortex
Complex partial seizures	
Formed hallucinations	Temporal neocortex or amygdaloid-hippocampal complex
Illusions	—
Dyscognitive experiences (déjà vu, dreamy states, depersonalization)	—
Affective states (fear, depression, or elation)	Temporal
Automatism (ictal and postictal)	Temporal and frontal
Absence	Frontal cortex, amygdaloid-hippocampal complex, reticular-cortical system
Bilateral epileptic myoclonus	Reticulocortical

Source: Modified from Penfield and Jasper.

9 years of age and takes the form of clonic contractions of one side of the face and body with high-voltage spikes in the opposite lower rolandic area. The seizures tend to disappear during adolescence. Epilepsia partialis continua is characterized by clonic movements of one group of muscles, most often of the face, hand, or foot, repeated at regular intervals of a few seconds. It may last for days or months on end, without spreading to other parts. It is related to a cortical-subcortical lesion of the opposite side and responds poorly to anticonvulsant medication.

Somatosensory seizures, either focal or "marching," point to a lesion in or near the opposite postcentral gyrus. Other focal sensory seizures—visual, auditory, olfactory, vertiginous—also have discrete localizing value (Table 15-1).

Seizure discharges arising in the temporal lobe are unique in that the initial event in the seizure, i.e., the aura, is often a hallucination or perceptual illusion, such as a feeling of familiarity, strangeness, fear, visceral sensation, and so forth. If these subjective experiences constitute the entire attack, they are classified as simple partial seizures. If they are followed by a period of unresponsiveness and altered behavior (lip smacking, chewing or swallowing movements, and walking in a daze, so-called automatisms), the seizures are classified as complex partial seizures.

It should be emphasized that any focal seizures may evolve into a generalized convulsion. If this happens rapidly or if the initial focal symptom is not recognized, the seizure is indistinguishable from grand mal.

Common Clinical Problems

Medical care will be sought in the clinical circumstances listed below. Each type of seizure problem requires a somewhat different approach. Initially, one must always ask whether the patient has indeed had a seizure or seizures and not some other neurologic disorder (syncope, episodic disturbances of behavior or confusion and stupor of various types, migraine). If the disorder was a seizure, one must ascertain the clinical setting in which it occurred. And finally, the type of seizure needs to be determined, a distinction that will help in localization of the discharging lesion (Table 15-1) and deciding upon therapy (Table 15-2).

1. For the pediatrician, neonatal seizures are a special problem, for they may be brief and fragmentary—a forced deviation of the head and eyes, an apneic episode, a stiffening of a limb, or a clonic twitching of several limbs and trunk. A skilled interpreter of neonatal EEGs can often settle the issue. Seizures in these circumstances are usually of dire significance, often being due to birth injury or metabolic disease. Blood gases, glucose, and Ca should be measured. Phenobarbital is the most useful anticonvulsant.
2. In an infant or young child, there may be episodes of a few seconds duration of massive flexion myoclonus (salaam or jacknife seizures). These may follow neonatal seizures. If hypsarrhythmia is present, a trial of ACTH or other anticonvulsant is mandated. The seizures tend to subside by 5 or 6 years, but the child remains mentally retarded in 90 to 95 percent of cases.
3. Febrile states are accompanied by one or more generalized seizures in one of every 20 young children. This tendency disappears after 5 to 6 years. Often there is a positive family history of this disorder. Quick recovery and a normal

TABLE 15-2 Common Antiepileptic Drugs

Generic name	Trade name	Usual daily dosage: Children	Usual daily dosage: Adults, mg	Principal therapeutic indications	Serum half-life, hours	Effective blood level, μg/mL
Phenobarbital*	Luminal	3–5 mg/kg (8 mg/kg infants)	60–200	Tonic-clonic seizures; simple and complex partial seizures; absence	96 ± 12	10–40
Phenytoin*	Dilantin	4–7 mg/kg	300–400	Tonic-clonic seizures; simple and complex partial seizures	24 ± 12	10–20
Carbamazepine	Tegretol	20–30 mg/kg	600–1200	Tonic-clonic seizures; complex partial seizures	12 ± 3	4–10
Primidone	Mysoline	10–25 mg/kg	750–1500	Tonic-clonic seizures; simple and complex partial seizures	12 ± 6	5–15
Ethosuximide	Zarontin	20–40 mg/kg	750–2000	Absence	40 ± 6	50–100
Methsuximide	Celontin	10–20 mg/kg	500–1000	Absence	40 ± 6	40–100
Diazepam	Valium	0.15–2 mg/kg (IV)	10–150	Status epilepticus		
Lorazepam	Ativan	0.1 mg/kg (IV)		Status epilepticus		
ACTH	—	40–60 units/day		Infantile spasms		
Valproic acid	Depakene	30–60 mg/kg	1000–3000	Absence and myoclonic seizures; as an adjunctive drug in tonic clonic and complex partial seizures	8 ± 2	50–100
Clonazepam	Clonopin	0.01–0.2 mg/kg	1.5–20	Absence; myoclonus	18–50	0.01–0.07

* Dosages differ in treatment of status epilepticus; see text.

neurologic examination and EEG are the general rule. Treatment of the infection and administration of barbiturates usually suffice. Some of the cases will prove later to be examples of focal or secondary epilepsy. The seizures will then continue throughout life, often changing to temporal lobe in type and requiring carbamazepine, phenytoin, or other medications.

4. A child or adolescent may present in status epilepticus. It is often the first manifestation of idiopathic epilepsy but may be caused by meningitis or encephalitis. Appropriate diagnostic steps are undertaken after a therapeutic regimen for status has been instituted (see further on).
5. A child or adolescent has had his first major generalized seizure and has a normal neurologic examination. An EEG and a CT scan or MRI should be obtained. If normal, the problem is whether to wait and observe the patient or administer anticonvulsant medication. The latter is more clearly indicated if the EEG is paroxysmally abnormal.
6. A child or adult known to be epileptic may still be having seizures despite medication. One must check the patient's compliance and the dosage and blood levels of the drug. If the level is low, the dosage is adjusted; if normal or high, the medication is changed in accordance with the type of seizure (see Table 15-2). The EEG should be checked.
7. The first appearance of a focal or partial seizure disorder requires a neurologic investigation with LP, EEG, and CT scan or MRI. Treatment is directed at both the primary lesion and the seizures. See Table 15-3 for the likely causes of such seizures at different ages.
8. A burst of generalized or multifocal seizures raises a number of diagnostic possibilities, again depending on the age at which they occur (Table 15-3): withdrawal from alcohol, barbiturate, or other sedative drug; abuse of cocaine or other drugs; recovery phase from hypoxia or ischemia with coma; hypo- or hyperglycemia, hypocalcemia, hypomagnesemia; uremia; septic shock; encephalitis; brain tumor; rarely porphyria or an aminoaciduria.
9. A patient who continues to have frequent complex partial and generalized seizures, despite protracted trials of all known medications, should be referred to an epilepsy center, where a search for cortical epileptogenic lesions is made by special techniques. If found, surgical excision or other procedures may be considered.
10. The most serious seizure problem is the recurrence of generalized convulsions at a frequency that does not allow consciousness to be regained in the interval between sei-

TABLE 15-3 Causes of Recurrent Seizures in Different Age Groups

Age of onset	Probable cause
Neonatal	Congenital maldevelopment, birth injury, anoxia, metabolic disorders (hypocalcemia, hypoglycemia, vitamin B_6 deficiency, phenylketonuria, and others)
Infancy (1–6 months)	As above; infantile spasms
Early childhood (6 months–3 years)	Infantile spasms, febrile convulsions, birth injury and anoxia, infections, trauma
Childhood (3–10 years)	Perinatal anoxia, injury at birth or later, infections, thrombosis of cerebral arteries or veins, or indeterminate cause ("idiopathic" epilepsy)
Adolescence (10–18 years)	Idiopathic epilepsy, including genetically transmitted types, trauma
Early adulthood (18–25 years)	Idiopathic epilepsy, trauma, neoplasm, withdrawal from alcohol or other sedative-hypnotic drugs
Middle age (35–60 years)	Trauma, neoplasm, vascular disease, alcohol or other drug withdrawal
Late life (over 60 years)	Vascular disease, tumor, degenerative disease, trauma

Note: Meningitis and its complications may be a cause of seizures at any age. In tropical and subtropical countries, parasitic infection of the CNS is a common cause.

zures—grand mal status epilepticus (SE). Treatment must be undertaken at once, because persistent SE has a mortality rate of about 10 percent, and many survivors are left with brain damage. An IV line is established with normal saline, and blood is drawn for serum chemistries and antiepileptic drug concentrations. The first drug to be administered should be a benzodiazepine, preferably *lorazepam,* 0.1 mg/kg by IV push (<2 mg/min). If the seizures continue, *phenytoin* is given, 20 mg/kg by slow IV push (<50 mg/min), blood pressure and ECG being closely monitored during the infusion. Additional doses of phenytoin, 5 mg/kg, are given if necessary to a maximum of 30 mg/kg. If status persists, the patient should be intubated and *phenobarbital* administered, 20 mg/kg by IV push (<100 mg/min). Failing all these measures, the patient should be anesthetized with *pentobarbital,* 5 mg/kg as an initial IV dose, and then maintained on a dose of 0.5 to 2 mg/kg/h. The rate of infusion is slowed every few hours to determine whether seizures have stopped.

In the majority of patients with seizures, medical therapy is the mainstay. It consists of eliminating causative factors, instituting sound physical and mental hygiene, and the administration of drugs of appropriate type and in adequate amounts. Table 15-2 lists the most commonly used drugs, along with their dosages, principal therapeutic indications, effective blood levels, and serum half-life.

For a more detailed discussion of this topic, see Adams and Victor: *Principles of Neurology*, 4th ed, pp 249–272.

ADDITIONAL READING

Annegers JF, Hauser WA, Shirts SB, Kurland LT: Factors prognostic of unprovoked seizures after febrile convulsions. *N Engl J Med* 316:493, 1987.

Browne TR, Feldman RG: *Epilepsy*. Boston, Little, Brown, 1983.

Engel J, Jr: *Seizures and Epilepsy*. Philadelphia, Davis, 1989.

Kutt H: Interactions between anticonvulsants and other commonly prescribed drugs. *Epilepsia* 25(suppl 2):188, 1984.

Pedley TA: Discontinuing antiepileptic drugs. *N Engl J Med* 318:982, 1988.

Penfield W, Jasper HH: *Epilepsy and Functional Anatomy of the Human Brain*. Boston, Little, Brown, 1954.

Porter RJ: *Epilepsy: 100 Elementary Principles,* 2nd ed. Philadelphia, Saunders, 1989.

Rocca WA, Sharbrough FW, Hauser A, et al: Risk factors for complex partial seizures: A population-based case-control study. *Ann Neurol* 21:22, 1987.

Thomas JE, Regan TJ, Klass DW: Epilepsia partialis continua: A review of 32 cases. *Arch Neurol* 34:266, 1977.

Treiman DM: The role of benzodiazepines in the management of status epilepticus. *Neurology* 40(suppl 2), 32, 1990.

16 Coma and Related Disorders of Consciousness

Coma and lesser degrees of impaired consciousness are arresting and alarming neurologic emergencies. If persistent, the conditions that cause them often end fatally or, even worse, leave the patient irreparably damaged, mentally and physically.

Coma is the equivalent of loss of consciousness, which in practical terms means a loss of awareness of and an inability to respond to external stimuli or inner needs. Coma differs from natural sleep in that the patient is unarousable; syncope differs by virtue of its brevity and natural resolution (see Chap. 17).

Different degrees of coma are distinguishable. In profound coma, all stimuli, even the most severely painful ones, have no effect. A somewhat lighter state of coma ("semicoma") is manifested by groaning, stirring, quickening of respiration, or a brief opening of the eyes when the patient is pinched or shaken. Still lesser degrees of impaired consciousness, through which the patient may pass as he sinks into or emerges from coma, are designated as stupor and confusion. A stuporous patient will open his eyes and make some simple response to loud voice or manipulation of his body but does not speak. A confused patient reveals in conversation an inability to respond and think with customary speed and clarity.

Notable is the fact that the foregoing states of impaired consciousness include *both* a reduced receptivity to stimulation and a reduced responsivity. When only the latter defect exists, the patient being paralyzed but alert and aware of his surroundings, the condition is referred to as the *"locked-in" syndrome* (also as "de-efferented state" or "pseudocoma"). It is due most often to a lesion of the basis pontis, which interrupts the descending motor pathways but spares the ascending sensory pathways, both the somatosensory pathways and the ones responsible for arousal and wakefulness. If the patient lacks the impulse to move, though not paralyzed, the condition is one of *catatonia* or *abulia* (also spoken of, in its most severe form, as "*akinetic mutism*"); it has no specific anatomic basis but is often observed with bilateral medial-orbital frontal lesions. *A persistent vegetative state* is observed in patients who have barely emerged from coma or have progressed into a state of profound dementia.

The patient is awake, blinks to threat, and is capable of a few primitive postural and reflex movements but is otherwise without awareness and responsiveness.

Profound coma, with total unreceptivity of all forms of stimulation and total unresponsivity, is often accompanied by loss of all brainstem and spinal reflexes. The pupils are fixed and dilated. Spontaneous breathing and blink, vestibulo-ocular, and oropharyngeal reflexes are abolished. In the absence of hypothermia or the severe effects of depressant medication and the presence of an isoelectric EEG, the condition conforms to *brain death*, as defined by the Harvard criteria. Such patients rarely survive for more than a few days, even with respiratory support; and if natural respiration is regained, a persistent vegetative state is inevitable.

The EEG provides a delicate confirmation and, with minor exceptions, an objective means of differentiating various degrees of altered consciousness and several of their causes. It also correlates with the different stages of sleep (see Chaps. 2 and 18).

MECHANISMS WHEREBY CONSCIOUSNESS IS DISTURBED BY DISEASE

Consciousness depends on the normal functioning of the reticular formations of the midbrain and thalamus and their connections with all parts of the cerebral cortex, to which they send and from which they receive fibers. From this it follows that a diffusely decorticate person is comatose. But the smallest lesions that produce coma are always to be found in the upper brainstem reticular formation; they deactivate the cerebral cortex. Lesser degrees of impairment of these structures cause drowsiness, inattentiveness, and an inability to sustain mental activity.

The following are the mechanisms by which the reticular activation of the cerebral cortex can be impaired:

1. *A generalized seizure,* in which the sudden excessive neuronal discharge originates in or spreads to and temporarily paralyzes deep central neuronal structures.
2. *Cerebral concussion,* in which a swirling motion of the brain and torque of the upper brainstem temporarily impairs neuronal function in the diencephalic-midbrain regions.
3. *Drugs,* particularly anesthetics, alcohol, barbiturates, and other sedatives, which paralyze these neurons, each by its own chemical pathology.
4. *Metabolic derangements,* as in uremia, diabetic or other acidoses, hepatic failure, hypoglycemia, and hypercapnia.
5. *Destructive lesions*—tumor, infarction, and hemorrhage—

directly involving the upper brainstem and thalamic reticular formation.

6. *Massive lesion of one cerebral hemisphere*—tumor, hemorrhage, contusion, or a subdural or epidural hematoma—which displaces the high midbrain and diencephalic reticular formations, usually with temporal lobe-tentorial herniation.
7. Critical *decline in blood pressure* (below 70 mm systolic in normotensive individuals), e.g., from blood loss and myocardial infarction.

Most Frequent Causes of Coma In the series of Plum and Posner, from the New York Hospital, approximately one-third of the patients admitted in coma proved to be suffering from drug poisoning, one-third from metabolic disease, and one-third from cerebrovascular disease (see Table 16-1). These were patients in whom the initial diagnosis was uncertain, so that obvious poisonings were underrepresented. Also, cases of traumatic coma are not included in this series since the cause was usually apparent, and the patients were transferred to the neurosurgical service. Encephalitis and brain abscess were infrequent, being found in only 29 of 500 cases.

CLINICAL APPROACH TO THE COMATOSE PATIENT

It is essential, when the patient is first seen, to obtain information as to the events that led up to the coma. But one must first make certain that the patient's airway is clear, that he is able to sustain respiration, and that his blood pressure is adequate. If not, cardiorespiratory resuscitative measures are undertaken. As indicated below, if shock, bleeding, or airway obstruction have supervened, the immediate institution of certain therapeutic measures takes precedence—insertion of an endotracheal tube, administration of O_2, pressor agents, blood, or glucose. There follows a complete medical and neurologic examination, including a CT scan and examination of the CSF, if there is any suspicion of meningitis. The demonstration of focal brain disease or meningeal irritation with pleocytosis permits the categorization of the diseases that cause coma into one of three groups and is particularly helpful in differential diagnosis. The diseases that constitute each of these groups and their main clinical and laboratory features are summarized in Table 16-2.

MANAGEMENT OF THE COMATOSE PATIENT

This requires the services of a well-coordinated team of nurses under the constant guidance of a physician. Treatment must start at once, even before the necessary diagnostic steps are completed. The principles of management are listed below;

TABLE 16-1 Final Diagnosis in 500 Patients Admitted to the Hospital with "Coma of Unknown Etiology"

Supratentorial mass lesions	101
Intracerebral hematoma	44
Subdural hematoma	26
Epidural hematoma	4
Cerebral infarct	9
Thalamic infarct	2
Brain tumor	7
Pituitary apoplexy	2
Brain abscess	6
Closed-head injury	1
Subtentorial lesions	65
Brainstem infarct	40
Pontine hemorrhage	11
Brainstem demyelination	1
Cerebellar hemorrhage	5
Cerebellar tumor	3
Cerebellar infarct	2
Cerebellar abscess	1
Posterior fossa subdural hemorrhage	1
Basilar migraine	1
Metabolic and other diffuse disorders	326
Anoxia or ischemia	87
Hepatic encephalopathy	17
Uremic encephalopathy	8
Pulmonary disease	3
Endocrine disorders (including diabetes)	12
Acid-base disorders	12
Temperature regulation	9
Nutritional	1
Nonspecific metabolic coma	1
Encephalomyelitis and encephalitis	14
Subarachnoid hemorrhage	13
Drug poisoning	149
Psychiatric disorders	8

Note: Listed here are only those patients in whom the initial diagnosis was uncertain and a final diagnosis was established. Thus, obvious poisonings and closed-head injuries are underrepresented.
Source: Plum and Posner.

details of management of shock, fluid and electrolyte imbalance, and other complications to which the insensate patient is subject (e.g., pneumonia, urinary tract infections, phlebothrombosis) can be found in *Harrison's Principles of Internal Medicine*.

1. The management of shock, if present, takes precedence over all other diagnostic and therapeutic measures.
2. Shallow and irregular respirations, stertorous breathing (indicating obstruction to inspiration), and cyanosis require the establishment of a clear airway and delivery of oxygen. The

TABLE 16-2 Important Points in the Differential Diagnosis of the Common Causes of Coma

General group	Specific disorder	Important clinical findings	Important laboratory findings	Remarks
Coma *with* focal or lateralizing signs of brain disease	Brain tumor	Stertorous breathing, neurologic signs dependent on location, papilledema	CT scan +; CSF pressure elevated; protein often > 100 mg percent	Steady progression of signs and symptoms
	Cerebral hemorrhage	Stertorous breathing, hypertension, flushed skin, hemiplegia	CT scan +; CSF grossly bloody and under increased pressure	Sudden onset, elderly patients
	Cerebral thrombosis	Unilateral or bilateral paralysis of abrupt onset	CT scan + after several days; CSF normal or protein modestly elevated	Stupor or coma
	Cerebral embolism	Sudden onset of paralysis	Same as above; occasionally up to 5000 RBC/mm^3 in CSF	Evidence of heart disease
	Fracture or concussion	Signs of skin trauma	CT scan ±; skull fracture by x-ray; CSF bloody and under increased pressure	Bleeding from nose or ears; history of trauma
	Subdural hematoma	Slow respiration, rising blood pressure, hemiparesis, dilated pupil	CT scan +; normal or increased CSF pressure; xanthochromia with relatively low protein	History of trauma; progressively severe headache, drowsiness, and confusion

	Brain abscess	Neurologic signs depending on location; symptoms and signs of increased intracranial pressure	CT scan +; fever, leukocytosis; increased pressure, protein and white cells, but normal glucose in CSF	Subacute evolution of headache and neurologic signs on background of sinus, ear, or lung infection or septicemia
	Hypertensive encephalopathy	Headache, severe hypertension, retinopathy, and convulsions	CT scan ±; CSF pressure normal or increased; protein 50–200 mg	Confusion, stupor, or coma evolving over several days
Coma *without* focal or lateralizing signs, *with* signs of meningeal irritation	Meningitis	Stiff neck, positive Kernig sign, fever, headache	CT scan ±; pleocytosis, increased protein, low glucose in CSF	Subacute or acute onset
	Subarachnoid hemorrhage	Stertorous breathing, hypertension, stiff neck, positive Kernig sign	CT scan may show blood and aneurysm; bloody or xanthochromic CSF under increased pressure	Sudden onset with headache
Coma *without* focal neurologic signs or meningeal irritation; CT scan and CSF normal	Alcohol intoxication	Hypothermia, hypotension, flushed skin, alcohol breath	Elevated blood alcohol	
	Barbiturate intoxication	Hypothermia, hypotension	Barbiturate in urine and blood; EEG often shows fast activity	History of intake of intoxicating substance
	Opiate intoxication	Slow respiration, cyanosis, constricted pupils		Administration of naloxone causes withdrawal signs

(*continued*)

TABLE 16-2 Important Points in the Differential Diagnosis of the Common Causes of Coma (*continued*)

General group	Specific disorder	Important clinical findings	Important laboratory findings	Remarks
Coma *without* focal neurologic signs or meningeal irritation; CT scan normal	Carbon monoxide intoxication	Cherry-red skin	Carboxyhemoglobin	
	Anoxia	Rigidity, decerebrate postures, fever, seizures, involuntary movements	CSF normal; EEG may be isoelectric or show high-voltage delta	Abrupt onset following cardiopulmonary failure; damage permanent if anoxia exceeds 3–5 min
	Hypoglycemia	Same as in anoxia	Low blood glucose; coeliac angiography may disclose insulinoma	Characteristic slow evolution through stages of nervousness, hunger, sweating, flushed face; then pallor, shallow respirations and seizures
	Diabetic coma	Signs of extracellular fluid deficit, hyperventilation with Kussmaul respiration, "fruity" breath	Glycosuria, hyperglycemia, acidosis; reduced serum bicarbonate; ketonemia and ketonuria	History of polyuria, polydipsia, weight loss, or diabetes

Uremia	Hypertension; sallow, dry skin, uriniferous breath, twitch-convulsive syndrome	Protein and casts in urine; elevated BUN and serum creatinine; anemia, acidosis, hypocalcemia	Progressive apathy, confusion, and asterixis precede coma
Hepatic coma	Jaundice, ascites, and other signs of portal hypertension	Elevated blood NH_3 levels; CSF yellow with normal protein	Onset over a few days or after paracentesis or hemorrhage from varices; confusion, stupor, asterixis, and characteristic EEG changes precede coma
Hypercapnia	Papilledema, diffuse myoclonus, asterixis	Increased CSF pressure; Pco_2 may exceed 75 mmHg; EEG theta and delta activity	Advanced pulmonary disease; profound coma and brain damage uncommon
Severe infections (septic shock); heat stroke	Extreme hyperthermia, rapid respiration	Vary according to cause	Evidence of a specific infection or exposure to extreme heat
Idiopathic epilepsy	Episodic disturbance of behavior or convulsive movements	Characteristic EEG changes	History of previous attacks

patient should be placed in a lateral position so that secretions and vomitus do not enter the tracheobronchial tree. Usually the pharyngeal reflexes are suppressed so that an endotracheal tube can be inserted without difficulty. Secretions should be removed by suctioning as soon as they accumulate; otherwise they will lead to atelectasis and bronchopneumonia. Oxygen can be administered by mask in a 100% concentration for 6 to 12 h, alternating with 50% concentration for 5 to 6 h. The depth of respiration can be increased by the use of 5 to 10% carbon dioxide for periods of 3 to 5 min every hour. Atropine should not be given; edema of the lungs and fluid in the tracheobronchial passages are not glandular secretions. Also, atropine thickens this fluid and may disturb temperature regulation. Aminophylline is helpful in controlling Cheyne-Stokes breathing. Respiratory paralysis dictates the use of endotracheal intubation and a positive pressure respirator.

3. Concomitantly, an IV line is established and blood samples are drawn for measurement of the blood elements, glucose, toxins, and electrolytes and for tests of liver and kidney function. Arterial blood gases should also be measured. Naloxone, 0.5 mg, should be given IV if a narcotic overdose is a diagnostic possibility.
4. With massive cerebral lesions it is common practice for a neurosurgeon to place a pressure-measuring device in the skull. This provides constant monitoring of intracranial pressure. When the pressure is elevated, mannitol, 50 g in a 20% solution, should be given IV over 10 to 20 min. Corticosteroids help to maintain the reduction in intracranial pressure. Repeated CT scans allow the physician to follow the size of the lesion and degree of localized edema and to detect herniations of cerebral tissue.
5. An LP should be performed if meningitis or subarachnoid hemorrhage is suspected, keeping in mind the risks of this procedure and the means of dealing with them (p. 17). A CT scan may have disclosed a subarachnoid hemorrhage, in which case an LP is not necessary.
6. Convulsions should be controlled by measures outlined in Chap. 15.
7. Gastric aspiration and lavage with normal saline may be useful in some instances of coma due to drug ingestion. Salicylates, opiates, and anticholinergic drugs (tricyclic antidepressants, phenothiazines, scopolamine), all of which induce gastric atony, may be recovered many hours after ingestion. Caustic materials should not be lavaged because of the danger of perforation. Lavage of strychnine and other analeptic drugs carries the danger of precipitating seizures

and cardiac arrhythmias. Induction of emesis by ipecac or apomorphine should be reserved for alert patients.

8. The temperature-regulating mechanisms may be disturbed, and extreme hypothermia, hyperthermia, or poikilothermia may occur. In hyperthermia, the use of a cooling mattress is indicated.
9. The bladder should not be permitted to become distended; if the patient does not void, he needs to be fitted with an external drainage apparatus or a retention catheter. Decompression of a greatly distended bladder should be carried out slowly, over a period of hours. Urine excretion should be kept between 500 and 1000 mL/day. The patient should not be permitted to lie in a wet or soiled bed.
10. Diseases of the central nervous system may upset the control of water, glucose, and salt. The unconscious patient can no longer adjust the intake of food and fluids by hunger and thirst. Both salt-losing and salt-retaining syndromes have been described with brain disease. Water intoxication and severe hyponatremia may of themselves prove fatal. If coma is prolonged, the insertion of a stomach tube will ease the problems of feeding the patient and maintaining fluid and electrolyte balance.
11. Aspiration pneumonia is avoided by prevention of vomiting (stomach tube), proper positioning of the patient, and restriction of oral fluids. Should it occur, corticosteroid therapy is beneficial. The legs should be examined each day for signs of phlebothrombosis and, if found, treated by anticoagulants or surgical measures. Deep vein thrombosis, which is a common occurrence in comatose and hemiplegic patients, often does not manifest itself by clinical signs. If can be prevented by the administration of low doses of warfarin (Coumadin) (maintaining a prothrombin time of 15 s) or by the use of inflatable boots or stockings.
12. If the patient is capable of moving, suitable restraints should be used to prevent falling out of bed.

Prognosis

Deep coma that lasts for 48 to 72 h carries a grave prognosis; many such patients fall into the category of brain death, usually with fatal outcome in a few days. A small number of these patients emerge into the category of persistent vegetative state, the prognosis of which is almost equally grave. Exceptionally, patients survive in a persistent vegetative state for years, but in most cases (about 90 percent) survival is measured in weeks or months. The absence of pupillary and corneal reflexes and ocular movements after 1 and 3 days of coma predicts to a high degree

TABLE 16-3 Glasgow Coma Scale*

Eyes open	
Never	1
To pain	2
To verbal stimuli	3
Spontaneously	4
Best verbal response	
No response	1
Incomprehensible sounds	2
Inappropriate words	3
Disoriented and converses	4
Oriented and converses	5
Best motor response	
No response	1
Extension (decerebrate rigidity)	2
Flexion abnormal (decorticate rigidity)	3
Flexion withdrawal	4
Localizes pain	5
Obeys	6
	3–15

*Circle the appropriate number and compute the total.

a fatal issue or a vegetative state. Low scores on the Glasgow coma scale, reproduced in Table 16-3, may be of help in predicting the outcome, particularly in cases due to cerebral trauma.

For a more detailed discussion of this topic, see Adams and Victor: *Principles of Neurology*, 4th ed, pp 273–290.

ADDITIONAL READING

Caronna JJ, Simon RP: The comatose patient: A diagnostic approach and treatment. *Int Anesthesiol Clin* 17(2/3):3, 1979.

Fisher CM: The neurological examination of the comatose patient. *Acta Neurol Scand Suppl* 36, 1969.

Guidelines for the detection of brain death in children. *Ann Neurol* 21:616, 1987.

Jennett B, Plum F: Persistent vegetative state after brain damage. *Lancet* 1:734, 1972.

Levy DE, Caronna JJ, Singer BH, et al: Predicting outcome from hypoxic-ischemic coma. *JAMA* 253:1420, 1985.

Plum F, Posner JB: *Diagnosis of Stupor and Coma,* 3rd ed. Philadelphia, Davis, 1980.

Ropper AH: Lateral displacement of the brain and level of consciousness in patients with an acute hemispheral mass. *N Engl J Med* 314:953, 1986.

17 | Faintness and Syncope

Syncope is synonymous with the common faint. In most cases, it is a transitory, spontaneously reversible state. A lesser form, a feeling as though one is about to faint, is referred to as faintness, or *presyncope*. Most otherwise healthy individuals have experienced the latter and many have at some time fainted.

CLINICAL FEATURES

In the common (vasovagal) type of faint, the person is assailed by a sense of weakness, as though all energy has been drained from the body. He feels uneasy and queasy and has a sense of giddiness and swaying. Headache, dimness of vision, and ringing in the ears are common accompaniments, and it may be impossible for the person to think clearly. Color drains from the face; a cold sweat breaks out. Pallor of the face coincides with pallor of the brain, which is the mechanism common to all types of faint. Signs of autonomic overactivity—salivation, nausea, and sometimes vomiting and sweating—are prominent and represent the body's attempts to counteract the fall in blood pressure.

The victim, who is usually standing or sitting, looks for a place to lie down. If unable to lie down promptly, he loses consciousness and falls to the ground. Breathing and pulse are imperceptible or barely perceptible. The appearance is one of death. Once horizontal for a few seconds or minutes, the patient stirs, opens his eyes, and quickly takes in the situation. Strength and color soon return as well. The patient is embarrassed, and his frightened companions are relieved by the rapid recovery.

Such an episode has at some time been witnessed by most people, but there are variations which may cause uncertainty. If unconsciousness persists for 15 to 20 s or the patient, for some reason, is maintained upright as the faint comes on, the limbs and trunk may jerk several times or stiffen, as in a seizure. Or the patient may not lose consciousness completely; he can hear voices of those around him but his responses betray confusion ("grayout"). Syncope of cardiac origin may be so abrupt that the fall results in injury, even a concussion. In general, however, the loss of strength and consciousness, though of sudden onset, provide sufficient warning to avoid a hurtfull fall. Sphincteric incontinence is also exceptional.

With these characteristics in mind, the distinction between a faint and a seizure should rarely occasion difficulty. Only the akinetic (astatic) seizure resembles a faint, but usually the former comes without warning or facial pallor. Even the seizure-like clonic jerking or tonic spasm of limbs and trunk that sometimes complicate a protracted faint is usually attended by the other manifestations of hypotension.

CAUSES OF SYNCOPE AND FAINTNESS

In Table 17-1 are listed the many types of syncope and faintness based on their established or presumed physiologic mechanisms.

In practice, only a small proportion of the conditions listed in the table are encountered with any degree of frequency. Moreover, the fundamental mechanism in all of them is the same: an inadequacy of blood flow to the brain, which in turn may be due to (1) a *loss of reflex peripheral constriction* with fall in blood pressure, as in vasopressor, or vasovagal, syncope (strong emotion, painful injury, prolonged standing still, orthostatic hypotension); (2) *diminished cardiac output,* as in heart block (Stokes-Adams attack) or cardiac arrhythmia or as a result of diminished venous return to the heart (Valsalva phenomenon); or (3) an *altered state of the blood* itself, in which insufficient oxygen or glucose is delivered to the brain.

Details of the clinical features and mechanisms of the various types of syncope will be found in the *Principles.*

CLINICAL APPROACH TO SYNCOPE

If on the scene of a common vasovagal faint, one need only ensure that the patient remain recumbent until the vasodepressor inadequacy has corrected itself. For the patient who reports one or more faints and is normal when seen, one must ascertain, from the descriptions of the episode, that it was a faint and not a seizure or an attack of anxiety, transient ischemia, or hypoglycemia. Having satisfied one's self on this point, one attempts to determine the mechanism of the faint and the likelihood of its recurrence. Some types of syncope, such as those of cardiac and orthostatic origin, must be taken seriously; others are obviously benign. An otherwise healthy adolescent or young adult who faints at the scene of an accident or when sitting or standing still in an overheated atmosphere needs no further study—only an explanation of the nature of vasovagal syncope and the admonition to avoid situations that are known to induce fainting.

TABLE 17-1 Causes of Episodic Faintness and Syncope

- I. Circulatory (deficient quantity of blood to the brain and extracranial structures)
  - *A.* Inadequate vasoconstrictor mechanisms
    1. Vasodepressor (vasovagal)
    2. Postural hypotension
    3. Primary autonomic insufficiency
    4. Sympathectomy (surgical or pharmacologic, i.e., due to antihypertensive medications)
    5. Peripheral and central nervous system diseases
    6. Carotid sinus irritability (see also bradyrhythmias, below)
  - *B.* Hypovolemia
    1. Blood loss
    2. Addison disease
  - *C.* Mechanical reduction in venous return to heart
    1. Valsalva maneuver
    2. Cough
    3. Micturition
    4. Atrial myxoma (ball-valve thrombus)
  - *D.* Reduced cardiac output
    1. Obstruction to left ventricular outflow: aortic stenosis, hypertrophic subaortic stenosis
    2. Obstruction to pulmonary flow: pulmonic stenosis, tetralogy of Fallot, primary pulmonary hypertension, pulmonary embolism
    3. Myocardial: massive myocardial infarction with "pump" failure
    4. Pericardial: cardiac tamponade
  - *E.* Cardiac arrhythmias
    1. Bradyrhythmias
       - *a.* Atrioventricular (AV) block (second and third degree) with Stokes-Adams attacks
       - *b.* Ventricular asystole
       - *c.* Sinus bradycardia, sinoatrial block, sinus arrest, sick-sinus syndrome
       - *d.* Carotid sinus syncope (see also inadequate vasoconstrictor mechanism, above)
       - *e.* Vagoglossopharyngeal neuralgia (and other painful states)
    2. Tachyrhythmias
       - *a.* Episodic ventricular fibrillation with or without associated bradyrhythmias
       - *b.* Ventricular tachycardia
       - *c.* Supraventricular tachycardia without AV block
- II. Other causes of episodic faintness and syncope
  - *A.* Altered state of blood to the brain
    1. Hypoxia
    2. Anemia
    3. Diminished CO_2 due to hyperventilation (faintness common, syncope rare)
    4. Hypoglycemia (faintness frequent, syncope rare)
  - *B.* Emotional disturbances
    1. Hysterical fainting
    2. Anxiety attacks (presyncope common, syncope rare)

A person convalescing from illness or one with a peripheral vasoconstrictor inadequacy (orthostatic hypotension, diabetic neuropathy, Parkinson disease, striatonigral degeneration and Shy-Drager syndrome) requires investigation of the underlying disease and the institution of certain corrective measures to help avoid future attacks. The latter include elevating the head of the bed by 8 to 12 in, arising slowly from a recumbent position, the use of a snug elastic abdominal binder and stockings, increasing salt intake to expand blood volume, and the administration of flurocortisone acetate (Florinef), 0.01 to 0.02 mg/day in divided doses.

In patients with cardiac syncope, it may be necessary to monitor cardiac rhythm for several days or weeks or even longer. The drug treatment of the various arrhythmias that induce syncope and the need for a pacemaker require consultation with a cardiologist. The treatment of carotid sinus syncope can be difficult. Atropine or ephedrine should be tried in patients whose attacks are associated with bradycardia or hypotension, respectively. If these medications fail and the attacks are incapacitating, surgical denervation of the carotid sinus or the placement of a demand pacemaker in the right ventricle needs to be considered.

Tussive syncope, micturition syncope, and "weight-lifter's syncope" simply require the use of antitussive medicines and treatment of tracheobronchitis, instruction to urinate while sitting, and interdiction of straining and heavy lifting, as the case may be. In patients who are fainting because of hypovolemia or the effects of antihypertensive drugs, it may suffice to restore the blood volume or discontinue or adjust the dosage of the offending drug(s).

A number of simple maneuvers may help to clarify the medical problem of syncope. Measurement of blood pressure while the patient is lying down and after standing relaxed for 3 min may disclose a fall of 20 to 30 mm or more, supporting the hypothesis of faulty vasoconstriction. An even better method is to study postural changes in blood pressure after the patient has been subjected to an 80° head-up tilt for 10 min. Combining an isoproterenol infusion with the upright-tilt test is a particularly useful method of reproducing neurally mediated syncopal spells (see Almquist et al). The presence of symptoms and signs of peripheral neuropathy, an autonomic neuropathy, or an extrapyramidal or cerebellar degeneration also points in the direction of defective vasoconstriction. Exhaling vigorously against resistance in the performance of the Valsalva maneuver may provoke a significant fall in cardiac output and presyncopal symptoms. Gentle massage of first one and then the other carotid sinus, while recording pulse and blood pressure, may reproduce carotid sinus syncope. Hyperventilation for 3 min often induces the initial part of an anxiety attack.

In some cases, even after all these tests, one may not be sure of having discovered the basis of the patient's syncopal attacks. The plan then is to have the patient avoid situations that induce postural hypotension and to make further observations of the circumstances surrounding future attacks.

For a more detailed discussion of this topic, see Adams and Victor: *Principles of Neurology*, 4th ed, pp 291–301.

ADDITIONAL READING

Almquist A, Goldenberg IF, Milstein S, et al: Provocation of bradycardia and hypotension by isoproterenol and upright posture in patients with unexplained syncope. *N Engl J Med* 320:346, 1989.

Kapoor WN, Karpf M, Wieand S, et al: A prospective evaluation and follow-up of patients with syncope. *N Engl J Med* 309:197, 1983.

Lipsitz LA: Orthostatic hypotension in the elderly. *N Engl J Med* 321:952, 1989.

Meissner L, Wiebers DO, Swanson JW, O'Fallon WM: The natural history of drop attacks. *Neurology* 36:1029, 1986.

Ross RT: *Syncope*. Philadelphia, Saunders, 1988.

Silverstein MD, Singer DE, Mulley AG, et al: Patients with syncope admitted to intensive care units. *JAMA* 248:1185, 1982.

18 Sleep and Its Abnormalities

Sleep laboratories throughout North America have greatly advanced our knowledge of the physiology of sleep and have given physicians new insights into the nature of many common sleep abnormalities.

Normal sleep obeys an elemental 24-h (circadian) rhythm, the neural control of which is thought to lie in the anterior hypothalamus. Nocturnal sleep is of two types: *nonrapid eye movement sleep (NREMS)* and *rapid eye movement sleep (REMS)*. The former is divided into four stages on the basis of its depth and accompanying physiologic, endocrine, and EEG changes. REMS occurs as a single phase and normally follows NREMS. Together they form a predictable sequence or cycle that lasts 70 to 100 min and repeats itself four to six times per night. The number of cycles and the proportions of NREMS and REMS vary with age. The total hours of sleep also are age linked—16 to 20 h in the newborn, 10 to 12 h in the child, 7 to 8 h in the adolescent, and less during late adult life—but there are wide individual variations.

As one falls asleep, one passes from an alert to a drowsy state and then into stage 1 NREMS, wherein muscles are relaxed, breathing is slowed, and eyelids are closed; low-voltage, mixed-frequency waves replace the alpha rhythm in the EEG. In stage 2, sleep spindles (12 to 14 Hz) and high-amplitude, sharp slow-wave (K) complexes appear in the EEG. Stages 3 and 4 are characterized by deep sleep and high-amplitude, delta waves (1 to 2 Hz) in the EEG. After 80 to 90 min, REMS interrupts the cycle, with bursts of rapid eye movements, stirring of the limbs, changes in blood pressure and respiration, and low-voltage, fast-frequency waves in the EEG; if the subject is awakened at this time, he reports dreams. After a period of 5 to 10 min of REMS, NREMS recurs. However, with succeeding cycles, the four discrete stages of NREMS can no longer be recognized, and in the latter portion of a night's sleep the cycles consist essentially of two alternating stages—REMS and stage 2 (spindle-K complex) sleep.

Experimental physiologists have proposed that the alternations of sleep and wakefulness depend upon the reciprocal interaction of excitatory (cholinergic) and inhibitory (aminergic) neurotransmitters produced by two interconnected neuronal populations in the pontine reticular formation. Details of this theoretical construct should be sought in the references listed at the end of the chapter.

SLEEP DISORDERS

Insomnia

Insomnia, strictly defined, is a chronic (more than 3 weeks) inability to sleep at times when sleep normally comes, but the term is commonly used to designate any short- or long-term disturbance in the depth, duration, or restorative powers of sleep. There may be delay in falling asleep, easy awakening during the night, or early morning awakening.

Apart from *pseudoinsomnia,* in which an individual expresses dissatisfaction with his sleep despite its normal depth and duration, there are two major types of insomnia, primary and secondary.

In primary insomnia there is a chronic derangement of the sleep mechanism, affecting the quantity and quality of sleep in the absence of any medical or psychiatric illness. It may be a lifelong condition. Unlike the rare individual who functions adequately on 3 to 4 hours of sleep, the primary insomniac complains of the effects of sleep deprivation. Moreover, sleep-laboratory recordings verify the inadequacy of his sleep.

Secondary (situational) insomnia is most often related to worry and anxiety (difficulty in falling asleep), depression (early morning awakening), and the abuse of alcohol and other drugs. Of course, breathing difficulty (chronic obstructive pulmonary disease) and painful medical or surgical conditions (e.g., pain in the spine, abdominal pain from peptic ulcer or carcinoma) are conducive to abnormal wakefulness. In addition, there are a number of special conditions in which a disturbance of sleep is the main abnormality and a source of distress to the patient. These are (1) *the "restless legs" syndrome* (anxietas tibiarum), unpleasant sensations of aching and formication of the legs, which provoke continuous movements of the legs and delay the onset of sleep; (2) *nocturnal leg movements,* which occur every 20 to 40 s for long periods during sleep and cause partial or full arousals; (3) *acroparesthesias of the hands,* due to tight carpal ligaments; (4) *cluster headaches,* described in Chap. 9; and (5) *nightmares and night terrors,* which usually occur in children who are also sleepwalkers but which may persist into adult life.

Of the more strictly neurologic diseases, acute confusional

states and deliria are known to derange sleep. In their most severe form, e.g., delirium tremens, the patient may be sleepless for days on end. During the inexhaustible activity of mania and hypomania, the patient seems to require little sleep to restore energy. Pontine infarction may reduce the amount and pattern of sleep (little or no REMS and reduced NREMS). This may also be observed in some cases of Huntington chorea, certain cerebellar degenerations, striatonigral degeneration, and progressive supranuclear palsy.

Treatment If the insomnia is of secondary type, it stands to reason that treatment needs to be directed to the underlying disease (antianxiety or antidepressant drugs or analgesics). In the patient with restless legs, a benzodiazepine (diazepam, clonazepam) at bedtime may be helpful. In some cases, the α-adrenergic blocker tolazoline (Priscoline) has been helpful. Baclofen (20 to 40 mg at bedtime) may reduce the sleep disturbance due to periodic leg movements.

The management of primary insomnia is difficult. In general, the long-term use of sedative-hypnotic drugs is not the answer to the problem. Barbiturates, short or long acting, should not be used because of the danger of addiction and of rebound insomnia (i.e., a worsening of the sleep disorder compared to the pretreatment state) when the drug is discontinued. The danger is less, but still exists, with drugs such as diazepam and chloral hydrate, and their nightly use has a cumulative effect, causing daytime drowsiness. The drugs with the least tendency to the development of tolerance and dependence are the benzodiazepines flurazepam (Dalmane) in doses of 15 to 30 mg at bedtime and triazolam (Halcion) in doses of 0.25 to 0.5 mg. In each case, the lesser dose should be used if possible.

Hypersomnic States

Of the hypersomnic states, two are of particular importance, because of their frequency and disturbing effects on the life of the patient: the narcolepsy-cataplexy syndrome and sleep apnea with daytime hypersomnolence. Some depressed patients sleep excessively as do patients with severe hypothyroidism and hypercapnia.

Narcolepsy-cataplexy syndrome This is a disease of obscure cause and pathology, characterized by frequently recurring (two to six per day) attacks of sleepiness. The unique features of narcoleptic attacks are their irresistibility, their occurrence in unusual circumstances (while standing, eating, or conversing, for example), and their polygraph findings, which show the attacks to represent episodes of REMS. The majority of narcoleptics also have occasional attacks of *cataplexy,* i.e., a sudden loss of muscle tone, which is provoked by hearty laughter or other strong emotion. The cataplexy is momentary and may affect only certain muscles, such as those of the jaw or arms, or it may be complete, with a fall to the ground but with retention of consciousness and immediate recovery. *Sleep paralysis*—a brief powerlessness of muscles occurring during the period of falling asleep or awakening—and *vivid hallucinations,* which may be associated, complete the tetrad that constitutes this syndrome.

This condition usually begins in adolescence or early adult years and, once begun, is lifelong. The prevalence in the general population is approximately 40 per 100,000, and males are more often affected than females. A genetic cause has been postulated but a mendelian pattern is not firmly established. However, positivity for HLA-DR2 antigen is nearly universal.

The *treatment* of narcolepsy consists of taking strategically spaced naps during the day and analeptic drugs—dextroamphetamine (Dexedrine), 5 to 20 mg/day; or methylphenidate (Ritalin), 10 to 30 mg/day; and imipramine (Tofranil), 25 mg tid for cataplexy. These drugs act by inhibiting REMS. Cataplexy, which is neither as frequent nor as troublesome as narcolepsy, can be avoided by the wary patient.

Sleep apnea and daytime hypersomnolence In certain individuals, notably those with upper airway obstruction or decreased respiratory drive, sleep may induce repeated episodes of prolonged (> 10 s) apnea. The *apnea of obstructive type,* especially in males, is often associated with obesity and adenotonsillar hypertrophy and less often with micrognathia, myotonic dystrophy, acromegaly, and hypothyroidism. The anatomy and physiology of the *central, or primary, type* is poorly understood, but a severe form of this disorder has been identified as *idiopathic central hypoventilation* (Ondine's curse). The central form has also been observed in patients with medullary lesions, e.g., lateral medullary infarction, syringobulbia, bulbar poliomyelitis, olivopontocerebellar degeneration.

Periods of obstructive apnea usually occur during REMS. Because of the repeated interruptions of nocturnal sleep, there is increased drowsiness throughout the day. In fact, the occurrence of persistent daytime drowsiness should raise the suspicion of obstructive sleep apnea, especially in males.

The treatment of obstructive sleep apnea consists of weight reduction and surgical measures that relieve nasopharyngeal obstruction. In primary sleep apnea, medroxyprogesterone and protriptyline are thought to be beneficial.

Other hypersomnic states Midbrain-diencephalic encephalitis, known during the decade that followed World War I as "encephalitis lethargica," produced hypersomnolence that could last for months on end. In central Africa, trypanosomiasis is the cause of a similar disorder. Patients with severe hypothyroidism may sleep for 15 to 20 h a day.

Periodic hypersomnia is part of the rare and obscure Kleine-Levin syndrome, in which adolescent boys lapse into a state of somnosis, with greatly increased appetite (bulimia), negativism, and social withdrawal. Its cause is unknown. Hypothalamic tumors are a rare cause of hypersomnolence, but usually other hypothalamic and pituitary symptoms are present.

Other Sleep Disorders

Benign parasomnic phenomena Numbered among these disorders are *somnolescent starts,* i.e., sudden, massive jerks of the legs or trunk at the moment of falling asleep; *sensory paroxysms*—flash of light, clanging sound, explosive sensation in the head ("exploding head syndrome")—also occurring as the individual dozes off and often associated with a somnolescent start; and *postdormital paralysis,* a brief state of paralysis on awakening "too soon."

Somnambulism and sleep automatism This is a condition in which a child, less often an adult, sleepwalks. In children it may be associated with enuresis and night terrors. Somnambulism occurs almost exclusively during stages 3 and 4 of NREMS. Children usually outgrow this disorder.

Nocturnal epilepsy is a well-established entity and is easily recognized if the seizure is generalized. If the seizure is of psychomotor (temporal lobe) type, it must be distinguished from night terrors, nightmares, and somnambulism.

Nocturnal enuresis (bed wetting) occurs in approximately 10 percent of children 4 to 14 years of age. It is more frequent in boys than in girls. The child does not awaken to relatively high intravesicular pressures, which usually occur during the first part of the night; an enuretic episode is most likely to occur about 4 h after the onset of sleep. Imipramine (Tofranil), 25 mg at bedtime, has proved to be an effective medication. Diseases of the bladder or its innervation, diabetes mellitus, diabetes insipidus, epilepsy, and sickle cell anemia, must be excluded but are seldom found.

For a more detailed discussion of this topic, see Adams and Victor: *Principles of Neurology,* 4th ed, pp 302–319.

ADDITIONAL READING

Brownell LG, West P, Sweatman P, et al: Protriptyline in obstructive sleep apnea. *N Engl J Med* 307:1037, 1982.

Gillin JC, Byerley WF: The diagnosis and management of insomnia. *N Engl J Med* 322:239, 1990.

Guilleminault C, Dement WC: 235 cases of excessive daytime sleepiness: Diagnosis and tentative classification. *J Neurol Sci* 31:13, 1977.

Hobson JA, Brazier MAB (eds): *The Reticular Formation Revisited*. New York, Raven Press, 1980.

Kramer RE, Dinner DS, Braun WE, et al: HLA-DR2 and narcolepsy. *Arch Neurol* 44:853, 1987.

Kryger MH, Roth T, Dement WC (eds): *Principles and Practice of Sleep Medicine*. Philadelphia, Saunders, 1988.

SECTION V
DERANGEMENTS OF INTELLECT, BEHAVIOR, AND LANGUAGE DUE TO DIFFUSE AND FOCAL CEREBRAL DISEASE

19 Delirium and Other Confusional States

The term *confusion* is used here in a general sense, to embrace all states in which patients are unable to think with customary speed, clarity, and coherence. Disorientation, impaired attentiveness and ability to concentrate, an inability to register immediate events and recall them later, and a general reduction in all mental activity are its most prominent features; reduced perceptiveness, sometimes with visual and auditory illusions and even hallucinations, is another variable feature.

By contrast, we use the term *delirium* to denote a special type of confusional state, the predominant features of which are a disorder of perception (misinterpretations and misidentifications), vivid and terrifying hallucinations and dreams, a kaleidoscopic array of strange and absurd fantasies and delusions, intense emotional experiences, insomnia, and a tendency to convulse. Delirium is also distinguished by a state of heightened alertness, i.e., an increased readiness to respond to stimuli, and by an evident overactivity of psychomotor and autonomic nervous system functions.

Some authors use the word *delirium* to designate all psychotic episodes resulting from acute cerebral disease, i.e., they make no distinction between delirium and any other confusional state. We separate them, in the belief that the pathogenesis of delirium differs from that of other confusional states.

ACUTE CONFUSIONAL STATES ASSOCIATED WITH REDUCED ALERTNESS AND PSYCHOMOTOR ACTIVITY

Some features of this syndrome have already been described in Chap. 16, under "Coma." In the most typical of these states—

due to drug intoxications and metabolic disorders—all mental functions are reduced to some degree, but alertness and the ability to grasp all elements of the immediate situation, to keep in mind recent happenings, and to react quickly and decisively are affected most of all. The patient is inattentive and easily distracted and cannot converse for long on any one topic. Illusory phenomena and hallucinations are variably present. There is a tendency to doze. As the confusion deepens, alertness and responsivity diminish until stupor supervenes.

The causes are listed in Table 19-1. As to the morbid anatomy and pathophysiology, all that has been said on the subject in Chap. 16 is applicable to at least one subgroup of the confusional states. In the majority of cases no consistent pathology is found. In the more severe forms of this syndrome, the EEG is almost invariably abnormal; high-voltage slow waves in the theta or delta range are the usual findings.

DELIRIUM

This syndrome is most perfectly depicted in the chronic alcoholic patient with delirium tremens. Upon cessation of drinking, over a period of 2 to 3 days, the patient becomes restless, apprehensive, and tremulous (fast-frequency kinetic tremor), sleeps poorly, and may have visual and auditory illusions and hallucinations. One or several generalized convulsions precede or initiate the delirium in almost 30 percent of cases. These symptoms rapidly give way to the full-blown syndrome of delirium—the patient is grossly tremulous, profoundly disoriented, distractible, and preoccupied with his hallucinations. He talks incessantly and incoherently. Sleep is impossible. The temperature may be elevated. With concomitant illnesses, such as pneumonia, meningitis, liver failure, or cranial trauma, psychomotor activity is depressed, in which case the line that separates delirium from other confusional states becomes indistinct.

In most instances, recovery from delirium tremens is complete in a matter of several days. Exceptionally, the delirium persists for weeks on end. More importantly, about 5 percent of cases end fatally, as a result of circulatory collapse or hyperthermia. Associated medical and surgical diseases add to the number of fatalities.

In the most typical cases, the EEG, if it can be obtained in such restless patients, may show either fast activity or nonfocal 5- to 7-per-second theta activity. No consistent cellular pathology has been observed in fatal cases, which is not surprising, for with resolution of the delirium, recovery is complete.

Other types of delirium, listed in Table 19-1, differ in minor ways from delirium tremens.

TABLE 19-1 Classification of Delirium and Acute Confusional States

I. Delirium

- *A.* In a medical or surgical illness (no focal or lateralizing neurologic signs; CSF usually clear)
  1. Typhoid fever
  2. Pneumonia
  3. Septicemia, particularly erysipelas and other streptococcal infections
  4. Postoperative and postconcussive states
  5. Thyrotoxicosis and ACTH intoxication (rare)
- *B.* In neurologic diseases that cause focal or lateralizing signs or changes in the CSF
  1. Vascular, neoplastic, or other diseases, particularly those involving the temporal and parietal lobes and upper part of the brainstem
  2. Cerebral contusion and laceration (traumatic delirium)
  3. Encephalitis due to viral (e.g., herpes simplex, infectious mononucleosis) and to unknown causes
- *C.* The abstinence states, exogenous intoxications, and postconvulsive states; signs of other medical, surgical, and neurologic illnesses absent or coincidental
  1. Withdrawal of alcohol (delirium tremens), barbiturates, and nonbarbiturate sedative drugs, following chronic intoxication (Chaps. 39 and 40)
  2. Drug intoxications: e.g., scopolamine, atropine, amphetamine, cocaine
  3. Postconvulsive delirium

II. Acute confusional states associated with psychomotor underactivity

- *A.* Associated with a medical or surgical disease (no focal or lateralizing neurologic signs: CSF clear)
  1. Metabolic disorders; hepatic stupor, uremia, hypoxia, hypercapnea, hypoglycemia, porphyria
  2. Infective fevers, especially typhoid
  3. Congestive heart failure
  4. Postoperative, posttraumatic, and puerperal psychoses
- *B.* Associated with drug intoxication (no focal or lateralizing signs; CSF clear): e.g., opiates, barbiturates and other sedatives, Artane, etc.

III. Confusional states associated with diseases of the nervous system (with focal or lateralizing neurologic signs and/or CSF changes)

- *A.* Cerebral vascular disease, tumor, abscess (especially of the *right* parietal, inferofrontal, and temporal lobes)
- *B.* Subdural hematoma
- *C.* Meningitis
- *D.* Encephalitis
- *E.* Subarachnoid hemorrhage

IV. Beclouded dementia, i.e., senile or other brain disease in combination with infective fevers, drug reactions, heart failure, or other medical or surgical diseases

BECLOUDED DEMENTIA

By this term we denote the acute confusional states of elderly persons in whom a pre-existing brain disease, most often Alzheimer disease, is complicated by some medical or surgical illness. It is the most common mental disorder seen on the wards of a general hospital.

In such a person almost any complicating illness may precipitate the confusional state, but certain ones stand out: concussive brain injuries; infections (particularly of lungs and bladder); operations (most often cardiotomy, prostatectomy, and removal of cataracts); congestive heart failure and chronic obstructive pulmonary disease; and severe anemia, notably pernicious anemia. The most readily identified causative factors are fever, intoxication with one or more drugs, dehydration, electrolyte imbalance, and alcoholism. Frequently, more than one of these factors is operative.

It often happens that the occurrence of this type of confusional state first draws attention to a pre-existing mental impairment, one that may have passed unnoticed or may have been attributed by the patient's family to the benign effects of aging. Upon recovery from the medical illness(es), the patient returns to his or her premorbid mental state, but the family may now be more aware of the patient's deficiencies.

MANAGEMENT OF THE CONFUSED OR DELIRIOUS PATIENT

This should be carried out in a general hospital rather than a psychiatric one, for the reasons that the confusional and delirious states are reversible, as a rule, and the primary need is the diagnosis and treatment of the underlying medical disorder(s).

The patient should be placed in relative isolation, so as not to disturb the rest of the ward. A well-lighted, quiet room and constant reassurance and explanation of all procedures are helpful. A family member or nurse should be in constant or near-constant attendance. All drugs which could possibly be causative should be discontinued, and any infection identified and treated with appropriate antibiotics. Any suspicion of meningitis requires a CSF examination. Fluid intake and output should be carefully recorded and fluid and electrolyte abnormalities corrected. Where the restlessness and agitation of delirium require the use of drugs, chlordiazepoxide (Librium) is the most favored drug, but diazepam and some of the older sedatives, such as paraldehyde and chloral hydrate, are equally safe and effective if given in adequate doses. The purpose of sedation in these circumstances is not to suppress the agitation completely but only to the point where nursing care is facilitated.

In Table 19-1 are listed the causes of the delirious and confusional states, classified according to their main clinical relationships.

For a more detailed discussion of this topic, see Adams and Victor: *Principles of Neurology,* 4th ed, pp 323–333.

ADDITIONAL READING

Medina JL, Rubino FA, Ross A: Agitated delirium caused by infarction of the hippocampal formation, fusiform and lingual gyri. *Neurology* 24:1181, 1974.

Mesulam M-M: Attention, confusional states, and neglect, in Mesulam M-M (ed), *Principles of Behavioral Neurology*. Philadelphia, Davis, 1985, pp 125–168.

Mori E, Yamadori A: Acute confusional state and acute agitated delirium. *Arch Neurol* 44:1139, 1987.

20 Dementia and the Amnesic (Korsakoff) Syndrome

In medicine, the term *dementia* is used conventionally to denote a chronic deterioration of intellectual, or cognitive, functions, such as learning and remembering, verbal facility, numerical skill, visual-spatial perception, and the capacity to make proper deductions from given premises and to analyze and solve problems. Because these functions are clinically separable and may occur in several combinations, it is evident that dementia may assume a variety of forms. Moreover, the anatomic substrates of the many diseases causing intellectual decline lie in different parts of the cerebral cortex and their related thalamic nuclei, and often in the basal ganglia as well. It is not surprising, therefore, that these diseases also evoke a number of noncognitive disturbances, such as loss of emotional control, changes in behavior and personality, and even disturbances of posture, movement, and coordination.

The very existence of the many dementia syndromes signifies that in humans all parts of the cerebrum are not equipotential in function. The occipital lobes are essential for visual perception, the temporal for auditory perception, the parietal for somatosensory function and transmodal associations, the posterior frontal for motor function, the left perisylvian region for language function, and the hippocampi and medial thalamic nuclei for learning and retentive memory. Yet it is a mistake to assume an absolutely strict localization of these functions, since lesions in each of these regions also have subtle and more general effects on intelligence, behavior, and personality.

For these reasons, we object to the all-inclusive term dementia and prefer to speak of the *dementia syndromes* or the *dementing diseases,* each of which may reflect a disproportionate affection of a certain function or part of the brain.

The student or physician who has more than a passing interest in these aspects of cerebral neurology would do well to review the discussions of perception, thinking, emotion, mood, impulse, and insight in *Principles of Neurology* or some other textbook of neurology and psychiatry and become skilled in the bedside examination of mental disorders of all types (a simplified mental status examination can be found at the end of this chapter).

THE NEUROLOGY OF DEMENTIA

Table 20-1 lists the dementing diseases, which are subdivided into three categories on the basis of their neurologic signs and associated clinical and laboratory signs of medical disease.

The special clinical and pathologic features of the dementing diseases will be discussed in subsequent chapters, but several general points should be made here. An inspection of Table 20-1 discloses that some dementing diseases are treatable, a fact that places a premium on accurate diagnosis. *The treatable forms of dementia are those due to neurosyphilis, cryptococcosis, subdural hematoma, brain tumor, chronic drug intoxication, normal-pressure hydrocephalus, pellagra, vitamin B_{12} deficiency and other deficiency states, hypothyroidism, and other metabolic and electrolyte disorders.* Obviously, the correct diagnosis of these diseases is of greater practical importance than the diagnosis of the untreatable ones. Unfortunately, approximately two-thirds of all dementias are due to untreatable degenerative diseases of the brain, usually Alzheimer disease.

Dementia Due to Degenerative Diseases

It is in this category of disease that a generic syndrome of dementia can most readily be discerned.

Here the earliest signs are subtle and easily overlooked. An employer or observant family member may remark on a reduction in the level of mental and physical activity, a certain lack of initiative and interest, a disinclination to converse, a neglect of routine tasks, and an abandonment of pleasureable activities. There follows a more obvious forgetfulness not only of proper names but also of appointments and assigned tasks. The patient asks the same question repeatedly, the answer being quickly forgotten. A febrile illness, infection, or excess of medication may provoke a state of more severe confusion. The patient becomes increasingly distracted by passing incidents or unreasonably preoccupied with some unimportant event. Complex activities can no longer be accomplished. Because of difficulty in calculation, the checkbook can no longer be balanced, and household finances need to be removed from the patient's responsibility.

Emotions are labile, often with outbursts of irritability and unreasonable anger. Those who are by nature suspicious may become frankly paranoid. Judgment is increasingly impaired. Loss of social graces comes late. All this happens with the patient making little or no complaint and seemingly unaware of the changes (lack of insight).

TABLE 20-1 Bedside Classification of the Dementing Diseases

I. Diseases in which dementia is associated with clinical and laboratory signs of other medical disease
   - *A.* Hypothyroidism
   - *B.* Cushing syndrome
   - *C.* Nutritional deficiency states such as pellagra, the Wernicke-Korsakoff syndrome, and subacute combined degeneration of spinal cord and brain (vitamin B_{12} deficiency)
   - *D.* Chronic meningoencephalitis: general paresis, meningovascular syphilis, cryptococcosis
   - *E.* Hepatolenticular degeneration, familial and acquired
   - *F.* Chronic drug intoxications

II. Diseases in which dementia is associated with other neurologic signs but not with other obvious medical disease
   - *A.* Invariably associated with other neurologic signs
     1. Huntington chorea (choreoathetosis)
     2. Schilder disease and related demyelinative diseases (spastic weakness, pseudobulbar palsy, blindness)
     3. Amaurotic familial idiocy and other lipid-storage diseases (myoclonic seizures, blindness, spasticity, cerebellar ataxia)
     4. Myoclonic epilepsy (diffuse myoclonus, generalized seizures, cerebellar ataxia)
     5. Subacute spongiform encephalopathy (one type of Creutzfeldt-Jakob disease) (myoclonic dementia)
     6. Cerebrocerebellar degeneration (cerebellar ataxia)
     7. Cerebral-basal ganglionic degenerations (apraxia-rigidity)
     8. Dementia with spastic paraplegia
     9. Progressive supranuclear palsy
     10. Certain hereditary metabolic diseases (Chap. 38)
   - *B.* Often associated with other neurologic signs
     1. Thrombotic or embolic cerebral infarction
     2. Brain tumor (primary or metastatic) or abscess
     3. Brain trauma, such as cerebral contusion, midbrain hemorrhage, chronic subdural hematoma
     4. Marchiafava-Bignami disease (often with apraxia and other frontal lobe signs)
     5. Communicating (normal-pressure) or obstructive hydrocephalus (usually with ataxia of gait)
     6. Progressive multifocal leukoencephalitis

III. Diseases in which dementia is usually the only evidence of neurologic or medical disease
   - *A.* Alzheimer disease
   - *B.* Pick disease
   - *C.* AIDS dementia
   - *D.* Alcoholic dementia
   - *E.* Degenerative disease of unspecified type

As the condition progresses, all intellectual faculties gradually fail, memory most of all. The patient's language functions deteriorate sooner or later. Vocabulary becomes restricted.

There is groping for proper names, and even simple ideas can no longer be conveyed in properly constructed phrases or sentences. Writing shows similar faults. There is also increasing inability to comprehend complex spoken or written requests. As language function deteriorates, palilalia and echolalia may appear. Agnosias and apraxias become increasingly prominent, and eventually the patient requires help in all activities, even the most personal ones.

There is also physical deterioration. Unused muscles become flabby and wasted. At first, food intake is sometimes increased, but then it diminishes gradually with loss of weight. Walking becomes more difficult and the patient sits in idleness much of the time. Later, bed is preferred. Grasping and sucking reflexes becomes easily evoked. By contrast, somatic sensation, vision, hearing, and capacity for movement are retained until near the end. The final stage is one of cerebral paraplegia in flexion, in which the patient lies curled up, immobile and mute, until pneumonia or some other intercurrent infection mercifully terminates life. The duration of the entire illness is 5 to 10 years.

Problems in diagnosis Many of the diseases listed in Table 20-1 alter the configuration of the dementing syndrome described above and also its temporal profile. In *Huntington chorea,* an altered mood, particularly depression, or changes in personality and character (heightened irritability, suspiciousness, impulsive behavior, and other emotional disturbances) may precede the memory loss. In *multi-infarct dementia,* the effects of one or more strokes may be added—hemiparesis, hemisensory loss, pseudobulbar palsy, homonymous hemianopia, or an early aphasia. As noted in Table 20-1, many of the dementing diseases have other identifying neurologic characteristics. An important example is *normal-pressure hydrocephalus,* in which a gait disorder is early and prominent, coming on before or with only slight mental change, and well before incontinence. An *endogenous depression* may simulate a type of progressive dementia. The patient's lack of interest and unwillingness to participate in tests of mental status makes clinical evaluation difficult. Complaints by the patient of loss of memory, the presence of a sad facial expression, crying, talk of dying, discrepancies in memory tests, intactness of language function and capacity for calculation, and a history of previous depression in the patient or in family members are helpful in differential diagnosis.

More than one factor may contribute to the dementia syndrome. Many patients with the Alzheimer-senile dementia complex may have one or more strokes. A considerable proportion of older parkinsonian patients develop senile dementia, and the patient with advanced Alzheimer disease may move stiffly and walk with small steps.

When the underlying disease (stroke, tumor, subdural hematoma) involves primarily one part of the brain, i.e., a frontal occipital, parietal, or temporal lobe, the early symptoms will be referable to that part. These focal cerebral symptoms are summarized in the next chapter.

The Amnesic Syndrome (Korsakoff Psychosis; Amnesic or Amnestic Confabulatory Syndrome)

These terms denote a special form of cognitive impairment in which learning and memory are deranged out of proportion to all other intellectual functions. Two features distinguish this category of disease: (1) an inability to recall events and other information that had been well established for months or years before the onset of the illness (*retrograde amnesia*) and (2) an inability to learn and retain new information, such as verbal, topographic, and motor skills (*anterograde amnesia*). The level of general intelligence is affected very little, and language function, ability to calculate, and previously learned skills are retained (no aphasia, apraxia, or agnosia). While a global amnesia is the main symptom, there are other subtle abnormalities. Psychometric tests disclose an impairment in concentration and visual and verbal abstraction and difficulty in changing from one task to another. Most patients with the amnesic syndrome are apathetic, indifferent to their surroundings, and lacking in initiative, spontaneity, and insight. Confabulation, i.e., fabrication of past events, is variably present in this syndrome and is not a requisite for the diagnosis.

The common diseases causing an amnesic syndrome are classified in Table 20-2. These diseases can be identified by their mode of onset and clinical course, the associated neurologic signs, and ancillary findings. It will be recognized that the structures commonly damaged by these diseases are the diencephalon (more specifically the medial thalamic nuclei) and the hippocampal formations. This is not to say that these structures form a "memory center" or that large hemispheric lesions do not impair memory, but only that the smallest lesions in diencephalic-hippocampal structures have the most devastating effects upon memory.

The diseases that cause an amnesic syndrome are discussed in the appropriate chapters. Also, special amnesias, e.g., verbal, are discussed with the aphasias and acalculia with parietal-occipital lesions. *Transient global amnesia,* which cannot with assurance be included with the epilepsies or other standard categories of disease, is described below.

TABLE 20-2 Classification of Diseases Characterized by an Amnesic Syndrome

I. Amnesic syndrome of sudden onset—usually with gradual but incomplete recovery
   A. Bilateral hippocampal infarction due to atherosclerotic-thrombotic or embolic occlusion of the posterior cerebral arteries or their inferior temporal branches
   B. Infarction of the basal forebrain due to occlusion of anterior cerebral-anterior communicating arteries
   C. Trauma to the diencephalic, inferomedial temporal, or orbitofrontal regions
   D. Spontaneous subarachnoid hemorrhage (mechanism of amnesia not understood)
   E. Carbon monoxide poisoning and other hypoxic states (rare)
II. Amnesia of sudden onset and short duration
   A. Temporal lobe seizures
   B. Postconcussive states
   C. "Transient global amnesia"
III. Amnesic syndrome of subacute onset with varying degrees of recovery, usually leaving permanent residua
   A. Wernicke-Korsakoff syndrome
   B. Herpes simplex encephalitis
   C. Tuberculous and other forms of meningitis characterized by a granulomatous exudate at the base of the brain
IV. Slowly progressive amnesic states
   A. Tumors involving the floor and walls of the third ventricle and limbic cortical structures
   B. Alzheimer disease (early stage) and other degenerative disorders with disproportionate affection of the temporal lobes

Transient Global Amnesia

This is the term given by Fisher and Adams to an acute syndrome in elderly patients who suddenly lose their immediate temporal and spatial orientation for several hours. Notable characteristics are a retrograde amnesia for events that had occurred in the hours or days before the amnesia began and a retained capacity, during the attack, to calculate, perform complex tasks, and recognize old friends and family. In this respect, the condition differs from the transient disorder of consciousness and the apparent amnesia (actually a failure of registration) that attends temporal lobe seizures, concussion, hypoxia, and other confusional states. The EEG may show a slight slowing in temporal leads during the attack.

The exact mechanism is unclear. A transient ischemia and seizure have both been postulated, but proof of either is lacking. When followed for years, the patient is no more liable to stroke than his age-matched peers. No treatment is needed, as a rule.

In only a small percentage of cases has the condition recurred, up to five or more times. In the older patients who later have a stroke, the amnesic state has not been reproduced as part of the stroke.

Management of the Demented Patient

The demented patient should be admitted to the hospital for the purpose of fully assessing the clinical state and determining the presence or absence of the treatable causes of dementia, which have been enumerated above. In addition to the history (which should always include information from a person other than the patient) and the neurologic and mental status examinations (see below), a number of ancillary examinations can be carried out. The latter include blood counts, vitamin B_{12} and drug levels, evaluation of endocrine and liver functions and cardiovascular status, CSF examination for neurosyphilis, and special tests of CNS function—EEG, CT scan, and, more and more, MRI.

Once it is established that the patient has an untreatable dementing disease, the cooperation of a responsible family member, who is apprised of the situation, is essential, for the latter must decide upon time of retirement, the assumption of legal/financial responsibility, the need for an attendant, placement in a nursing home, etc. Since most of the underlying diseases are slowly progressive and incurable, this can be done in a series of unobtrusive steps. Adjustments to work, home life, and driving a car depend largely on the patient's circumstances, the degree of disability, and treatability of an associated disease(s).

Medical treatment is indicated at times. Antidepressant medication (amitriptyline, 25 to 75 mg at bedtime) helps alleviate mood change and insomnia. Severe paranoia may be controlled with thorazine (10 to 25 mg tid); afternoon hallucinations are suppressed in some patients by caffeine and dexedrine at lunch time and nocturnal wandering by diazepam or chloral hydrate. A sudden worsening in the mental state should always raise suspicion of an infection, an electrolyte imbalance, a cardiac or cerebral vascular event, or pulmonary embolism.

THE MENTAL STATUS EXAMINATION

This must be systematic and at a minimum should include the following:

1. *Insight* (patient's replies to questions about the chief symptoms): What is your difficulty? Are you ill? When did your illness begin?
2. *Orientation* (knowledge of personal identity and present situa-

tion): What is your name, your address, current location (building, city, state)? What is your occupation? Are you married?

Place: What is the name of the place where you are now (building, city, state)? How did you get here? On what floor is it? Where is the bathroom?

Time: What is the date today (year, month, day of the week and of the month)? What time of the day is it? What meals have you had? When was the last holiday?

3. *Memory*

Remote: Tell me the names of your children and their birth dates. When were you married? What was your mother's maiden name? What was the name of your first school teacher? What jobs have you held?

Recent past: Tell me about your recent illness (compare with previous statements). What did you have for breakfast today? What is my name (or the nurse's name)? When did you see me for the first time? What tests were done yesterday? What were the headlines of the newspaper today? Give the patient a simple story, oral or written, and ask him to retell it after 3 to 5 min.

Immediate recall ("short-term memory"): Repeat these numbers after me (give series of 3, 4, 5, 6, 7, 8 digits at speed of one per second). Now when I give a series of numbers, repeat them in reverse order.

Memorization (learning): The patient is given four simple data (examiner's name, date, time of day, and a fruit, structure, or trait, such as honesty) and is asked to repeat them until he or she can do so without prompting. The capacity to reproduce them at intervals after committing them to memory is a test of *retentive memory span.*

Visual span: Show the patient a picture of several objects; then ask him to name the objects and note any inaccuracies.

4. *General information:* Ask about names of the current president, first president, and recent presidents, well-known historic dates, the names of large rivers, of large cities, number of weeks in a year, definition of an island.

5. *Capacity for sustained mental activity:* Crossing out all the a's on a printed page; counting forward and backward; saying the months of the year forward and backward; naming 12 flowers, 12 trees, or 12 vegetables.

Calculation: Test ability to add, substract, multiply, and divide. Substraction of serial 7's from 100 is a good test of calculation as well as of concentration.

Construction: Draw a clock and place hands at 7:45; map of United States; floor plan of your house; copy a cube.

Abstract thinking: See if the patient can detect similarities and differences between classes of objects (orange and apple, horse and dog, desk and bookcase) or explain a proverb or a fable.

6. *General behavior:* Attitudes, general bearing, stream of thought, attentiveness, mood, manner of dress.
7. *Special tests of localized cerebral functions:* Grasping, sucking, aphasia battery, praxis with both hands, and cortical sensory function.

The many formal psychologic tests for dementia yield quantitative data of comparative value but in themselves cannot be used for diagnostic purposes. A comparison of the Wechsler Adult Intelligence Scales (WAIS) and the Wechsler Memory Scale is useful in distinguishing the amnesic state from a more general dementia (a discrepancy of 25 or more points between the two tests). The Mini-Mental Status of Folstein et al is a useful bedside method of scoring cognitive impairment and following its progress.

For a more detailed discussion of this topic, see Adams and Victor: *Principles of Neurology,* 4th ed, pp 334–346.

ADDITIONAL READING

Deutsch JA (ed): *The Physiological Basis of Memory,* 2nd ed. New York, Academic, 1983, pp 199–268.

Fisher CM, Adams RD: Transient global amnesia. *Acta Neurol Scand,* 40 (suppl 9), 1964.

Folstein M, Folstein S, McHugh PR: "Mini-mental status." A practical method for grading the cognitive state of patients for the clinician. *J Psychiatr Res* 12:189, 1975.

Mayeux R, Stern Y: Subcortical dementia. *Arch Neurol* 44:129, 1987.

Mishkin M: A memory system in the monkey. *Phil Trans R Soc Lond* B298:85, 1982.

Victor M, Adams RD, Collins GH: *The Wernicke-Korsakoff Syndrome,* 2nd ed. Philadelphia, Davis, 1989.

Wells C (ed): *Dementia.* Philadelphia, Davis, 1977, p 250.

21 Neurologic Syndromes Caused by Lesions in Particular Parts of the Cerebrum

For the most part, the dementing diseases discussed in Chap. 20 are diffuse or multifocal in nature, implicating the association cortex and several lobes of the brain. Presented here are the symptoms and syndromes that are related more specifically to particular parts of the cerebrum, i.e., cerebral cortex and subcortical white matter. These focal syndromes are described in terms of the conventional lobular divisions of the cerebrum, but it is obvious that most diseases do not respect these boundaries. Hence the syndromes by which these diseases express themselves may overlap or occur in a number of combinations.

It needs to be remembered that all parts of the cerebrum are widely connected with other parts via tracts in the central white matter and with the thalamic nuclei via corticothalamic and thalamocortical pathways. Even though localized lesions give rise to certain syndromes manifested as disorders of thinking, speaking and behavior, one must guard against the presumption of overly discrete localization of function in the cerebral cortex. Surprising also is the magnitude of many cerebral lesions that result in no cerebral symptoms or signs whatsoever. In general, the degree of intellectual deficit correlates with the amount of brain destroyed by a lesion.

The lobular division of the cerebrum is illustrated in Fig. 21-1, which is a photograph of the (left) lateral surface of the brain, imprinted with the names of the important sulci and gyri. Fig. 21-2 is a map of the surfaces of the cerebral cortex, numbered according to the different cytoarchitectonic areas recognized by Brodmann. The cortical surface can also be subdivided into broad functional zones, as depicted in Fig. 21-3. These schemes are the ones that are conventionally used in discussing the functional anatomy of the human brain.

SYNDROMES CAUSED BY LESIONS OF THE FRONTAL LOBES

The frontal lobes are often conceived to be man's supreme evolutionary attainment. They lie anterior to the central (rolandic) sulcus and superior to the sylvian fissure and consist of several

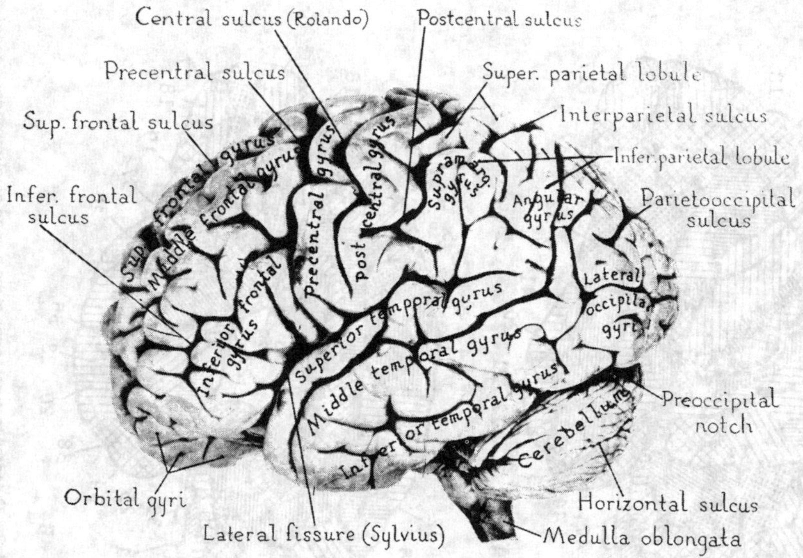

Fig. 21-1 Photograph of lateral surface of the human brain. (*From MB Carpenter and J Sutin, Human Neuroanatomy, 8th ed, Baltimore, Williams & Wilkins, 1982.*)

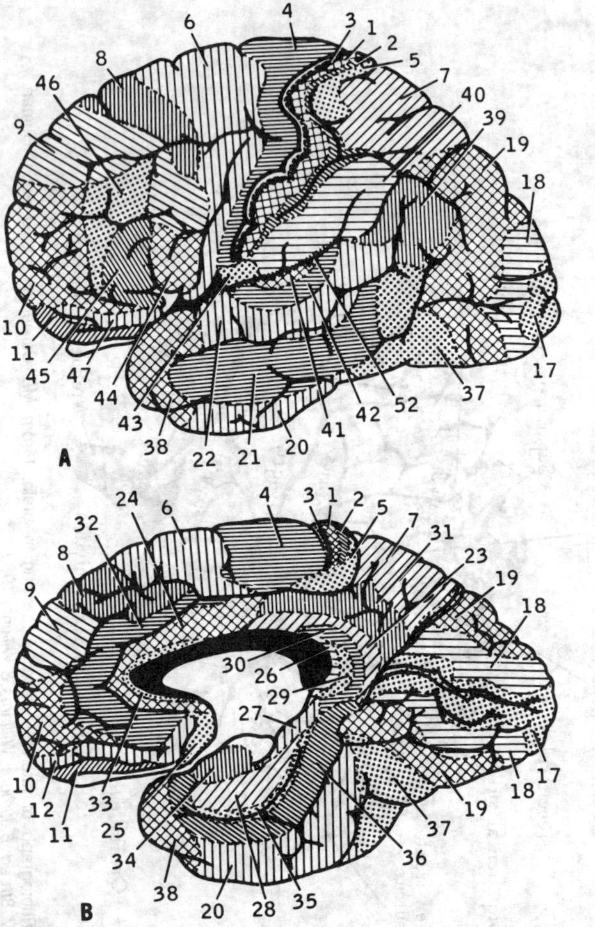

Fig. 21-2 Cytoarchitectural zones of the human cerebral cortex according to the scheme of Brodmann. *A*. Lateral surface. *B*. Medial surface.

functionally different parts, as indicated in Figs. 21-1, 21-2, and 21-3.

The posterior parts of the frontal lobes are specifically related to motor function. Voluntary movement depends on the integrity

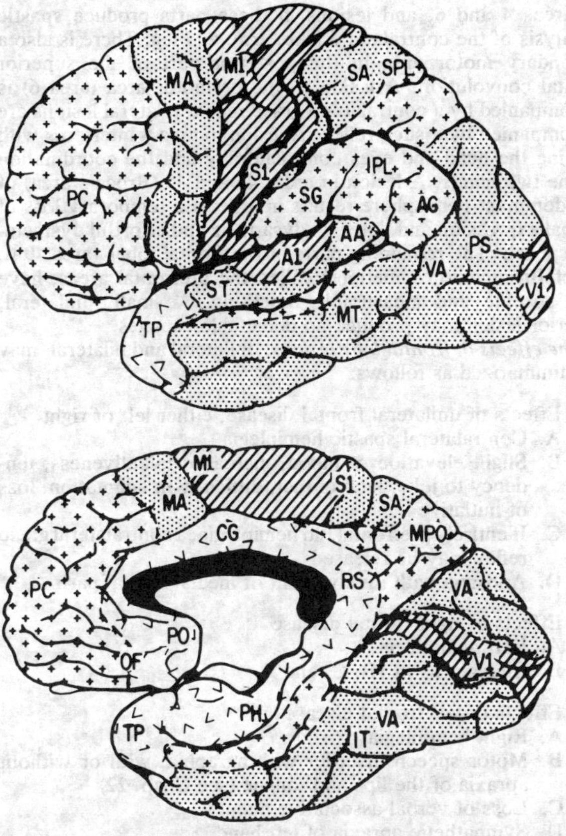

Fig. 21-3 Approximate distribution of functional zones on lateral (above) and medial (below) aspects of the cerebral cortex. Abbreviations: AA, auditory association cortex; AG, angular gyrus; A1, primary auditory cortex; CG, cingulate cortex; INS, insula; IPL, inferior parietal lobule; IT, inferior temporal gyrus; MA, motor association cortex; MPO, medial parieto-occipital area; MT, middle temporal gyrus; M1, primary motor area; OF, orbitofrontal region; PC, prefrontal cortex; PH, parahippocampal region; PO, parolfactory area; PS, peristriate cortex; RS, retrosplenial area; SA, somatosensory association cortex; SG, supramarginal gyrus; SPL, superior parietal lobule; ST, superior temporal gyrus; S1, primary somatosensory area; TP, temporopolar cortex; VA, visual association cortex; V1, primary visual cortex. (*Redrawn from M-M Mesulam.*)

of areas 4 and 6, and lesions in these parts produce spastic paralysis of the contralateral face, arm, and leg. There is also a secondary motor area in the posterior part of the superior frontal convolution. A lesion of the premotor area (area 6) is accompanied by a contralateral grasp reflex; bilateral lesions are accompanied by a suck reflex. A lesion in area 8 interferes with turning the head and eyes contralaterally and the coordination of the two hands. A lesion in areas 44 and 45 (Broca's area) of the dominant hemisphere results in at least a temporary loss of verbal expression and, later, in dysarthric and effortful dysmelodic speech. The remaining parts of the frontal lobes (areas 9 to 12 of Brodmann), sometimes called the prefrontal areas, have less specific and measurable functions. A small, unilateral, anterior lesion may produce no detectable changes.

The effects of frontal lobe lesions, unilateral and bilateral, may be summarized as follows:

I. Effects of unilateral frontal disease, either left or right
   - A. Contralateral spastic hemiplegia
   - B. Slight elevation of mood, increased talkativeness, tendency to joke, lack of tact, difficulty in adaptation, loss of initiative
   - C. If entirely prefrontal, no hemiplegia; a contralateral grasp reflex may be released
   - D. Anosmia with involvement of medial-orbital parts

II. Effects of right frontal disease
   - A. Left hemiplegia
   - B. Changes as in 1B, C, and D

III. Effects of left frontal disease
   - A. Right hemiplegia
   - B. Motor speech disorder with agraphia, with or without apraxia of the lips and tongue (see Chap. 22)
   - C. Loss of verbal associative fluency
   - D. Sympathetic apraxia of left hand
   - E. Changes as in 1B, C, and D

IV. Effects of bifrontal disease
   - A. Bilateral hemiplegia
   - B. Spastic bulbar (pseudobulbar) palsy
   - C. If prefrontal, abulia or akinetic mutism, lack of ability to sustain attention and solve complex problems, rigidity of thinking, bland affect, labile mood, personality change, and varying combinations of grasping, sucking, decomposition of gait, and sphincteric incontinence. Rarely, with superior-frontal lesions, there may be hyperactivity.

SYNDROMES CAUSED BY LESIONS OF THE TEMPORAL LOBES

The sylvian fissure separates the superior and lateral surfaces of the temporal lobe from the frontal lobe and from the anterior part of the parietal lobe (Fig. 21-1). Posteriorly, the temporal lobe merges with the occipital lobe and superolaterally, with the parietal lobe. The temporal lobe includes the superior, middle, and inferior temporal, fusiform, and hippocampal convolutions and, on its superior surface, the transverse gyri of Heschl. The latter constitute the auditory receptive area. Hearing is represented bilaterally so that the Heschl gyri of both temporal lobes need to be affected to cause cortical deafness. The hippocampal convolution, once thought to be related to olfactory function, is now known to be of critical importance in learning and memory. A lesion in the superior convolution of the dominant temporal lobe (areas 41 and 42) results in a failure to understand the spoken word (auditory verbal agnosia) and is an important component of Wernicke aphasia (Chap. 22). Finally, the temporal lobes include a large part of the limbic system, which subserves the emotional and motivational aspects of behavior and vegetative functions ("visceral brain," Chap. 24).

The lower fibers of the geniculocalcarine pathway (from the inferior retina) swing in a wide arc over the temporal horn of the ventricle en route to the occipital lobes, and lesions that interrupt them produce a contralateral upper homonymous quadrantanopia.

The effects of lesions in one or both temporal lobes are tabulated below:

I. Effects of unilateral disease of the dominant temporal lobe
   A. Homonymous upper quadrantanopia
   B. Impaired comprehension of verbal material presented through the auditory sense (Wernicke aphasia)
   C. Dysnomia or amnesic aphasia
   D. Impaired reading and writing of music

II. Effects of unilateral disease of nondominant temporal lobe
   A. Homonymous upper quadrantanopia
   B. Inability to judge spatial relationships in some cases
   C. Impairment in tests of visually presented nonverbal material
   D. Agnosia for steady state harmonic sounds

III. Effects of disease of either hemisphere
   A. Auditory illusions and hallucinations
   B. Psychotic behavior (aggressivity)

IV. Effects of bilateral disease
   A. Korsakoff amnesic defect (hippocampal formations)
   B. Apathy and placidity

C. Increased sexual activity (B and C constitute the Kluver-Bucy syndrome)
D. "Sham rage"
E. Failure to recognize familiar tunes

SYNDROMES CAUSED BY LESIONS IN THE PARIETAL LOBES

Anteriorly this lobe is bordered by the rolandic sulcus and inferiorly by the sylvian fissure. Posteriorly it has no definite boundary. The postcentral convolution (areas 1, 3, and 5) is the terminus of somatosensory pathways from the opposite half of the body. However, destructive lesions here cause mainly a defect in sensory discrimination (position sense, stereognosis, localization of stimuli) and only variable impairment of primary sensation ("cortical sensory syndrome"). Also, with bilateral simultaneous stimulation the patient may perceive only the stimuli from one side ("extinction"). With a large lesion of the nondominant parietal lobe, the patient is often unaware of his hemiplegia and hemianesthesia (anosognosia). Lack of recognition of the left arm and leg and neglect of the left side of the body (as in grooming and dressing) and of external space are related phenomena. These disorders are observed only infrequently with left-sided lesions.

With lesions of the dominant angular gyrus the patient may lose the ability to read (alexia). Additionally, in some patients there is loss of ability to write (agraphia), to calculate, and to identify fingers (finger agnosia). This constellation of abnormalities is known as the Gerstmann syndrome.

Effects of parietal lobe lesions may be summarized as follows:

I. Effects of unilateral disease of the parietal lobe, right or left
   A. Cortical sensory syndrome and sensory extinction (or total hemianesthesia with large acute lesions of white matter)
   B. Mild hemiparesis, unilateral muscular atrophy in children
   C. Homonymous hemianopia (incongruent) or visual inattention and sometimes anosognosia, neglect of the opposite one-half of the body and of extrapersonal space (more frequent with right than with left parietal lesions)
   D. Abolition of optokinetic nystagmus to one side (when striped drum is rotated toward the side of the lesion)

II. Effects of unilateral disease of the dominant parietal lobe (left hemisphere in righthanded patients); *additional* phenomena include
   A. Disorders of language (especially alexia)
   B. Gerstmann syndrome
   C. Tactile agnosia (bimanual astereognosis; see Chap. 8)

   D. Bilateral ideomotor and ideational apraxia (Chap. 22)

III. Effects of unilateral disease of the nondominant (right) parietal lobe
   A. Topographic memory loss
   B. Anosognosia and dressing apraxia. These disorders may occur with lesions of either hemisphere but have been observed more frequently with lesions of the nondominant one.

SYNDROMES CAUSED BY LESIONS OF THE OCCIPITAL LOBES

The medial surface of the occipital lobe is demarcated from the parietal lobe by the parietal-occipital fissure; on the lateral surface there is no sharp demarcation from the posterior temporal or parietal lobe. On the medial surface, the calcarine fissure, which courses in an anteroposterior direction, is the major landmark; the calcarine cortex is the terminus of the corresponding geniculocalcarine pathway. The main function of the occipital lobe and the temporoparietal association areas is the reception of visual stimuli (area 17) and their recognition (areas 18 and 19). Like the other lobes of the cerebrum it is connected through the corpus callosum with the corresponding lobe of the other hemisphere.

As indicated in Chap. 12, a destructive lesion in one occipital lobe results in a contralateral homonymous hemianopia, i.e., a loss of vision in part or all of the corresponding, or homonymous, fields (nasal field of one eye and temporal field of the other). Occasionally there may be changes in the form and contour of visually perceived objects (*metamorphopsia*) or illusory displacement of images from one side of the visual field to the other (*visual allesthesia*) or abnormal persistence of the visual image after the object has been removed (*palinopsia*). Visual illusions and elementary (unformed) hallucinations may also occur. Bilateral lesions cause "cortical" blindness, a state of blindness without change in the optic fundi or pupillary reflexes.

Lesions in Brodmann areas 18 and 19 of the dominant hemisphere (Fig. 21-2) cause an inability to recognize objects presented visually (visual object agnosia) even though by tests of visual acuity and perimetry the individual appears to see sufficiently well to do so; such individuals are able to recognize objects by tactile or other nonvisual senses. *Alexia,* or inability to read, represents a visual verbal agnosia, or "word blindness"; patients can see letters and words but do not know their meaning, although they can still recognize them through tactile or auditory senses. Other types of agnosia—e.g., for recognition of faces (*prosopagnosia*), for a complex of objects the elements of which are perceived but not the whole (*simultanagnosia*), and for color—and the Balint syndrome (inability to look at and grasp an object, visual ataxia, and visual inattention) are observed with bilateral ventromesial occipitotemporal lesions.

The details of these *occipital syndromes* can be found in the *Principles* and are summarized below:

I. Effects of unilateral disease, either right or left
   A. Contralateral (congruent) homonymous hemianopia, which may be central (splitting the macula) or peripheral; also homonymous hemiachromatopsia
   B. Irritative lesions—elementary (unformed) visual hallucinations
II. Effects of left occipital disease
   A. Right homonymous hemianopia
   B. If deep white matter or splenium of corpus callosum is involved, alexia and color-naming defect
   C. Object agnosia
III. Effects of right occipital disease
   A. Left homonymous hemianopia
   B. With more extensive lesions, visual illusions (metamorphopsias) and hallucinations (more frequent with right-sided than left-sided lesions)
   C. Loss of topographic memory and visual orientation
IV. Bilateral occipital disease
   A. Cortical blindness (pupils reactive)
   B. Loss of perception of color
   C. Prosopagnosia, simultanagnosia
   D. Balint syndrome

DISCONNECTION SYNDROMES

Focal lesions of the cerebral white matter, which separate different parts of one hemisphere (*intrahemispheric*) or one hemisphere from another (*interhemispheric* or *commissural*), have certain definable effects. These are called disconnection syndromes and are illustrated in Fig. 21-4.

When the corpus callosum is sectioned surgically or destroyed (anterior four-fifths) by an anterior cerebral artery occlusion, the language and perceptual areas of the left hemisphere are isolated from those of the right. If blindfolded, such a patient is unable to match an object held in one hand with that in the other, nor can he match an object seen in the right half of the visual field with one in the left half. If given verbal commands, he performs correctly with the right hand but not with the left. Without vision, objects placed in the right hand are named correctly but not those in the left.

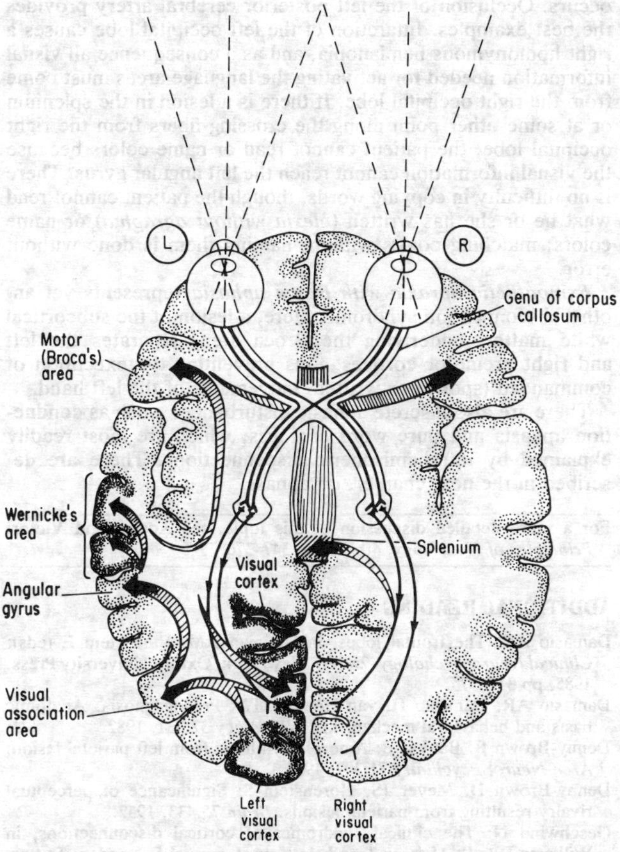

Fig. 21-4 Connections involved in naming a seen object and in reading. The visual pattern is transferred from the visual cortex and association areas to the angular gyrus, which arouses the auditory pattern in the Wernicke area. The auditory pattern is transmitted to the Broca area where the articulatory form is aroused and transferred to the contiguous face area of the motor cortex. With destruction of the left visual cortex and splenium (or intervening white matter), words perceived in the right visual cortex cannot cross over to the language areas and the patient cannot read.

In lesions confined to the posterior fifth of the corpus callosum (splenium), only the visual part of the disconnection syndrome occurs. Occlusion of the left posterior cerebral artery provides the best examples. Infarction of the left occipital lobe causes a right homonymous hemianopia, and as a consequence all visual information needed for activating the language areas must come from the right occipital lobe. If there is a lesion in the splenium or at some other point along the crossing fibers from the right occipital lobe, the patient cannot read or name colors because the visual information cannot reach the left angular gyrus. There is no difficulty in copying words, though the patient cannot read what he or she has written (*alexia without agraphia*) or name colors; matching colors without naming them is done without error.

Sympathetic apraxia with Broca aphasia represents yet another disconnection syndrome. Here, a lesion of the subcortical white matter, underlying the Broca area, separates the left and right premotor cortices, thus preventing the execution of commanded (spoken or written) movements of the left hand.

There are also discrete aphasic disturbances, such as conduction aphasia and pure word deafness, which are most readily explained by intrahemispheric disconnections. These are described in the next chapter, on aphasia.

For a more detailed discussion of this topic, see Adams and Victor: *Principles of Neurology*, 4th ed, pp 347–376.

ADDITIONAL READING

Damasio AR: The frontal lobes, in Heilman KM, Valenstein E (eds): *Clinical Neuropsychology*, 2nd ed. New York, Oxford University Press, 1985, pp 339–375.

Damasio AR, Damasio H, van Hoesen GW: Prosopagnosia: Anatomic basis and behavioral mechanisms. *Neurology* 32:331, 1982.

Denny-Brown B, Banker B: Amorphosynthesis from left parietal lesion. *Arch Neurol Psychiatry* 71:302, 1954.

Denny-Brown D, Meyer JS, Horenstein S: Significance of perceptual rivalry resulting from parietal lesions. *Brain* 75:433, 1952.

Geschwind N: The clinical syndromes of cortical disconnections, in Williams D (ed): *Modern Trends in Neurology*, vol 5. London, Butterworth, 1970, p 29.

Hubel D: Exploration of the primary visual cortex. *Nature* 299:515, 1982.

Lilly R, Cummings SL, Benson F, Frankel M: The human Kluver-Bucy syndrome. *Neurology* 33:1141, 1983.

Mesulam M-M (ed): *Principles of Behavioral Neurology*. Philadelphia, Davis, 1985.

Walsh K: *Neuropsychology: A Clinical Approach*, 2nd ed. New York, Churchill Livingstone, 1987.

22 Affections of Speech and Language

Man's ability to substitute word symbols for objects and ideas is the basis of his extraordinary communicative skill, which, together with his manual facility, set him above all other members of the animal kingdom. All thinking and other aspects of inner psychic life also take place in terms of word symbols, and literate men and women use them to record their ideas and experiences for others to read. In a much narrower sense, language is the means by which the patient makes known his complaints and the physician gathers information as to the status of the nervous system and the manifestations of its diseases.

Speech and language depend upon elaborate mechanisms that evolve over the first two decades of life and come to be localized in particular (perisylvian) parts of the left cerebral hemisphere (Fig. 22-1). Right-hand dominance usually develops in parallel. We know this from the experiments of nature, wherein speech and language functions are lost when these parts of the brain are destroyed. This statement requires qualification only insofar as in a small proportion of left-handed individuals the right cerebral hemisphere is dominant for language, and lesions there cause aphasia. In either hemisphere, language functions have their sensory and motor aspects, for certain restricted lesions may interfere more with one than the other.

TERMINOLOGY

Aphasia or *dysphasia* may be defined as a loss of production or comprehension of spoken or written language, or both, due to an acquired disease of the brain. A failure to name objects is called *anomia*. *Alexia* (or visual verbal agnosia) refers to an inability to read by a person who was literate. *Agraphia* is a loss of ability to write. *Auditory verbal agnosia* or *word deafness* specifies a loss of understanding of spoken words. *Dysarthria* (or the more severe *anarthria*) is a pure motor disorder of the muscles of articulation, language function being intact. *Aphonia* or *dysphonia* signifies an inability to vocalize, articulation and language being unaffected.

CLINICAL VARIETIES OF APHASIA

Despite the complexity of language mechanisms and the bewildering nomenclature that has characterized writings on this subject, most instances of aphasia will be found, on systematic examination, to fall into a relatively small number of recurring, identifiable types, tabulated below. More than 80 percent of all aphasias fall into the first (major) group. Frequently, there is an overlapping of syndromes.

A. Major aphasic syndromes
   1. Global aphasia
   2. Broca aphasia
   3. Wernicke aphasia
   4. Anomic aphasia

B. Minor, or restricted (disconnection), syndromes
   1. Conduction aphasia
   2. Transcortical aphasias, motor and sensory
   3. Modality specific aphasias
      a. "Pure" word blindness
      b. "Pure" word deafness
      c. "Pure" word mutism
      d. Agraphia

Global, or Total, Aphasia

Here, all language functions, both receptive and expressive, are lost. Although awake, able to regard and follow the examiner with the eyes, move the tongue and lips, and swallow, the patient emits no words or at most a stereotyped, repetitive utterance or expletive. Nor is there any understanding of words spoken or written by the examiner. Moreover, the patient is unable to express himself by writing with the left hand if the right is paralyzed (as it often is). The lesion is usually large, and there may be a hemiplegia and hemisensory defect and a tendency to turn and look to the left. Drowsiness, inattentiveness, and profound apathy (abulia) may also be present.

The usual cause is an embolic occlusion of the stem of the middle cerebral artery or embolic or thrombotic occlusion of the internal carotid artery. Large hemorrhages may have a similar effect but are more likely to cause stupor and coma, so that the language disorder is not in evidence. Widespread tumor invasion, involving both the Broca and Wernicke areas, may rarely progress to the point of abolishing all language functions. Global aphasia of vascular causation tends to recover to some degree and may come to resemble Broca aphasia.

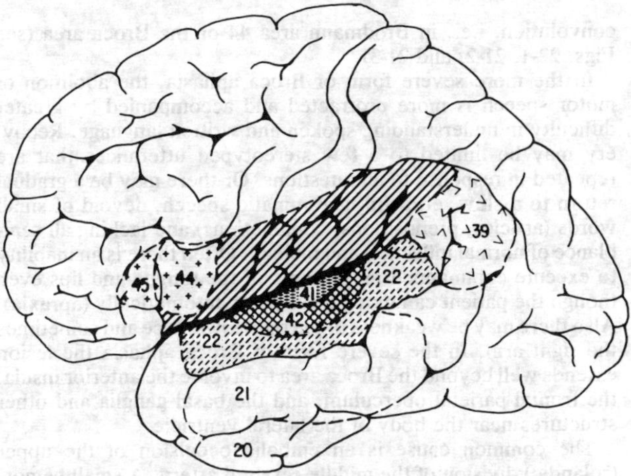

Fig. 22-1 Lateral surface of the left cerebral hemisphere, showing the classic language areas, numbered according to Brodmann. The auditory association areas of Wernicke (areas 41 and 42) actually lie on the superior surface of the temporal lobe, deep within the sylvian fissure. The elaboration of speech and language probably involves a much larger area of cerebrum, including all of the shaded zone of cortex and subcortical areas. (The latter are not shown.)

Broca Aphasia

Here the primary deficit is in language output or production, hence the synonyms *motor*, or *expressive*, *aphasia*. The latter term is not apt, since all aphasic patients have some difficulty expressing themselves.

Broca aphasia varies greatly in severity. In the milder forms, the capacity to speak (and to write) is impaired while other language functions (the understanding of written and spoken words) are little affected. However, if the patient's comprehension is stringently tested (e.g., with complex spoken commands), it will be found to be variably impaired almost without exception. Rarely, the patient may be mute, despite the preserved understanding of the written and spoken word, a condition originally referred to as "aphemia." As a rule, the mutism gives way to a sparse, effortful, and frequently dysarthric speech and then to full recovery. Mohr points out that the lesion in this recoverable type of aphasia is relatively small and restricted to a zone in and immediately around the posterior part of the inferior frontal convolution, i.e., in Brodmann area 44 or the Broca area (see Figs. 22-1, 21-2, and 21-3).

In the more severe form of Broca aphasia, the abolition of motor speech is more protracted and accompanied by greater difficulty in understanding spoken and written language. Recovery may be limited to a few stereotyped utterances that are repeated in response to all questions. Or there may be a gradual return to a slow, effortful, agrammatic speech, devoid of small words (articles, prepositions, conjunctions) and lacking all semblance of normal inflection and melody. Often there is an inability to execute commanded movements of the tongue and lips even though the patient can move these parts automatically (apraxia). Also there may be weakness of the right lower face and sometimes the right arm. In the severe form of Broca aphasia the lesion extends well beyond the Broca area to involve the anterior insula, the frontal-parietal operculum, and the basal ganglia and other structures near the body of the lateral ventricle.

The common cause is an embolic occulsion of the upper (rolandic) division of the middle cerebral artery. A small hemorrhage, traumatic lesion, or inflammatory focus may have the same effect but is less frequent.

Wernicke, or Sensory, Aphasia

This syndrome is comprised of two main elements: (1) an inability to understand spoken or written words, even though hearing and vision are normal, and (2) a fluently articulated but paraphasic speech. By paraphasia is meant the distortion of words by substituting unwanted phonemes or syllables, e.g., *frem* for *friend* (literal paraphasia) or the substitution of one word for another, such as *father* for *brother* (verbal paraphasia). Neologisms (words that are not part of the language) may also appear. Despite the fluency and normal inflection of the patient's speech, it is devoid of meaning and may be entirely incomprehensible (jargon aphasia). The patient, however, is usually unaware or not fully aware of his deficit. In addition, there are invariable defects in reading, writing, naming, and repetition, which parallel in severity the defect in comprehension. The lesion involves the posterior perisylvian region (superior temporal, angular, and supramarginal convolutions). Varying degrees of right homonymous hemianopia may accompany the language disorder. The most frequent cause is an embolic occlusion of the posterior temporal branch or inferior division of the left middle cerebral artery.

Anomic (Amnesic, Nominal) Aphasia

Some degree of word-finding and naming difficulty is observed in all forms of aphasia. Only when the patient's main deficit is in naming does the term *anomic aphasia* apply. Such patients have little receptive or expressive difficulty and can immediately repeat a spoken word, but they have lost the ability to name objects. There are also pauses in speech, groping for words, circumlocution, and the substitution of another word, phrase, or gesture which conveys the meaning.

Anomic aphasia has been associated with lesions in disparate parts of the language areas—deep in the basal portion of the posterior temporal lobe, in the frontal lobe, and in the angular gyrus. It may be a manifestation of early Alzheimer disease or of confusional states due to metabolic or infectious disease, in which instances it has no localizing value. Finally, anomic aphasia may be the only residual abnormality after recovery from Wernicke, conduction, or transcortical aphasia.

Dissociative Language Syndromes

This term denotes certain language disorders resulting not from lesions of the cortical language areas themselves but presumably from lesions that interrupt association pathways, thus separating primary receptive areas or the more strictly receptive parts of the language mechanisms from the motor ones (*conduction aphasia*) or the entire perisylvian language areas from other parts of the cerebral cortex (*transcortical aphasias*). (See Fig. 21-4)

Conduction aphasia In *conduction aphasia* (also called *central aphasia*), the patient comprehends spoken and written language but is unable to repeat what is heard; spontaneous speech is fluent but paraphasic. The Wernicke language area in the temporal lobe is said to be separated from the Broca area, probably by a lesion of the arcuate fasciculus, although such a discrete lesion has not been demonstrated pathologically.

Transcortical aphasias As a result of widespread anoxic damage or infarction, the intact motor-sensory language areas may be isolated from the surrounding cortex. In the *sensory type* of transcortical aphasia, information from the damaged (parietal-occipital) cortex cannot be transferred to the Wernicke area for conversion into verbal form. The disorder of language is much like that of Wernicke aphasia, except for the *remarkable preservation of repetition*. In extreme degree, this takes the form of echoing, parrot-like, words, phrases, and songs that are heard (*echolalia*). In transcortical motor aphasia (observed with partially recovered Broca aphasia and with abulic states due to frontal lobe damage) the patient, who spontaneously produces only a few grunts and syllables, can faultlessly repeat phrases that are heard or read, and even sentences of some length.

Several modality specific aphasias have also been classified as dissociative or disconnection syndromes. In *pure word mutism*, a syndrome that also goes by many other names, the patient loses all capacity to speak while retaining perfectly the ability to write, to understand spoken words, and to read silently with comprehension. This syndrome is probably closely related to what Mohr has called "small Broca's aphasia."

In *pure word deafness*, the patient can hear but cannot comprehend spoken language. Expressive speech remains normal. This disorder has been attributed to a lesion of the dominant temporal lobe, undercutting the Wernicke area and separating it from the Heschl gyri as well as from the contralateral auditory region (by interrupting fibers that cross in the corpus callosum).

Pure word blindness (visual verbal agnosia, alexia without agraphia) has been described in Chap. 21, with other commisural syndromes. *Pure agraphia* is a great rarity and its pathologic basis is uncertain.

DISORDERS OF ARTICULATION AND PHONATION

The act of speaking involves an intricate and highly coordinated sequence of contractions of the respiratory musculature, larynx, pharynx, palate, tongue, and lips. These structures are innervated by the phrenic, vagal, hypoglossal, and facial nerves; and the nuclei of these nerves are controlled by both motor cortices through the corticobulbar tracts. As with all motor activity, there are also extrapyramidal influences from the basal ganglia and cerebellum.

Phonation, or the production of vocal sounds, is a function of the larynx, more particularly of the vocal cords. The modulation of vocal sounds by contractions of the pharynx, palate, tongue, and lips constitutes *articulation*.

Dysarthria and Anarthria

With pure disorders of articulation (dysarthria or anarthria) language functions are intact. The only exception occurs with a restricted left frontal lesion and "small" Broca aphasia, in which there occurs, with recovery from mutism, a cortical aphasic dysarthria (see above). The latter is distinguished from nonaphasic (upper motor neuron) dysarthria by its variability and normalization in the pronunciation of automatic words and phrases. Defects in articulation are of several types, depending on the location of the causative lesion.

A. *Lower motor neuron dysarthria (atrophic bulbar paralysis):* Tongue weak and withered; difficulty speaking, vocalizing, swallowing; lingual (la-la-la) and labial (mi-mi-mi) consonants poorly enunciated. Usual cause: progressive bulbar palsy.

B. *Spastic and rigid dysarthria:* Upper motor neuron lesion with slow slurred speech, spastic masseters, and pseudobulbar palsy (see Chap. 3); dysphonia and dysphagia; no atrophy of tongue; hyperactive jaw jerk and facial reflexes. Usual causes: multiple strokes, amyotrophic lateral sclerosis.

In Parkinson disease and choreoathetotic disorders, speech is also affected in characteristic ways. In the former, speech is rapid, uninflected, and hypophonic. Choreoathetotic speech is slow, halting, uneven in volume, and accompanied by grimacing because of the superimposition of involuntary movements of the face, tongue, pharynx, and larynx upon voluntary movements.

C. *Ataxic dysarthria:* With cerebellar lesions, the speech is slow, slurred, scanning (unnatural separation of syllables), and of variable volume, syllables being uttered with lesser or greater (explosive) force than intended.

Defects in phonation With paralysis of both vocal cords, the patient can speak only in whispers. There may be an inspiratory stridor, due to failure of the vocal cords to separate during inspiration. Whispering speech is also a feature of advanced Parkinson disease, certain frontal lobe lesions, and stuporous states. With paralysis of only one vocal cord, the voice is low pitched and rasping and its range is reduced.

A restricted dystonia of bulbar muscles underlies the strained, effortful speech of so-called spastic dysphonia (see Chap. 4).

EXAMINATION OF SPEECH AND LANGUAGE

This begins with one's first encounter with the patient—by listening to his spontaneous utterances and engaging him in conversation. One takes note of his choice of words (an indication of the level of education); the volubility and fluency of his conversation or the lack of it; the inflection and melody of speech; and the speed of utterance and pressure of speech. The inability to construct ideas in well-connected sequences is readily evident, as is any tendency to grope for words, to make grammatical errors out of keeping with the level of education, and to interject paraphasias and neologisms. A failure to understand questions and to give correct answers immediately raises questions as to defective hearing and the presence of a receptive aphasia.

One must then explore the language mechanism more pointedly by asking the patient to do the following:

1. Name common and uncommon objects, parts of objects, and parts of the body.

2. Repeat words, phrases, and full sentences after the examiner.
3. Read passages from a book and perform written commands.
4. Carry out one-, two-, and three-part spoken commands.
5. Write from dictation and copy printed passages and geometric figures.

From these data one should be able to determine the nature of the speech disorder (dysphonia, dysarthria, or aphasia) and, if an aphasia exists, whether any one of the special language functions—speaking, writing, reading, understanding spoken words, repeating, and naming—is disproportionately affected.

Developmental language disorders are described in Chap. 27, on growth and development.

For a more detailed discussion of this topic, see Adams and Victor: *Principles of Neurology*, 4th ed, pp 377–395.

ADDITIONAL READING

Benson DF: *Aphasia, Alexia, and Agraphia*. New York, Churchill Livingstone, 1979.

Damasio AR, Damasio H: The anatomic basis of pure alexia. *Neurology* 33:1573, 1983.

Geschwind N: Disconnection syndromes in animals and man. *Brain* 88:237, 585, 1965.

Gloning K: Handedness and aphasia. *Neuropsychologia* 15:355, 1977.

Kertesz A: *Aphasia and Associated Disorders*. New York, Grune & Stratton, 1979.

Levine DN, Calvanio R: Conduction aphasia, in Kirshner HS, Freeman FR (eds): *The Neurology of Aphasia*. Lisse, Swets and Zeitlinger, 1982.

Mohr JP, Pessin MS, Finkelstein S, et al: Broca aphasia: Pathologic and clinical. *Neurology* 28:311, 1978.

Naesser MA, Alexander MP, Helm-Estabrook N, et al: Aphasia with predominantly subcortical lesion sites. *Arch Neurol* 39:2, 1982.

SECTION IV
ANXIETY AND DISORDERS OF ENERGY, MOOD, EMOTION, AND AUTONOMIC FUNCTIONS

23 Lassitude and Fatigue, Nervousness, Irritability, Anxiety, and Depression

These phenomena are more abstruse than the cognitive abnormalities described in the preceding chapters and, in their least complicated forms, represent only slight aberrations of normal reactions to all manner of medical and neurologic diseases. Yet they may be expressions of disturbed neurologic function and the forerunners of important medical or psychiatric diseases. Their proper place in the semiology of neuropsychiatry is difficult to judge. We have placed them in this section of the book, in relation to limbic, autonomic, and hypothalamic diseases, of which they are not infrequently a part.

USE OF TERMS

The phenomena under consideration, by their very vagueness, require that special care be taken in their definition. Patients, in their attempts to describe these phenomena, use many different terms with various degrees of imprecision; always the physician must determine what the patient means by these terms if he is to assess their seriousness intelligently.

Lassitude, fatigue, lack of energy, listlessness, and *languor* are more or less synonymous terms, referring to weariness or a loss of the sense of well being that is typical of persons who are healthy in mind and body. *Weakness* is clearly a separate phenomenon, denoting a diminished power and endurance of muscle contraction, and is more appropriately considered in relation to neuromuscular diseases (Chaps. 44 and 46). *Nervousness* is the vaguest of all the terms in this group. It may be used by the lay person to describe feelings of restlessness, tension, apprehension, and irritability or more serious psychiatric symptoms (obsessions, phobias, delusions, etc.) or even tics and tremors. *Anxiety* is defined as an intermittent or sustained emotional disturbance characterized by feelings of fear and apprehension, usually with a topical content and associated with signs of autonomic overactivity. *Depression* as a symptom simply refers to a state of sadness, dejection, hopelessness, and despair; frequently it is combined with anxiety. The wider implications of anxiety and depression are considered in Chaps. 53 and 54.

The foregoing phenomena are notable for their frequency and in the great majority of patients they come and leave without explanation. But at times they persist and aggrandize to the point where they demand medical attention. It is a mark of high medical competence to know whether they are more or less normal reactions or require further investigation and treatment. Their more advanced and obvious forms and the syndromes of which they are a part will be elaborated in Chaps. 53 and 54, under the headings of anxiety neurosis and various types of depressive illness.

LASSITUDE AND FATIGUE

Of all the symptoms in this group, these are the most frequent. More than half of all hospitalized patients register a direct complaint of fatigability or admit to it when questioned. Of course, patients have their own way of stating their complaints—"tired all the time," "exhausted," "pooped out," "no pep," etc. Often they speak of "weakness" when they mean fatigability. Indeed, the distinction between the two is not always easy. Loss of endurance and muscle aching may occur in a number of ill-defined muscle diseases, described in Chap. 52, even though the testing of maximum strength, or "peak power," shows them to be normal. Surprisingly, in a number of neuromuscular diseases which actually weaken muscles, fatigability is not a complaint.

In approaching this clinical problem, the physician begins with a survey of the patient's daily schedule. Long hours of sustained work—sometimes from necessity, at other times because of certain notions of duty—is one cause, but most individuals recognize this state and do not seek medical advice for it. Chronic infection and neoplasia (carcinomatosis or lymphomatosis) are other causes which must be sought medically. Physical fatigue may for a long time be the only manifestation of Epstein-Barr (EB) virus infection, brucellosis, viral hepatitis, Lyme disease, and tuberculosis. Less common diseases that should be sought in the patient with chronic fatigue are hypothyroidism, adrenal insufficiency, diabetes mellitus, and severe anemia.

However, the majority of patients (>90 percent) who complain of chronic fatigue will be found to suffer some type of psychiatric illness. Formerly the condition was called *neurasthenia*. Because it is so regularly associated with other symptoms such as irritability, insomnia, headaches, palpitation, trembling, feelings of hopelessness, etc., the condition has come to be recognized for what it is—anxiety neurosis or depression.

NERVOUSNESS, IRRITABILITY, ANXIETY, AND DEPRESSION

Like lassitude and fatigue, nervousness, irritability, anxiety, and depression are among the most common symptoms encountered in office and hospital practice. Virtually everyone has experienced some degree of these symptoms when faced with a threatening event, a challenging task for which one feels inadequate, or some overwhelming personal problem. They should then be viewed as natural and transient reactions to the vicissitudes of life. Only when they occur without explanation or are unduly severe and prolonged are they brought into medical focus.

These symptoms are more likely to occur at certain times in life than at others. Adolescence rarely passes without a period of turmoil, as the young attempt to emancipate themselves from parental dominance and adjust to scholastic demands, a work situation, or the opposite sex. The menses are regularly accompanied by increased tension and moodiness, a state that is given its own name ("premenstrual tension"). In the postpartum period it is exceptional for the new mother not to experience transient anxiety and depression ("postpartum blues"), possibly due to hyperprolactinemia. Menopause is another time when emotional stability may be threatened. The irritability and peevishness of the aged is an accepted fact of life.

These symptoms, even in their simplest form, reveal themselves in a number of behavioral changes. Headaches increase in frequency and sleep is disturbed. Often there is a mild somberness of mood, an increased tendency to tears and anger, a fatigue that bears no proper relationship to activity and rest, a tendency to sweat, tremble, to feel lightheaded, and to be aware of palpitations. Some of the more prominent autonomic effects can be evoked by hyperthyroidism and hyperadrenocorticism.

Many of these symptoms are but an accompaniment of a major medical problem and as such require no more than explanation and reassurance. When more severe, they are readily identifiable as components of chronic anxiety neurosis and panic attacks; and intense feelings of worry, sadness, and self-concern are shared with endogenous depression. These latter conditions are more fully described in Chaps. 53 and 54.

For a more detailed discussion of this topic, see Adams and Victor: *Principles of Neurology*, 4th ed, pp 399–408.

ADDITIONAL READING

Cassidy WL, Flanagan NB, Spellman M, Cohen ME: Clinical observations in manic depressive disease. *JAMA* 164:1535, 1953.

Holmes GP, Kaplan JE, Glantz NM, et al: Chronic fatigue syndrome. A working case definition. *Ann Intern Med* 108:387, 1988.

Lader M: The nature of clinical anxiety in modern society, in Spielberger CD, Sarason IG (eds): *Stress and Anxiety*, vol 1. New York, Halsted, 1975, pp 3–26.

Snaith RP, Taylor CM: Irritability: Definition, assessment, and associated factors. *Br J Psychiatry* 147:127, 1985.

Swartz MN: The chronic fatigue syndrome—one entity or many? *N Engl J Med* 319:1726, 1988.

Wheeler EO, White PD, Reed EW, Cohen ME: Neurocirculatory asthenia (anxiety neurosis, effort syndrome, neurasthenia). *JAMA* 142:878, 1950.

24 The Limbic Lobes and the Neurology of Emotion

In medical parlance, much license is taken with the terms *emotional problem* and *stress*, which are applied indiscriminately to states of anxiety and depression, strong reactions to distressing life events, so-called psychosomatic diseases, and many other symptoms for which a ready explanation is not available. To some physicians, the terms are synonymous with *functional disorders*, the implication being that function of the brain can change without there being a physical basis for it. Our objections to this idea are set forth in the introduction to the section on psychiatric diseases.

By *emotion* we mean a condition of the organism involving certain bodily changes (mainly visceral ones, under the control of the autonomic nervous system) in association with a mental state of excitement or perturbation and leading usually to an impulse to action or to a certain type of behavior. Happiness, love, hate, fear, and anger are examples of primary emotions; gloom, anxiety, and amiability are thought to represent lesser degrees of emotion. If emotion is intense, there may ensue a disturbance of intellectual functions, viz., a measure of disorganization of ideas and actions, and a tendency toward a more automatic behavior of ungraded, stereotyped character.

The cerebral mechanisms that control emotion are located in the limbic system. The latter comprises the medial parts of the temporal, frontal, and parietal lobes and their central connections with the amygdaloid nuclei, septal region, preoptic area, hypothalamus, anterior thalamus, habenula, and central midbrain tegmentum (Fig. 24-1). The peripheral effector apparatus is the autonomic nervous system and the visceral and other structures under its control.

Details of the anatomy and physiology of the limbic system will be found in the *Principles*.

NEUROLOGY OF EMOTIONAL DISTURBANCES

The most studied and best-known derangements of emotion are the following:

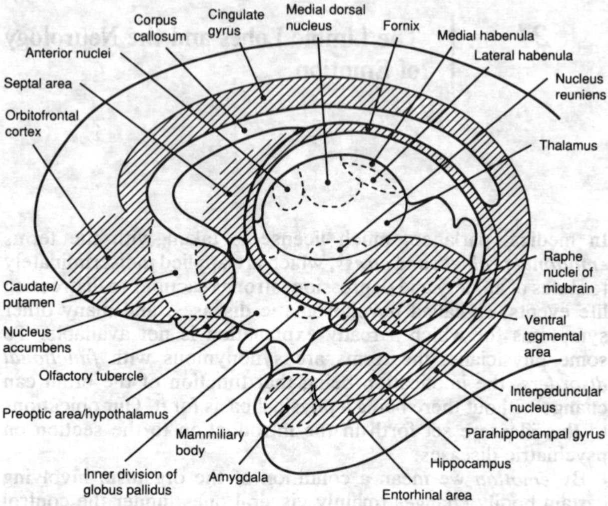

FIG. 24-1 Sagittal schematic of the limbic system. The location of the major limbic structures and the thalamus, hypothalamus, and midbrain tegmentum are shown. *(From Angevine and Cotman.)*

I. Disturbances of emotionality
  A. Due to perceptual abnormalities (illusions and hallucinations)
  B. Due to cognitive derangements (delusions)
II. Disinhibition of emotional expression
  A. Emotional lability
  B. Pathologic laughing and crying
III. Rage reactions and aggressivity
IV. Apathy and placidity
  A. Kluver-Bucy syndrome
  B. Other syndromes
V. Altered sexuality
VI. "Diencephalic" epilepsy
VII. Endogenous fear, anxiety, depression, and euphoria

EMOTIONAL LABILITY

The emotions of the infant and child are easily provoked and little inhibited. Their control is achieved gradually, through maturation of the brain and through learning and conditioning. To be "grown up" implies an ability to inhibit one's emotions; not that there is less feeling (affect) with maturation, but rather the outward expression of it is suppressed. The permissible display of emotion in adults varies between the sexes and in different cultures.

Any patient whose cerebrum has been extensively damaged by disease may lose fine emotional control. Tears come too easily; loud and prolonged laughter is evoked by mildly amusing remarks or happenings. Meeting an old friend or hearing the national anthem results in an embarrassing display of emotion. The response is more or less appropriate to the stimulus, and the affect is congruent with the visceral and motor components of emotional expression. The anatomic substrate is not known. To a slight degree the condition accompanies advanced age, but it is most prominent with diffuse degenerative and multifocal vascular lesions of the brain which do not lend themselves to clinicoanatomic correlation.

PATHOLOGIC (FORCED, SPASMODIC) LAUGHING AND CRYING

Here, as a consequence of cerebral disease, the patient is readily provoked to outbursts of uncontrollable laughter and crying, sometimes continuing to the point of exhaustion. In general, the reaction is consonant with the stimulus situation and the feeling or affect is appropriate, but often the relationships between stimulus, affect, and response are not evident. Characteristic of both pathologic laughter and crying is the invariability of the response and its excessive nature (the expression of mild degrees of pleasure or sadness is not possible). Clearly, the inhibition of the emotional mechanisms is enfeebled. All the facial, bulbar, respiratory, and visceral musculature, which provide the substrate of emotional expression and are normally under the control of centers in the lower brainstem, appear to be liberated from cerebral control. The condition is often a part of pseudobulbar palsy due to multiple vascular, demyelinative (multiple sclerosis), or motor system disease (amyotrophic lateral sclerosis) in which corticobulbar tracts are interrupted bilaterally. However, forced laughing and crying may be observed without discernible weakness of faciobulbar muscles, and vice versa.

In spasmodic laughing and crying and in emotionally labile states, imipramine or norpramine are often helpful in improving control.

AGGRESSIVITY, VIOLENCE, ANGER, AND RAGE

The control of these reactions is also achieved during the processes of maturation and "civilization." Raw emotion is sublimated into socially acceptable behavior patterns. Tantrums, uncontrollable rage reactions, violence, and aggressivity are turned into competitiveness in sports, scholastic activities, and boldness in business ventures. The rate at which this developmental sequence proceeds varies from one individual to another. In some, especially males, the process is not complete until 25 to 30 years of age, or even later, and until that time, the abnormal behavior is called sociopathic.

Individuals of this type, with little provocation, can change from a calm demeanor to a state of wild rage, with blindly furious impulse to violence and destruction. They appear out of contact with reality and are impervious to all argument and pleading. What is so obviously abnormal is the provocation of such behavior by some trifling event and a degree of reaction that is out of all proportion to the stimulus.

Rage reactions of this magnitude may be encountered in the following medical settings: (1) as part of a psychomotor seizure; (2) as a sociopathic disorder of obscure origin; or (3) as a manifestation of certain brain tumors or the aftermath of stroke or head injury. As many as 70 percent of the 410,000 patients suffering brain injury each year in the United States are left in an irritable, aggressive state. Alcoholism may be an aggravating factor. The location of the lesions in the few cases in which they have been identified is shown in Fig. 24-2.

In treatment, behavior modification techniques reduce violent outbursts in as many as 75 percent of cases. When violent behavior is secondary to psychotic ideation, antipsychotic drugs are the favored treatment. Some authors have reported success with propranolol.

PLACIDITY AND APATHY

A quantitative reduction in all psychomotor activity is the most common behavioral alteration in patients with cerebral disease. There are fewer thoughts, fewer words, and fewer movements per unit of time. That this is not a purely motor deficit is disclosed in conversation with the patient who shows a lack of ongoing psychic activity, a slowness in thinking, and a diminished perceptivity, inquisitiveness, and interest in his surroundings. Depending on how one views this state, there is a heightened threshold to stimulation, reduced attentiveness, an inability to focus the mind and maintain an alert attitude, a lack of drive or impulse (abulia), and apathy.

By collating the data of several neurologists, Poeck has charted the lesions associated with a state of placidity and apathy (Fig. 24-2).

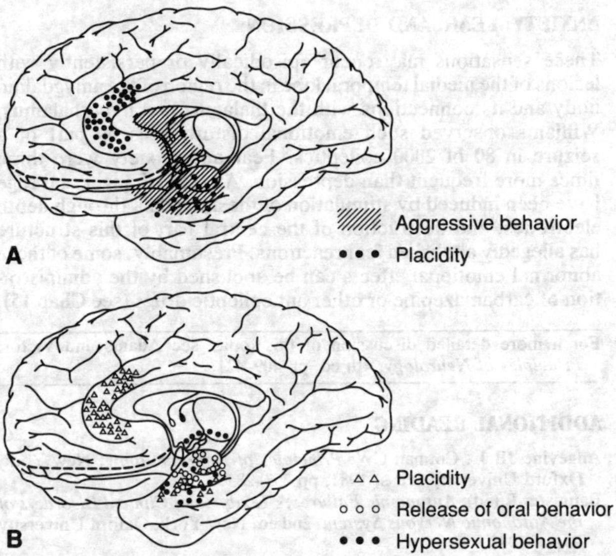

FIG. 24-2 *A.* Localization of lesions which, in humans, can lead to aggressive behavior and placidity. *B.* Localization of lesions which, in humans, can lead to placidity, release of oral behavior, and hypersexuality. *(From Poeck.)*

ALTERED SEXUALITY

The normal pattern of sexual behavior may be altered with diseases of the limbic system. Lesions of the orbital parts of the frontal lobes may remove moral-ethical restraints with indiscriminate hypersexuality. With superior prefrontal lesions, abulia and lack of impulse reduce sexual as well as other functions. We have observed an occasional case of marked hypersexuality in male and female patients with encephalitis and temporal lobe tumor, but the exact anatomy of the lesions was not ascertained. Stimulation of the ventral septal area has evoked sensations of pleasure and lust, and sexual arousal has been reported with psychomotor seizures arising from medial temporal foci. Hyposexuality and diminished libido are common manifestations of depressive illness. Most temporal lobe epileptics prove to be hyposexual.

ANXIETY, FEAR, AND DEPRESSION

These sensations may occur episodically or persistently with lesions of the medial temporal lobe in the region of the amygdaloid body and its connections with the thalamus and hypothalamus. Williams observed such emotional disturbances as part of a seizure in 80 of 2000 epileptics. Fear and anxiety were three times more frequent than depression. Attacks of anger and rage have been induced by stimulation of the amygdala through depth electrodes, and destruction of the central part of this structure has allegedly abolished fear reactions. Presumably, some of these abnormal emotional effects can be abolished by the administration of carbamazepine or other antiepileptic drugs (see Chap 15).

For a more detailed discussion of this topic, see Adams and Victor: *Principles of Neurology*, 4th ed, pp 409–421.

ADDITIONAL READING

Angevine JB Jr, Cotman CW: *Principles of Neuroanatomy*. New York, Oxford University Press, 1981, pp 253–283.

Bannister R (ed): *Autonomic Failure: A Textbook of Clinical Disorders of the Autonomic Nervous System*, 2nd ed. New York, Oxford University Press, 1988.

Geschwind N: The clinical setting of aggression in temporal lobe epilepsy, in Field WS, Sweet WH (eds): *The Neurobiology of Violence*, St. Louis, Warren H. Green, 1975.

Panksepp J: Mood changes, in Vinken PJ, Bruyn GW, Klawans HL (eds): *Handbook of Clinical Neurology*, vol 45. Amsterdam, North-Holland, 1985, chap. 21, pp 271–285.

Poeck K: Pathophysiology of emotional disorders associated with brain damage, in Vinken PJ, Bruyn GW (eds): *Handbook of Clinical Neurology*, vol 3. *Disorders of Higher Nervous Activity*. Amsterdam, North-Holland, 1969, chap. 20, pp 343–367.

Poeck K: Pathological laughter and crying, in Vinken PJ, Bruyn GW, Klawans HV (eds): *Handbook of Clinical Neurology*, vol 45. Amsterdam, North-Holland, 1985, chap. 16, pp 219–225.

25 Disorders of the Autonomic Nervous System

The visceral and homeostatic functions of the human organism, which are essential to life and survival of the species, are involuntary and under the control of the autonomic nervous system, acting in unison with the endocrine glands.

The autonomic nervous system consists of two parts: a craniosacral (parasympathetic) outflow and a thoracolumbar (sympathetic) one. The cerebral control of these two systems resides in the hypothalamus. These features are illustrated in Figs. 25-1 and 25-2. The outflow of sympathetic fibers from the spinal cord and their distribution are illustrated in Fig. 25-3. The anatomic details are described in the *Principles*.

The diseases that affect the autonomic nervous system will be summarized in this chapter, and those of the hypothalamus in Chap. 26.

TESTS FOR ABNORMALITIES OF THE AUTONOMIC NERVOUS SYSTEM

These tests are outlined in Table 25-1. The use of the simpler ones (the noninvasive bedside tests and the tests of pupillary innervation) coupled with clinical inquiry and examination permit the diagnosis of the following disorders.

Complete Autonomic Paralysis (Dysautonomic Polyneuropathy)

This is a relatively rare type of polyneuropathy characterized by the almost exclusive affection of sympathetic and parasympathetic postganglionic fibers. The condition occurs sporadically in adults and children and is thought to represent an autoimmune reaction similar to that of the Guillain-Barré syndrome. In a few cases it has been linked in some way to the Epstein-Barr virus.

Clinically, over a period of a week or a few weeks, the patient develops anhidrosis, orthostatic hypotension, paralysis of pupillary reflexes, impaired bladder and bowel function, gastric anacidity, and loss of lacrimation, salivation, and pilomotor and vasomotor reflexes in the skin. Somatic sensory and motor functions and tendon reflexes are preserved. The CSF protein is normal or elevated.

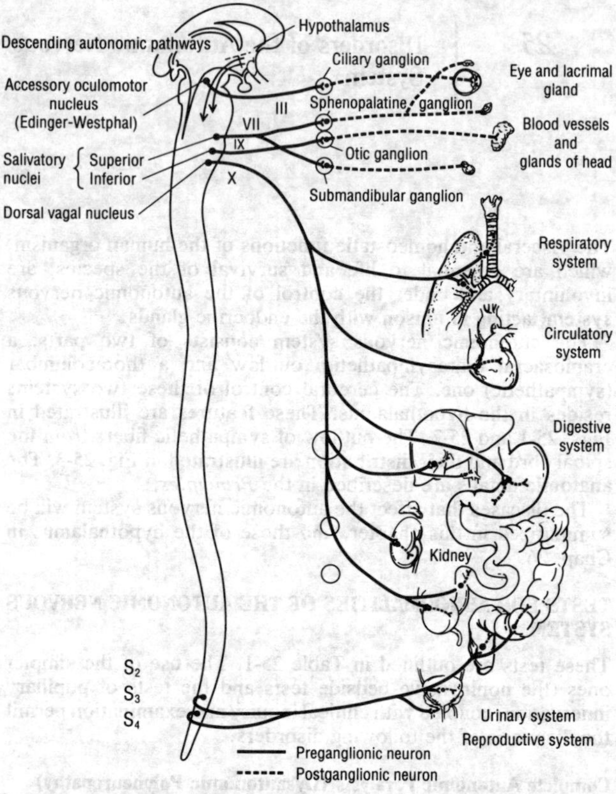

FIG. 25-1 The parasympathetic (craniosacral) division of the autonomic nervous system. Preganglionic fibers extend from nuclei of the brainstem and sacral segments of the spinal cord to peripheral ganglia. Short postganglionic fibers extend from the ganglia to the effector organs. The lateral-posterior hypothalamus is part of the supranuclear mechanism for the regulation of parasympathetic activities. The frontal and limbic parts of the supranuclear regulatory apparatus are not indicated in the diagram (see text). *(From CL Noback, R Demarest, The Human Nervous System, 3rd ed, New York, McGraw-Hill, 1981.)*

Recovery has occurred in all cases, so that the pathology is not known. Corticosteroid therapy may hasten recovery.

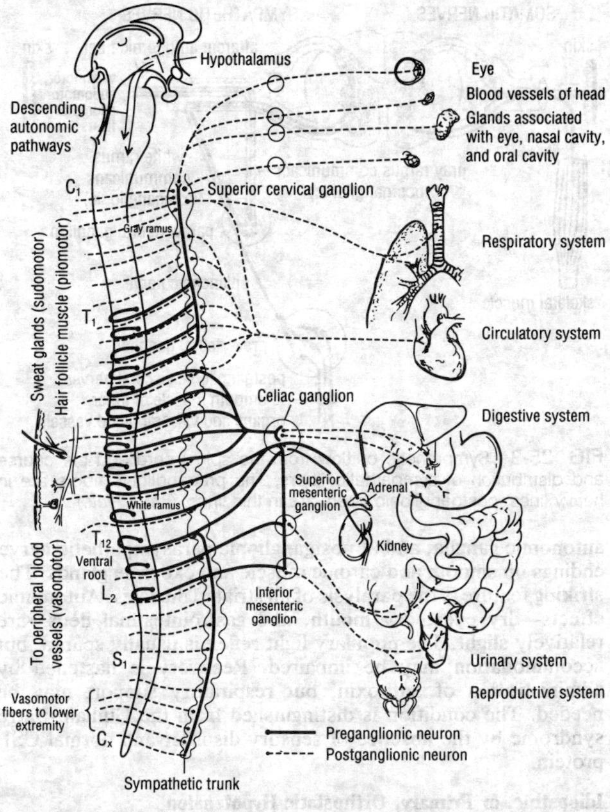

FIG. 25-2 The sympathetic (thoracolumbar) division of the autonomic nervous system. Preganglionic fibers extend from the intermediolateral nucleus of the spinal cord to the peripheral autonomic ganglia, and postganglionic fibers extend from the peripheral ganglia to the effector organs, according to the scheme in Fig. 25-3. *(From CL Noback, R Demarest, The Human Nervous System, 3rd ed, New York, McGraw-Hill, 1981.)*

Botulism

The clostridial toxin blocks the release of acetylcholine from presynaptic vesicles at the motor end plates, at synapses in all

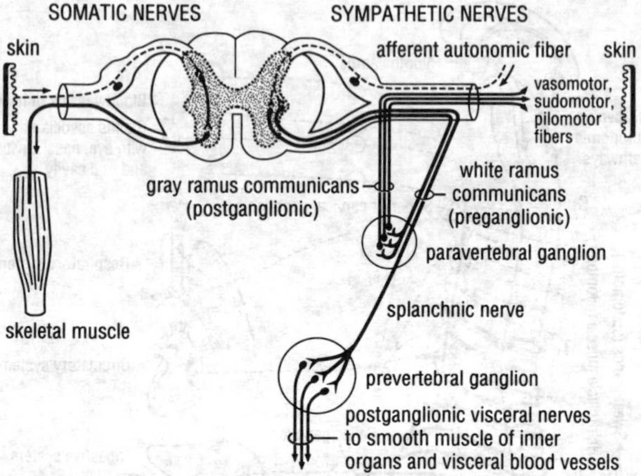

FIG. 25-3 Sympathetic outflow from the spinal cord and the course and distribution of sympathetic fibers. The preganglionic fibers are in heavy lines; postganglionic fibers are in thin lines. *(From Pick.)*

autonomic ganglia, and at postganglionic parasympathetic nerve endings on smooth and cardiac muscle and exocrine glands. The striking feature is the paralysis of all striated muscles. Autonomic effects—dry eyes, dry mouth, and gastrointestinal ileus—are relatively slight. The pupillary light reflex is usually spared, but accommodation may be impaired. Recovery is hastened by administration of antitoxin, but respiratory support may be needed. The condition is distinguished from the Guillain-Barré syndrome by the absence of sensory disorder and normal CSF protein.

Idiopathic, or Primary, Orthostatic Hypotension

Because of a failure of constriction of capacitance vessels in the lower extremities upon standing, venous return and cardiac output are diminished and blood pressure falls precipitously, often with syncope (see Chap. 17). Corrective vasomotor reflexes are incompetent and plasma catecholamine and renin fail to rise.

Two types of primary orthostatic hypotension have been identified:

1. The first type is believed to involve mainly the postganglionic sympathetic fibers, with sparing of the parasympathetic, somatosensory, and motor fibers. Orthostatic hypotension develops gradually, more often in middle-aged women. Cases are sporadic and the cause unknown.

2. The second type involves mainly the preganglionic neurons that originate in the spinal cord and may develop in conjunction with or be followed by Parkinson disease or striatonigral or pontocerebellar degeneration ("multisystem atrophy").

Anhidrosis, impotence, and atonicity of the bladder are common to both syndromes. The two types can be distinguished pharmacologically. In the peripheral postganglionic type, resting plasma norepinephrine levels are subnormal and fail to rise on standing; also denervation hypersensitivity to injected norepinephrine can be demonstrated. In the central preganglionic type, plasma norepinephrine levels also fail to rise on standing, but resting levels are normal, as is the sensitivity to administered norepinephrine.

Treatment follows along the lines indicated in Chap. 17.

Secondary Orthostatic Hypertension

In several types of polyneuropathy—diabetic, Guillain-Barré, chronic inflammatory, infectious mononucleosis, porphyric, alcoholic-nutritional—the autonomic fibers may be damaged and some of the symptoms of disordered autonomic function (impotence, anhidrosis or hyperhidrosis, atonic bladder, diarrhea or constipation, orthostatic hypotension) are then added to the more common neuropathic picture (see Chap. 44).

Riley-Day Syndrome

This is a familial disease of the autonomic nervous system, inherited as an autosomal recessive trait and observed mainly in Jewish infants and children. Postural hypotension, impaired temperature regulation, hyperhidrosis, insensitivity to pain, and denervation sensitivity of the pupils are the main clinical features. This disorder is described further in Chap. 44, with the inherited neuropathies.

PARTIAL OR RESTRICTED AUTONOMIC SYNDROMES

Horner and Stellate Ganglion Syndromes

The features of the Horner (Bernard-Horner) syndrome have been listed in Table 13-2. A lesion that involves the lateral medulla, the T2 spinal root, and the superior cervical or the postganglionic fibers that course along the carotid artery result in a Horner syndrome. A lesion of the inferior cervical (stellate) ganglion produces a Horner syndrome in combination with a paralysis of sympathetic reflexes in the arm (hand and arm are dry and warm)—*the stellate ganglion syndrome*. The latter may

TABLE 25-1 Clinical Tests of Autonomic Function

Test	Normal response	Part of reflex arc tested
	Noninvasive bedside tests	
Blood pressure response to standing or vertical tilt	Fall in BP ≧30/15 mmHg	Afferent and efferent limbs
Heart rate response to standing	Increase 11–29 beats per minute; 30:15 ratio ≧ 1.04	Afferent and efferent limbs
Isometric exercise	Increase in diastolic BP, 15 mmHg	Sympathetic efferent limb
Heart rate variation with respiration	Maximum-minimum heart rate ≧ 15 beats per minute; Expiration-inspiration ratio ≧ 1.2*	Vagal afferent and efferent limbs
Valsalva ratio	≧ 1.4*	Afferent and efferent limbs
Sweat tests	Sweating over all body and limbs	Sympathetic efferent limb
Axon reflex	Local piloerection, sweating	Postganglionic sympathetic efferent fibers
Plasma noradrenaline level	Rises on tilting from horizontal to vertical	Sympathetic efferent limb
Plasma vasopressin level	Rise with induced hypotension	Afferent limb
	Invasive tests	
Valsalva maneuver	Phase I: Rise in BP Phase II: Gradual reduction of BP to plateau; tachycardia Phase III: Fall in BP Phase IV: Overshoot of BP, bradycardia*	Afferent and efferent limbs

Baroreflex sensitivity	1. Slowing of heart rate with induced rise of BP* 2. Steady state responses to induced rise and fall of BP	1. Parasympathetic afferent and efferent limbs 2. Afferent and efferent limbs
Infusion of pressor drugs	1. Rise in BP 2. Slowing of heart rate	1. Adrenergic receptors 2. Afferent and efferent parasympathetic limbs
	Other tests of vasomotor control	
Radiant heating of trunk	Increased hand blood flow	Sympathetic efferent limb
Immersion of hand in hot water	Increased blood flow of opposite hand	Sympathetic efferent limb
Cold pressor test	Reduced blood flow	Sympathetic efferent limb
Emotional stress	Increased BP	Sympathetic efferent limb
	Tests of pupiliary innervation	
4% Cocaine	Pupil dilates	Sympathetic innervation
0.1% Adrenaline	No response	Postganglionic sympathetic innervation
1% Hydroxyamphetamine hydrobromide	Pupil dilates	Postganglionic sympathetic innervation
2.5% Methacholine, 0.125% pilocarpine	No response	Parasympathetic innervation

Note: BP = blood pressure.
* Age-dependent response.
Source: McLeod and Tuck.

involve the terminations of preganglionic fibers or the ganglion cells (postganglionic) or both. If the lesion is mainly postganglionic, denervation hypersensitivity to norepinephrine can be demonstrated. Trauma, tumor invasion, radiation injury, and subclavian aneurysm are the usual causes.

Approximately two-thirds of cases of oculosympathetic paralysis are due to brainstem strokes or other brainstem lesions (Keane). About 20 percent are preganglionic, due mainly to trauma or tumors of the neck and upper thorax, and a lesser number are postganglionic, due to a variety of causes (see Table 13-2).

Sympathetic and Parasympathetic Paralysis in Tetraplegia and Paraplegia

Complete lesions at the level of C4 or C5 or upper thoracic segments of the cord interrupt all suprasegmental control mechanisms of the spinal sympathetic and parasympathetic nervous system. Lower thoracic lesions affect mainly the sacral sympathetic outflow. Hypotension, loss of sweating and piloerection, gastric dilatation, paralytic ileus, and paralysis of bladder are the initial effects. Plasma adrenalin and noradrenalin are reduced. This state has a time course similar to that of spinal shock. Dissipation of the latter is followed by hyperactivity of autonomic reflexes and automatic bladder function (see Chap. 34).

Raynaud Phenomenon

Painful blanching of the fingers with emotional stress or exposure to cold is the main feature. In many cases, no cause can be discerned, but other ("secondary" cases) are due to partial obstruction of the brachial circulation, as occurs with cervical rib or thoracic outlet syndrome or with repeated trauma to the hands, as in sculling or use of a jackhammer. Prostaglandins have had a satisfactory therapeutic effect in some cases.

Disturbances of Bladder and Bowel Function

The storage and intermittent evacuation of urine are served by three components of the bladder: the large detrusor (smooth) muscle, which is the bladder itself; the closely related internal sphincter, and the external sphincter, which is composed of striated muscle (as is the anal sphincter). Afferent and efferent innervation of these structures is provided through the pudendal nerves and sacral segments 2, 3 and 4. These segments give rise to preganglionic fibers, which synapse in the parasympathetic ganglia in the bladder wall. The hypogastric plexus, derived from

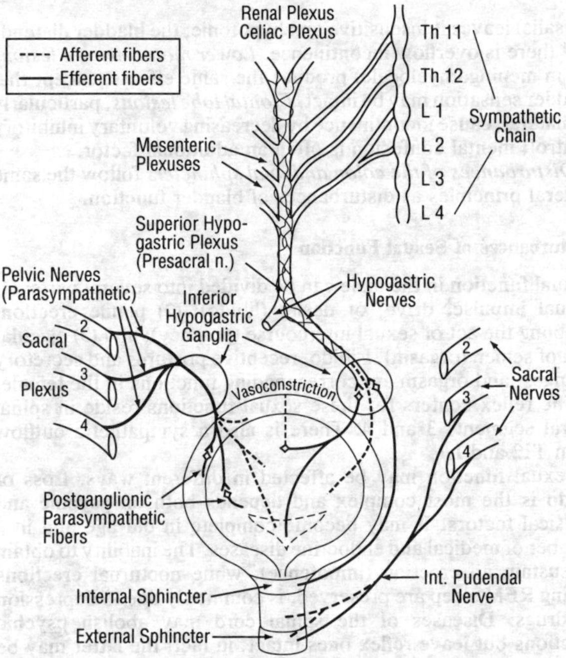

FIG. 25-4 Innervation of the urinary bladder and its sphincters.

T10, T11 and T12 segments, supplies sympathetic nerves to the dome of the bladder. The innervation of the bladder and its sphincters are illustrated in Fig. 25-4.

Suprasegmental control of the sacral segments comes from the pontomesencephalic tegmentum via reticulospinal tracts, which are both facilitatory and inhibitory, and from the motor cortex via tracts that descend in apposition to the corticospinal tracts and are inhibitory.

Acute lesions of the spinal cord at levels above the sacral segments cause spinal shock, inhibiting detrusor function and resulting in urinary retention with overflow incontinence. As spasticity of the legs gradually supervenes, the detrusor also becomes "spastic" (overactive); the detrusor cannot be inhibited, and the patient is intermittently incontinent as the bladder empties automatically. *Deafferentation* of the bladder (as in tabes dorsalis) leaves it insensitive and hypotonic; the bladder distends and there is overflow incontinence. *Lower motor neuron lesions* (as in meningomyelocele) produce the same effects, except that bladder sensation may be intact. *Frontal lobe lesions,* particularly if bilateral, cause incontinence by decreasing voluntary inhibitory control; mental confusion is often an additional factor.

Disturbances of the colon and anal sphincters follow the same general principles as disturbances of bladder function.

Disturbances of Sexual Function

Sexual function in the male can be divided into several parts: (1) sexual impulse, drive, or desire (libido): (2) penile erection, enabling the act of sexual intercourse (potency); and (3) ejaculation of semen (orgasm). Libido, receptive postures and secretory changes, and orgasm are corresponding functions in the female.

The reflex centers for these sexual functions reside in spinal sacral segments 3 and 4. There is also a sympathetic outflow from T12 and L1.

Sexual function may be affected in different ways. Loss of libido is the most complex and depends both on psychic and physical factors. It may become complete in old age and in a number of medical and endocrine diseases. The inability to obtain or sustain an erection (impotence), while nocturnal erections during REM sleep are preserved, is commonly due to depression or drugs. Diseases of the spinal cord may abolish psychic erections but leave reflex ones intact; in fact; the latter may be overactive and painful (priapism). Destructive lesions of the sacral segments and nerves (nervi erigentes and pudendal nerves) may abolish all genital sensation and response.

Loss of libido and inability to attain orgasm are more frequent in women than in men, especially in neurotic personalities. Fecundity and infertility are usually unrelated to the other aspects of sexuality.

For a more detailed discussion of this topic, see Adams and Victor: *Principles of Neurology*, 4th ed, pp 422–444.

ADDITIONAL READING

Appenzeller O: *Clinical Autonomic Failure: Practical Concepts*, Amsterdam, Elsevier, 1986.

Bannister R (ed): *Autonomic Failure: A Textbook of Clinical Disorders of the Autonomic Nervous System*, 2nd ed. New York, Oxford University Press, 1988.

Blaivas JG: The neurophysiology of micturition: A clinical study of 550 patients. *J Urol* 127:958, 1982.

Cohen J, Low P, Fealey R, et al: Somatic and autonomic function in progressive autonomic failure and multiple system atrophy. *Ann Neurol* 22:692, 1987.

Keane JR: Oculosympathetic paresis: Analysis of 100 hospitalized patients. *Arch Neurol* 36:13, 1979.

Low PA, Dyck PJ, Lambert EH: Acute panautonomic neuropathy. *Ann Neurol* 13:412, 1983.

McLeod JG, Tuck RR: Disorders of the autonomic nervous system. Part I. Pathophysiology and clinical features. Part II. Investigation and treatment. *Ann Neurol* 21:419, 519, 1987.

Pick J: *The Autonomic Nervous System*. Philadelphia, Lippincott, 1970.

Young RR, Asbury AK, Corbett JL, Adams RD: Pure pandysautonomia with recovery: Description and discussion of diagnostic criteria. *Brain* 98:613, 1975.

26 The Hypothalamus and Neuroendocrine Disorders

As was remarked in Chap. 25, the hypothalamus functions as the "head ganglion" of both the autonomic nervous system and the endocrine system, and the activity of the two is closely integrated. The hypothalamic nuclei release neurotransmitter peptides, which modulate neuronal activity in other parts of the nervous system and also the glandular cells of the anterior hypophysis. These neurotransmitters, of relatively recent discovery, are called hypophysiotropic hormones or hypothalamic releasing factors.

The nuclei of the hypothalamus, to which reference will be made in the text, are conventionally divided into three groups: the anterior group, including the supraoptic and paraventricular nuclei; the middle group, including the tuberal, arcuate, ventromedial, and dorsomedial nuclei; and the posterior group, including the mammillary and posterior hypothalamic nuclei. The anatomic relationships of these small aggregates of neurons, which lie between the thalamus and optic chiasm, are illustrated in Fig. 26-1. From the downward-bulging inferior surface of the hypothalamus (tuber cinereum) emerges the median eminence or infundibulum. The latter extends into the pituitary stalk, which contains the axonal fiber system connecting the anterior hypothalamus with the posterior lobe of the pituitary body (the pars nervosa or neurohypophysis). Coursing over the surface of the infundibulum is the hypophysial-portal system of veins, which convey releasing factors to the glandular or adenohypophysial cells.

HYPOTHALAMIC-PITUITARY DISEASES

Diabetes Insipidus

Diabetes insipidus (DI), the best known of the hypothalamic syndromes, is characterized by polyuria (the excretion of large quantities of low osmolar urine) and polydipsia (increased thirst and drinking of water). It is caused by lesions that prevent granules of *vasopressin* (antidiuretic hormone, or ADH), which are formed in the cells of the supraoptic and paraventricular nuclei, from being transported and released into the posterior lobe of the pituitary body, from which it is normally transferred into the blood stream and carried to the renal tubules. The cells

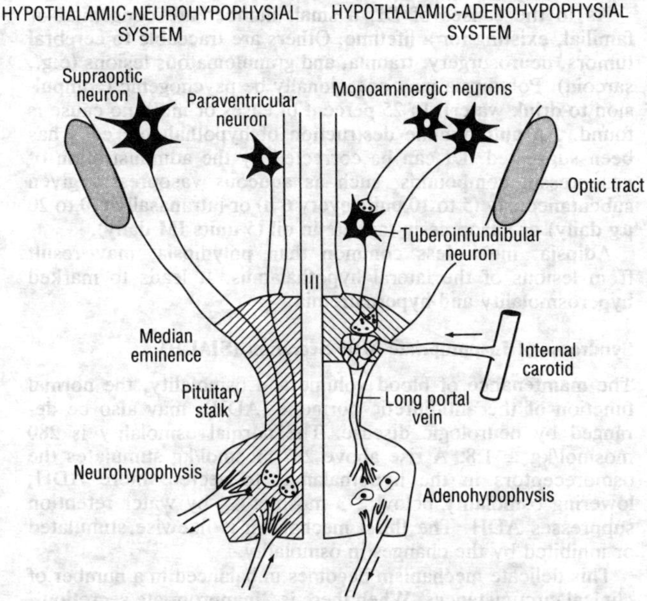

Fig. 26-1 Diagram of the hypothalamic-pituitary axis. Indicated on the left is the hypothalamic-neurohypophysial system consisting of supraoptic and paraventricular neurons, axons of which terminate on blood vessels in the posterior pituitary (neurohypophysis). The hypothalamic-adenohypophysial system is illustrated on the right. Tuberoinfundibular neurons, believed to be the source of the hypothalamic regulatory hormones, terminate on the capillary plexus in the median eminence. *(Courtesy of Dr. JB Martin.)*

of these nuclei also elaborate oxytocin, the principal hormonal stimulant to lactation and uterine contraction. The renal tubule cells control the amount of water that is excreted, and a congenital abnormality or destruction of the tubular cells (nephrogenic DI) has the same effect as a hypothalamic lesion.

The diagnosis of DI is suggested by the presence of polyuria (urine specific gravity of <1.005 even under conditions of fluid restriction) and polydipsia (drinking >3000 mL of fluid daily). Proof that the patient has DI and is not a compulsive water drinker is obtained by the injection of 5 pressor units of pitressin subcutaneously, which will diminish urine output and increase the osmolality of blood and urine.

As to the causes of DI, a small number are congenital or familial, existing for a lifetime. Others are traceable to cerebral tumors, neurosurgery, trauma, and granulomatous lesions (e.g., sarcoid). Polydipsia may occasionally be psychogenic (compulsion to drink water). In 25 percent of cases or more no cause is found. An autoimmune destruction of hypothalamic cells has been suggested. DI can be corrected by the administration of vasopressin compounds, such as aqueous vasopressin given subcutaneously (5 to 10 units every 6 h) or intranasally (10 to 20 μg daily) or vasopressin tannate in oil (5 units IM daily).

Adipsia, much less common than polydipsia, may result from lesions of the lateral hypothalamus. It leads to marked hyperosmolality and hypernatremia.

Syndrome of Inappropriate ADH Secretion (SIADH)

The maintenance of blood volume and osmolality, the normal function of the antidiuretic hormone (ADH), may also be deranged by neurologic disease. The normal osmolality is 280 mosmol/kg ± 1.8. A rise above 287 mosmol/kg stimulates the osmoreceptors in the hypothalamus to secrete more ADH; lowering osmolality below 273 mosmol/Kg by water retention suppresses ADH. The thirst mechanism is likewise stimulated or inhibited by the changes in osmolality.

This delicate mechanism becomes unbalanced in a number of clinical circumstances. When there is "inappropriate secretion" or ectopic production of ADH, blood volume rises and serum osmolality falls. Sodium levels fall with hypo-osmolality. If below 120 meq/L, hyponatremia poses a danger and should be corrected carefully (see Chap. 38). Merely reducing water intake to 400 to 600 mL/day is adequate for counteracting milder degrees of hyponatremia. The usual causes are lung tumors (ectopic ADH production), certain drugs (carbamazepine, chlorthiazide, chlorpromazine, vincristine), and a variety of acute intracranial diseases, not necessarily ones that affect the hypothalamus directly.

A salt-wasting syndrome, which may be mistaken for SIADH, causes a reduction in serum sodium and of plasma volume. It may occur with a number of different intracranial diseases. The distinction from SIADH is important because treatment consists of the administration of an increased amount of intravenous fluid and not of fluid restriction.

Other Hypothalamic Syndromes

Precocious puberty This disorder in males or females always prompts a neurologic and endocrinologic investigation. In males, the most frequent cause is a teratoma of the pineal gland (Chap. 29). In females, one should anticipate an estrogen-secreting tumor or hypothalamic hamartoma (i.e., a tumor-like collection of cells due to a developmental abnormality). The latter is often associated with neurofibromatosis or polyostotic fibrous dysplasia. Diagnosis is greatly facilitated by CT scanning and MRI.

Adiposogenital dystrophy (Froelich syndrome) This consists of obesity, growth retardation, and delayed sexual development. The nuclei in the medial part of the hypothalamus (tuberal nuclei) fail to stimulate the adenohypophysis to produce growth hormone (GH) and FSH. The usual causes are craniopharyngioma (suprasellar cyst), pituitary adenoma, cholesteatoma, and other rare tumors.

Abnormalities of growth A deficiency of growth hormone-releasing factor and therefore of GH may cause growth retardation. Or it may be caused by an inherently inactive GH molecule, in which case plasma levels of GH are actually high, as in dwarfism. Growth retardation may occur as a separate entity or in association with other hypothalamic defects (e.g., Froelich syndrome). The opposite may occur—gigantism—if an excess of GH is produced in childhood or adolescence. This has been reported with pituitary tumors and hypothalamic gangliocytomas.

Disturbances of regulation of temperature, appetite, and sleep Lesions of the posterior part of the hypothalamus result in hypothermia or poikilothermia and those of the anterior hypothalamus, in hyperthermia.

The hypothalamus also plays an important role in the regulation of appetite. However, extreme obesity or anorexia and aphagia with inanition have seldom been traced to lesions of the hypothalamus.

Sleep disturbances, usually hypersomnia, occur with lesions at the junction of the posterior hypothalamus and the midbrain.

For a more detailed discussion of this topic, see Adams and Victor: *Principles of Neurology*, 4th ed, pp 445–454.

ADDITIONAL READING

Breningstall, GN: Gelastic seizures, precocious puberty and hypothalamic hamartoma. *Neurology* 35:1180, 1985.

Martin JB, Reichlin S: *Clinical Neuroendocrinology*, 2nd ed. Philadelphia, Davis, 1987.

Stunkard AJ, Sorensen TIA, Hanis C, et al: An adoption study of human obesity. *N Engl J Med* 314:193, 1986.

III GROWTH AND DEVELOPMENT OF THE NERVOUS SYSTEM AND THE NEUROLOGY OF AGING

27 Development of the Nervous System and the Neurology of Aging

Disease must always be judged by comparing the patient to standards of normalcy. Only when a given function falls outside the range of natural individual variation does it become pathologic. This poses a problem for the neurologist because at each period up to adulthood, as maturation and development proceed, the standards change. The changes are most marked during embryonic and fetal life, but they continue at a rapid rate during infancy and early childhood and are not completed until late adolescence. Senescence—the process of growing old—proceeds for even a longer period, provided it is not interrupted by disease. Thus, for more than half the average life span, the standards of normal neurologic functioning are in inclination or declination. What is normal at one age is abnormal at another.

In order to evaluate intelligently the status of the nervous system, the neurologist must learn and fix in mind the normal standards of nervous functioning for every epoch of life. This is especially difficult in infancy and early childhood. Indeed, in these age periods, failures in attaining certain milestones of motility, language, and general behavior are far more useful indicators than the conventional signs of neurologic disease. Also, the neurologist must know which diseases are more likely and which are less likely to appear at any given age.

NORMAL AND ABNORMAL DEVELOPMENT OF THE NERVOUS SYSTEM

In the normal neonatal, infantile, and childhood periods (defined in Table 27-1), neurologic functions emerge in a reasonably predictable sequence. By examining large numbers of normal infants, pediatric neurologists and psychologists have been able to construct a statistically valid developmental timetable with due allowances for individual variations. By comparing the patient's age at the time of attainment of certain behaviors with the standard performance at his or her chronological age, one can derive a developmental quotient. Of course, due allowance must be made for the effects of intercurrent illness and social neglect. The main milestones are itemized in Tables 27-2 and 27-3.

TABLE 27-1 Time Scale of Stages in Human Growth and Development

Growth period	Approximate age
Prenatal	From 0 to 280 days
Ovum	From 0 to 14 days
Embryo	From 14 days to 9 weeks
Fetus	From 9 weeks to birth
Premature infant	From 27 to 37 weeks
Birth	Average 280 days
Neonate	First 4 weeks after birth
Infancy	First year
Early childhood (preschool)	From 1 to 6 years
Later childhood (prepubertal)	From 6 to 10 years
Adolescence	Girls, 8 or 10 to 18 years; boys, 10 or 12 to 20 years
Puberty (average)	Girls, 13 years; boys, 15 years

Source: Lowrey.

Exogenous and endogenous agents may have adverse effects on the nervous system long before birth. One can judge the time of their occurrence and to some extent the nature of the intrauterine diseases only after birth by comparing the physical findings and functional capacities with normal standards of brainstem and spinal reflexes for the neonate. Some knowledge of embryology helps in this regard—recognition of the stage at which development was arrested indicates the point at which the disease struck. Table 27-4 indicates the timing of major morphologic changes in the nervous system of the developing fetus and forms the basis of *teratology* (the science of congenital malformations).

The adaptations required of the fetus are most demanding during the parturitional period, when it is suddenly thrust into the outside world and forced to exist independently. At this time the brain is subjected to unusual forces as it passes through the birth canal. Once the umbilical cord is severed, the heart must circulate adequate quantities of oxygenated blood. This may prove to be inadequate, most often because of prematurity and sometimes because of failure of closure of the foramen ovale or ductus arteriosus, and the brain suffers irreversible hypoxic-ischemic damage. Later, such infants are observed to manifest cerebral palsy and mental retardation.

Departures from normal development take the form of either (1) a slowness or an arrest of development or (2) a regression from a functional level that had been achieved earlier. The former is an expression of a developmental failure of genetic type or the result of a nonprogressive disease. The latter, i.e., regression after a period of normal development, stands as the most reliable indicator of an ongoing disease process. The only exceptions to this principle are those cases in which injury or disease strikes at a time when the nervous system is insufficiently developed to manifest neurologic signs. At such a time, examination may disclose no abnormalities; the latter appear only at a later stage of development, when the injured structures are needed for normal functions. A congenital hemiplegia, for example, will usually not be evident until 5 to 6 months of age, when the corticospinal tract has become sufficiently myelinated and functional. This point is discussed further in Chap. 42.

RESTRICTIVE OR SELECTIVE DEVELOPMENTAL DISORDERS

A large number of abnormalities appear in the course of acquisition of speech and language, in learning ability and scholastic achievement, and in behavior and social adaptation. A single complex function is retarded in its development, and except for this one abnormality, the rest of the nervous system may be functioning normally. Since these special disorders can also be influenced by the patient's social and cultural surroundings, there is an ongoing controversy about the relative importance of purely genetic and environmental factors ("nature versus nurture"). Both are important, but the genetic aspect dominates current thinking on this subject.

Disorders of Speech and Language

The acquisition of speech and language begins in the first months of postnatal life with babbling and lalling and progresses successively through the stages of articulated words, phrases, and sentences, to reading and writing, enlargement of vocabulary, and knowledge of grammar and rhetorical skill. The process is not finalized until adulthood. Each successive stage depends on the continued maturation of the brain. For example, not until the sixth year of age are most children ready to be taught to read and write, i.e., to become literate. Educational opportunity is necessary for the full realization of these capacities.

In a considerable number of children, particularly those with family histories of speech defect, ambidexterity, and left handedness, there are specific types of delay in the timetable of language development. These restricted abnormalities appear more frequently in males than in females in a proportion of 4 : 1. Table 27-5 lists the common types of congenital language disorders in children who are otherwise normal, i.e., are neither deaf nor mentally retarded (nor impaired in any other way). It is obvious that in all the disorders of speech and language in children,

TABLE 27-2 Neurologic Functions and Disturbances in Infancy

Age	Normal functions	Pathologic signs
Newborn period	Blinking, tonic deviation of eyes on turning head, sucking, rooting, swallowing, yawning, grasping, brief extension of neck in prone position, incurvation response, Moro response, flexion postures of limbs; biceps reflexes present and others variable; infantile type of flexor plantar reflex; stable temperature, respirations, and blood pressure; periods of sleep and arousal; vigorous cry	Lack of arousal (stupor or coma); high-pitched or weak cry; abnormal (incomplete or absent) Moro response; opisthotonus; flaccidity or hypertonia; convulsions; tremulous limbs; failure of tonic deviation of eyes on passive movement of head or of head and body
2–3 months	Supports head; smiles; makes vowel sounds; adopts tonic asymmetric neck postures (tonic neck reflexes); large range of movements of limbs, tendon reflexes usually present; fixates on and follows a dangling toy; suckles vigorously; periods of sleep sharply differentiated from awake periods; support and stepping unelicitable; vertical suspension—legs flex, head up; optokinetic nystagmus elicitable	Absence of any or all of the normal functions; convulsions; hypotonia or hypertonia of neck and limbs; vertical suspension—legs extend and adduct
4 months	Good head support, minimal head lag; coos and chuckles; inspects hands; tone of limbs moderate or diminished; turns to sounds; rolls over from prone to supine; grasping, sucking, and tonic neck reflexes subservient to volition	No head support; motor deficits; hypertonia; no social reactions; tonic neck reflexes present; strong Moro response; absence of symmetric attitude

TABLE 27-2 Neurologic Functions and Disturbances in Infancy (*continued*)

Age	Normal functions	Pathologic signs
5–6 months	Babbles; reaches and grasps; vocalizes in social play; discriminates between family and strangers; Moro and grasp disappear; tries to recover lost object; begins to sit, no head lag on pull to sit; positive support reaction; tonic neck reflexes gone; Landau response (holds head above horizontal and arches back when held horizontally); begins to grasp objects with one hand, holds bottle	Altered tone; obligatory postures; cannot sit or roll over; hypo- or hypertonia; persistent Moro and grasp; persistent tonic neck reflexes; no Landau response
9 months	Creeps and pulls to stand, stands holding on; sits securely; babbles "Mama," "Dada," or equivalent; sociable, plays "pat-a-cake," seeks attention; drinks from cup; Landau present; parachute response present; grasps with thumb to forefinger	Fails to attain these motor, verbal, and social milestones; persistent automatisms and tonic neck reflexes or hypo- or hypertonia
12 months	Stands alone; may walk, or walks if led; tries to feed self; may say several single words, echoes sounds; plantar reflexes definitely flexor; throws objects	Retardation in attaining these milestones; functions at earlier level; persistence of automatisms
15 months	Walks independently (9–16 months), falls easily; moves arms steadily; says several words, scribbles with crayon; requests by pointing; interest in sounds, music, pictures, and animal toys	Retardation at earlier age level; persistent abnormalities of tone and posture; sensory discriminations defective

(*continued*)

TABLE 27-2 Neurologic Functions and Disturbances in Infancy (*continued*)

Age	Normal functions	Pathologic signs
18 months	Says at least 6 words; feeds self; uses spoon well; may obey commands; runs stiffly, seats self in chair; hand dominance; throws ball; plays several nursery games; uses simple tools in imitation; removes shoes and stockings; points to two or three parts of body, common objects, and pictures in book	Cannot walk; no words
24 months	Says 2- or 3-word sentences; scribbles; runs well, climbs stairs one at a time; bends over and picks up objects; kicks ball; turns knob; organized play; builds tower of 6 blocks; sometimes toilet trained	Retarded in all motor, linguistic, and social adaptive skills

Source: Modified from Gesell.

intelligence, vision and hearing, and the control of labial, lingual, palatal, and laryngeal movements should be tested.

Mixed forms of speech impairment are frequent. They tend to lessen with maturation, and milder forms may disappear in late adolescence and adulthood. These disorders are not psychogenic, but the child may develop a sense of inferiority or other neurotic tendencies because of the speech disorder.

Special drills and educational methods are helpful in correcting these maturational defects.

Learning Disorders

Academic achievement does not measure up to the level of intelligence in 10 to 15 percent of children. Psychosocial factors such as lack of scholastic opportunity, bad home environment, and ghetto life may play a role. In many instances, borderline intelligence or a particular inability to process information or marginal defects in reading and calculation are important. The hyperkinetic state, common to boys, may interfere with learning.

TABLE 27-3 Developmental Achievements of the Normal Preschool Child

Age	Observed items	Useful clinical tests
2 years	Runs well; goes up and down stairs, one step at a time; climbs on furniture; opens doors; helps to undress; feeds well with spoon; puts three words together; listens to stories with pictures	Pencil-paper test: scribbles, imitates horizontal stroke; folds paper once; builds tower of six blocks
2½ years	Jumps on both feet; walks on tiptoes if asked; knows full name, asks questions; refers to self as "I"; helps put away toys and clothes; names animals in book, knows 1 to 3 colors; can complete three-piece form board	Pencil-paper test: copies horizontal and vertical line; builds tower of eight blocks
3 years	Climbs stairs, alternating feet; talks constantly, recites nursery rhymes; rides tricycle; stands on one foot momentarily; plays simple games; helps in dressing; washes hands; identifies five colors	Builds nine-cube tower; builds bridge with three cubes; imitates circle and cross with pencil
4 years	Climbs well, hops and skips on one foot, throws ball overhand, kicks ball; cuts out pictures with scissors; counts four pennies; tells a story, plays with other children; goes to toilet alone	Copies cross and circle; builds gate with five cubes; builds a bridge from model; draws a human figure with two to four parts other than head; distinguishes short and long line
5 years	Skips; names four colors, counts ten pennies; dresses and undresses; asks questions about meaning of words	Copies square and triangle; distinguishes heavier of two weights; more detailed drawing of a human figure

Such children are overactive, impulsive, inattentive, distractible, impatient, and easily frustrated ("attention deficit disorder"). This, too, is a specific abnormality—a restricted, genetically determined developmental delay. Hypometabolism of the premotor and superior prefrontal cortex has recently been demonstrated.

Correction of learning disorders requires the concerted effort of family and special educators. Drugs such as methylphenidate,

TABLE 27-4 Timetable of Growth and Nervous System Development in the Normal Embryo and Fetus

Age, days	Size (crown-rump length), mm	Nervous system development
18	1.5	Neural groove and tube
21	3.0	Optic vesicles
26	3.0	Closure of anterior neuropore
27	3.3	Closure of posterior neuropore; ventral horn cells appear
31	4.3	Anterior and posterior roots
35	5.0	Five cerebral vesicles
42	13.0	Primordium of cerebellum
56	25.0	Differentiation of cerebral cortex and meninges
150	225.0	Primary cerebral fissures appear
180	230.0	Secondary cerebral sulci and first myelination appear in brain
240–270		Tertiary cerebral sulci and further myelination and growth of brain

TABLE 27-5 Developmental Disorders of Speech and Language

Type	Clinical manifestations
Developmental speech delay	Failure to speak words and short phrases by age 2 years (delay may be up to 3–4 years); normal understanding of spoken word and normal communication by gestures; speech later becomes normal or nearly so
Congenital word deafness (developmental receptive dysphasia)	Despite adequate hearing (response to sounds), an inability to distinguish word patterns or reproduce them in speech; idioglossia develops
Congenital inarticulation	Unable to coordinate vocal, articulatory, and respiratory movements for speaking; normal understanding of spoken words: lisping, lallation, cluttered speech, which are special types of articulatory defect
Congenital word blindness (developmental dyslexia and dysgraphia)	Inability to read, spell, and write words, despite ability to recognize letters; normal understanding of spoken word and of meaning of objects and diagrams; difficulty in copying and color naming; many variants thereof
Dyscalculia	Inability to learn basic arithmetic; may be combined with dyslexia
Stuttering-stammering	Intermittent, involuntary repetition of syllables or blocking; worse with excitement or stress; disappears or improves with maturity except in severe forms

5 to 10 mg tid, or dextroamphetamine, 2.5 to 5 mg tid, may be helpful in some cases of hyperactivity.

Impaired Social Development

Here the retardation is in the sphere of social adaptation, a long process that includes the successive harmonious adaptation to mother, family, teachers, and social peers. Easy frustration, disobedience, persistent tantrums, and inability to accept authority and curb one's impulses are flagrant manifestations. This may lead to truancy, family discord, and unlawful conduct, i.e., sociopathy (see Chap. 53). With maturation there is usually improvement.

THE NEUROLOGY OF AGING

At the other end of the life cycle there is a predictable decline in neurologic functioning. The aging process is based on neuronal loss in many systems, which begins in midadult life and proceeds until death. This decline is interrupted only by the premature termination of life by trauma, cancer, or vascular disease, which in themselves may be age-related but are not caused by senility alone. In many but not all systems of neurons the most obvious underlying morphologic changes are neuronal lipofuscinosis, gradual cell loss, and replacement gliosis. A volumetric change in the cerebrum with age is regularly displayed in CT scans and MRI, which show convolutional atrophy and enlarged ventricles. At a later stage, senile plaques and Alzheimer neurofibrillary changes are added, but there is still not full agreement as to whether this is simply an aging effect or an age-linked disease. We have taken the latter standpoint, and for this reason we discuss Alzheimer dementia with the degenerative diseases (Chap. 41).

The Neurologic Signs of Aging

The following are the most consistent signs:

1. A tendency to be self-centered, rigid, conservative, and hypercritical, or the opposite—unduly pliant, vacillating, and uncritically accepting of ideas.
2. An increased forgetfulness of proper names and a diminished facility with words (verbal amnesia).
3. Presbyopia.
4. Small pupils and sluggish pupillary reflexes.

5. Diminished range of upward gaze.
6. Presbycusis; increased tendency to vertigo.
7. Diminished sense of smell.
8. Impaired agility of movement and balance.
9. Diminished Achilles reflex.
10. Diminished vibratory sense in the feet.
11. Reduced muscle power and thinness of leg muscles.
12. Altered stance and gait (senile gait; see Chap. 6).

Any one or combination of these defects in old persons are more likely to be a manifestation of the aging process than of concurrent disease.

Apart from the nervous system, other organ systems also deteriorate with age, as shown in Table 27-6.

TABLE 27-6 Physiologic and Anatomic Deterioration with Age

System	Percentage of decrease
Brain weight	15
Blood flow to brain	20
Speed of return of blood acidity to equilibrium after exercise	83
Cardiac output at rest	35
Number of glomeruli in kidney	44
Glomerular filtration rate	31
Number of fibers in nerves	37
Nerve conduction velocity	10
Number of taste buds	64
Maximum 0_2 utilization with exercise	60
Maximum ventilation volume	47
Maximum breathing capacity	44
Power of hand grip	45
Maximum work rate	30
Basal metabolic rate	16
Body water content	18
Body weight (males)	12

Source: Shock.

For a more detailed discussion of this topic, see Adams and Victor: *Principles of Neurology*, 4th ed, pp 457–497.

ADDITIONAL READING

Albert ML (ed): *Clinical Neurology of Aging*. New York, Oxford Universiy Press, 1984.

Barlow C: *Mental retardation and related disorders*. Philadelphia, Davis, 1977.

Denckla MB: Autism, in Asbury AK, McKhann GM, McDonald WI (eds): *Diseases of the Nervous System*. Philadelphia, Saunders, 1986, chap 73, pp 906–913.

Fries JF, Crapo LM: *Vitality and Aging*. San Francisco, Freeman, 1981.

Gesell A (ed): *The First Five Years of Life: A Guide to the Study of the Pre-school Child*. New York, Harper & Row, 1940.

Katzman R, Terry RD: *The Neurology of Aging*. Philadelphia, Davis, 1983.

Kinsbourne M: Disorders of mental development, in Menkes JH (ed): *Textbook of Child Neurology*, 4th ed. Philadelphia, Lea & Febiger, 1990, pp 763–796.

Lowrey GH: *Growth and Development of Children*, 8th ed. Chicago, Yearbook Publishers, 1986.

Rapin I, Allen DA: Developmental language disorders. Nosologic considerations, in Kirk U (ed): *Neuropsychology of Language, Reading, and Spelling*. New York, Academic, 1983, pp 155–184.

IV THE MAJOR CATEGORIES OF NEUROLOGIC DISEASE

28 Disturbances of CSF Circulation and Intracranial Pressure

In the adult, the average intracranial volume is 1700 mL. The volume of the brain is approximately 1400 mL; that of the CSF is 150 mL; and that of the blood is 150 mL. The proportion of CSF in the ventricles, cisterns, and subarachnoid spaces varies with age. By CT scanning, the distance between the lateral ventricles gradually increases from 1.0 to 1.5 cm and the width of the third ventricle increases from 3 to 6 mm (by the age of 60 years).

The site of formation, the circulation, and absorption of CSF are described in detail in the *Principles*. The differential pressures between the lateral ventricles, the main site of formation, and the arachnoid villi, the sites of absorption, result in a slow rate of flow in this direction.

The CSF serves as a kind of water jacket in which the brain is suspended and thereby protected from blows to the head. Waste products of cerebral metabolism, such as CO_2, lactate, and H ions, diffuse into the CSF, from which they are absorbed into the blood stream ("sink action" of the CSF). The blood vessels offer a barrier between the blood and CSF (BCSFB), similar to the one between blood and brain (BBB).

The intact cranium and vertebral column and the relatively inelastic dura form a rigid container, and the volumes of blood, CSF, and brain are constant in conditions of health. An increase in the volume of any one of these components must be at the expense of the other two (Monro-Kellie hypothesis). These accommodative volume-pressure relationships are subsumed under the term *compliance* and are schematically portrayed in Fig. 28-1.

INCREASED INTRACRANIAL PRESSURE

There are three main mechanisms of raised intracranial pressure (ICP):

1. *Increased volume* (mass effect) due to cerebral tumor, abscess, hemorrhage, or massive infarction; to an epidural or subdural hematoma; or to acute diffuse brain swelling, as occurs in anoxic states, hypertensive encephalopathy, water intoxica-

tion, and Reye syndrome. The latter two conditions are observed mainly in children.

2. *Increased venous pressure* from heart failure or superior mediastinal obstruction, which increases the volume of blood in pial veins and dural sinuses and probably also interferes with CSF absorption.
3. *Obstruction to the flow and absorption of the CSF:* Obstruction in the ventricles or around the base of the brain causes a tension hydrocephalus. If absorption is blocked, a pseudotumor state develops. These are discussed below.

An increased ICP is present when the CSF pressure, normally 90 to 180 mmH_2O (6 to 13 mmHg), exceeds 200 mm. When a pressure-measuring device is placed into the epidural space with the head and trunk elevated to 45°, the pressure is 2 to 5 mmHg. During coughing, it rises to 20 mmHg and immediately falls to 10 mm. Steady levels up to 15 mmHg are harmless. Above that level, clinical signs of increased ICP begin to appear—headache, nausea and vomiting, drowsiness, ocular and gaze palsies, papilledema, visual obscurations, and eventually blindness. Ropper finds that pupillary dilatation, abducens palsies, drowsiness/stupor, raised systolic blood pressure, and bradycardia (presumably from medullary compression) do not bear a direct relationship to ICP. Patients maintain normal mental function and adequate cerebral circulation at pressures up to 40 mmHg, providing blood pressure is maintained. At 40 to 50 mmHg, cerebral blood flow is reduced; rhythmic rises in pressure (Lundberg waves) are superimposed and coma supervenes.

Preventing rises in ICP above 15 to 20 mmHg improves the outcome of diseases that cause increased ICP. Effective measures are elevation of the head and shoulders to 15° to 20°, restriction of fluids to 1000 mL/day (to maintain an osmolality of 305 to 315), mechanical respiration to reduce PCO_2 and the use of hyperosmolar agents. Reduction of PCO_2 causes vasoconstriction, which reduces cerebral blood volume, which in turn reduces ICP. Mannitol, given as an IV bolus of 0.25 g/kg every 3 to 4 h, is the most favored hyperosmolar agent. Some neurosurgeons prefer to use furosemide, glycerol, or ethacrynic acid.

TENSION HYDROCEPHALUS

This is due to an obstruction to the flow of CSF at some point between its main site of formation (within the lateral ventricles) and the basilar subarachnoid space. Because of the obstruction, CSF accumulates within the ventricles, dilating them, compressing the periventricular tissues, and slightly expanding the cerebral

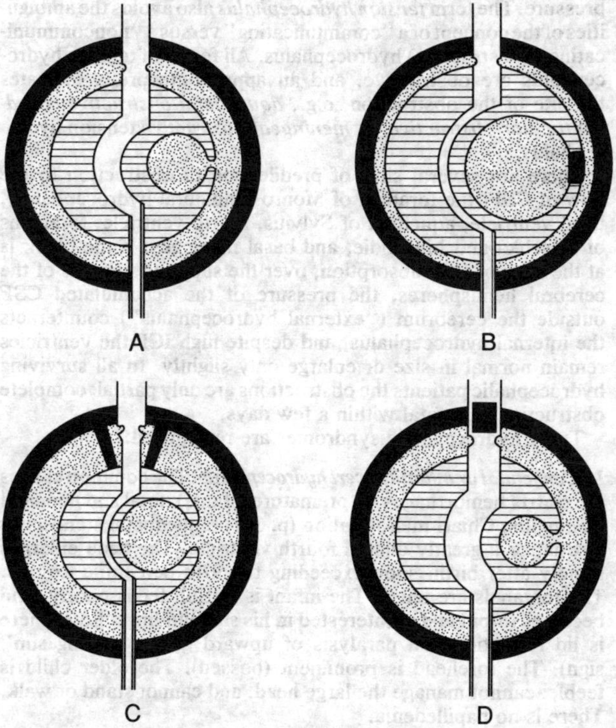

FIG. 28-1 *A*. Schematic representation of the three components of the intracranial contents: the incompressible brain tissue (*shaded*); the vascular system, open to the atmosphere; and the CSF (*dotted*). *B*. With ventricular obstruction. *C*. With obstruction at or near the points of outlet of the CSF. *D*. With obstruction of the venous outflow. *(Redrawn from Foley.)*

hemispheres. In an infant or young child (up to 2 years), whose cranial sutures are not fully closed, the head enlarges as well (*manifest or overt hydrocephalus*). Some degree of suture separation (diastasis) is also possible in older children.

Unfortunately, the term *hydrocephalus* is also used when the ventricles enlarge passively, as a result of brain atrophy (*hydrocephalus ex vacuo*). It is therefore preferable to use the qualifying adjective *tension* for the obstructive type of hydrocephalus, in which the CSF is or has been under increased pressure. The term *tension hydrocephalus* also avoids the ambiguities of the concept of a "communicating" versus a "noncommunicating" (obstructive) hydrocephalus. All forms of tension hydrocephalus are obstructive, and an appropriate prefix indicates the site of the obstruction, e.g., *aqueductal-obstructive, third-ventricular-obstructive,* or *meningeal-obstructive* tension hydrocephalus.

There are several sites of predilection of obstruction to the flow of CSF: the foramen of Monro (unilateral hydrocephalus), third ventricle, aqueduct of Sylvius, fourth ventricle, foramens of Luschka and Magendie, and basal meninges. If the block is at the sites of CSF absorption, over the superior surfaces of the cerebral hemispheres, the pressure of the accumulated CSF outside the cerebrum ("external hydrocephalus") counteracts the internal hydrocephalus, and despite high ICP the ventricles remain normal in size or enlarge only slightly. In all surviving hydrocephalic patients the obstructions are only partial; complete obstructions are fatal within a few days.

Three hydrocephalic syndromes are recognized:

1. Congenital or infantile overt hydrocephalus The common causes are matrix hemorrhages (in premature infants), fetal and neonatal meningitis, Chiari malformation (p. 361), aqueductal stenosis or atresia, or a greatly dilated fourth ventricle. The head enlarges rapidly after birth, soon exceeding the 97th percentile for age. The fontanels are tense. The infant is fretful, feeds poorly, and becomes torpid and uninterested in his surroundings. Later there is lid retraction and paralysis of upward gaze ("setting sun" sign). The forehead is prominent (bossed). The older child is feeble, cannot manage the large head, and cannot stand or walk. There is no papilledema.

2. Acquired occult tension hydrocephalus The usual causes are posterior fossa tumor, the late effects of ependymitis or subarachnoid hemorrhage, and decompensation of a congenital hydrocephalus. Bifrontal and bioccipital headaches, nausea, and vomiting are frequent manifestations. Papilledema is present. Slowness of response, inattentiveness, poverty of mental activity, and perseveration develop gradually. Gait becomes progressively impaired.

3. Normal-pressure hydrocephalus As a high-pressure, occult hydrocephalus gradually corrects itself (compensates) or as a *relatively* normal-pressure (180 to 200 mmH_20) hydrocephalus develops gradually, the greatly enlarged ventricles compress the cerebral white matter. Headache, if present originally, recedes and there is no papilledema. A subacutely or slowly developing unsteadiness of gait is the most prominent manifestation, followed by blunting of the intellect and incontinence of urine. The usual causes are the late effects of meningeal inflammation, subarachnoid hemorrhage from trauma or ruptured aneurysm, intraventricular tumors, and meningeal carcinomatosis.

The *treatment* of all forms of persistent symptomatic hydrocephalus is ventriculoatrial or ventriculoperitoneal shunting with a one-way valve. Lumboperitoneal shunts may be used for meningeal-obstructive hydrocephalus.

BENIGN INTRACRANIAL HYPERTENSION (PSEUDOTUMOR CEREBRI, MENINGEAL HYDROPS)

This is a syndrome of obscure origin observed most frequently but not exclusively in obese young women. Over a period of weeks the patient develops headaches and papilledema in the absence of ventricular enlargement or any other evidence of an intracranial mass lesion. Other neurologic signs are minimal. There is some evidence that the absorption of CSF is impaired.

The high CSF pressures, unless controlled, threaten vision and may result in permanent blindness. In some patients, the pressure can be reduced by lumbar punctures repeated every few days. Gradually the pressure may stabilize at a lower safe level (200 to 250 mmH_2O). Weight reduction may also be helpful but is difficult to accomplish. Prednisone (40 to 60 mg/day) or oral hyperosmotic agents such as glycerol (15 to 60 mg qid) or acetazolamide (500 mg bid) may be of value is some cases. Lumbar thecoperitoneal shunt is an effective and relatively safe surgical procedure. Patients who do not respond to any of these measures and are threatened with visual loss require surgical decompression of the optic nerve by opening the nerve sheath.

In addition to pseudotumor cerebri there is a large number of *other nontumorous causes of raised ICP*: heart failure, hypertensive encephalopathy, excessive doses of tetracycline and vitamin A in children, thrombosis of the lateral or superior sagittal venous sinuses, hypo- and hyperadrenalism, hypoparathyroidism, and hypercapnia.

INTRACRANIAL HYPOTENSION

The most frequent cause is lumbar puncture, which allows persistent leakage of CSF. Upon sitting or standing, which increases the negative intracranial pressure, a generalized headache develops within minutes, accompanied by pain and stiffness of the neck and sometimes by nausea and vomiting. Recumbency relieves these symptoms, as do bed rest and forced fluids. The leak stops after a few days (occasionally longer).

A rare syndrome of spontaneous intracranial hypotension may follow a strain or hurtful fall. A similar syndrome may occur in patients who have been shunted with a one-way valve; usually the valve setting is too low, and readjustment of the pressure setting relieves the symptoms.

For a more detailed discussion of this topic, see Adams and Victor: *Principles of Neurology*, 4th ed, pp 501–515.

ADDITIONAL READING

Adams RD, Fisher CM, Hakim S, et al: Symptomatic occult hydrocephalus with "normal" cerebrospinal fluid pressure: A treatable syndrome. *N Engl J Med* 273:117, 1965.

Black PM: *Idiopathic normal pressure hydrocephalus:* Results of shunting in 62 patients. *J Neurosurg* 53:371, 1980.

Durcan FJ, Corbett JJ, Wall M: The incidence of pseudotumor cerebri. *Arch Neurol* 45:875, 1988.

Fishman RA: *Cerebrospinal Fluid in Diseases of the Nervous System*. Philadelphia, Saunders, 1980.

Foley J: Benign forms of intracranial hypertension—"toxic" and "otitic" hydrocephalus. *Brain* 78:1, 1955.

Ropper AH, Kennedy SK (eds): *Neurological and Neurosurgical Intensive Care*, 2nd ed. Rockville, MD, Aspen, 1988.

29 | Intracranial Neoplasms

DEFINITIONS

Neoplasia of neural tissue is an evolving blastomatous lesion, the constituent cells of which multiply without restraint and form a mass within the cranial or spinal cavity. Two types occur: (1) *primary tumors*, made up of astrocytes, oligodendrocytes, ependymocytes, histiocytes, microgliocytes (together called *gliomas*); special arachnoidal fibroblasts (*meningiomas*); neuroblasts-medulloblasts and pineocytes; and (2) *secondary tumors*, i.e., metastatic carcinomas from lung, breast, etc., and lymphomas. Cerebral neoplasms need to be distinguished from *hamartomas*, which are tumor-like formations that have their basis in maldevelopment and undergo no significant growth in the lifetime of the host. Examples of hamartomas are the lesions of tuberous sclerosis, the central lesions of neurofibromatosis, teratomas of the pineal gland, suprasellar craniopharyngiomas, vascular malformations, lipomas, and cholesteatomas. Hamartomas may enlarge due to accumulation of the metabolic products of their cells or expansion of their constituent vessels and occasionally undergo neoplastic change (e.g., gliomatous transformation of central neurofibromas). Well-differentiated neurons never become neoplastic.

ETIOLOGY

Little is known. Familial occurrence is low, except in a few types that are associated with neurofibromatosis, tuberous sclerosis, von Hippel-Lindau disease, and carotid body tumors. Some lymphomas may be caused by the EB virus. Human polyoma virus has been implicated in the gliomatous changes that characterize the lesions of progressive multifocal leucoencephalopathy.The Bailey-Cushing classification, still in common use, is based on the theory that brain tumors arise from primitive nerve and glial cells; but it is now generally accepted that neoplastic transformation can occur in mature elements. The frequency of the different types of intracranial tumor is shown in Table 29-1.

TABLE 29-1 Types of Intracranial Tumor in the Combined Series of Zülch, Cushing, and Olivecrona, Expressed in Percentage of Total (Approximately 15,000 Cases)*

Tumor	Percentage of total
Gliomas†	
Glioblastoma multiforme	20
Astrocytoma	10
Ependymoma	6
Medulloblastoma	4
Oligodendrocytoma	5
Meningioma	15
Pituitary adenoma	7
Neurinoma (schwannoma)	7
Metastatic carcinoma	6
Craniopharyngioma, dermoid, epidermoid, teratoma	4
Angiomas	4
Sarcomas	4
Unclassified (mostly gliomas)	5
Miscellaneous (pinealoma, chordoma, granuloma)	3
	100

* In the large Latin American series reported by Polak, the frequency of tumor types is much the same, except for a somewhat higher proportion of metastatic tumors.

† In *children*, the proportions differ: astrocytoma, 48%; medulloblastoma, 44%; ependymoma, 8%.

PATHOPHYSIOLOGY

As a group, the gliomas arise in one or a few foci in the cerebral white matter, central gray matter, brainstem, or cerebellum. They cannot be completely excised. The well-differentiated tumor cells of an astrocytoma and oligodendroglioma infiltrate and displace the normal cells and myelinated fibers. Undifferentiated glial cells (glioblastoma multiforme, grade III astrocytoma) proliferate more rapidly, often outstripping their blood supply, and becoming necrotic and hemorrhagic in places.

With tumor growth there is compression of venules in the adjacent cerebral white matter and a weakening of the blood-brain barrier. Plasma proteins seep into the brain tissue, causing *vasogenic* or *localized cerebral edema*. This is evidenced by increased protein levels in the CSF, decreased attenuation on CT scanning, and an increase in T_2 signal intensity in MRI.

As the mass in the cerebrum or cerebellum increases in size, intracranial pressure rises and adjacent normal brain is displaced. Because of the compartmentalization of the cranial cavity by dura (falx, tentorium), pressure from a mass in one compartment

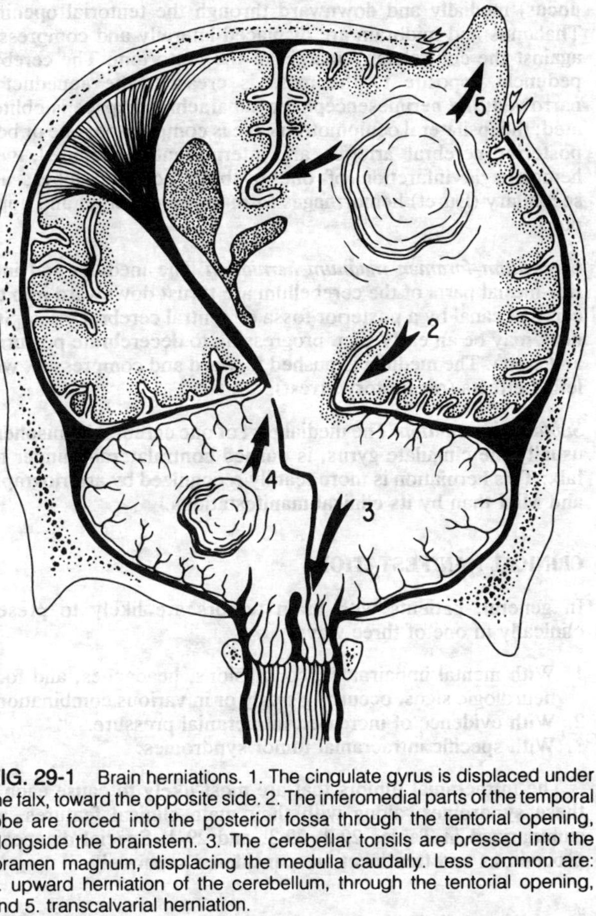

FIG. 29-1 Brain herniations. 1. The cingulate gyrus is displaced under the falx, toward the opposite side. 2. The inferomedial parts of the temporal lobe are forced into the posterior fossa through the tentorial opening, alongside the brainstem. 3. The cerebellar tonsils are pressed into the foramen magnum, displacing the medulla caudally. Less common are: 4. upward herniation of the cerebellum, through the tentorial opening, and 5. transcalvarial herniation.

causes a shift or herniation of brain tissue into another compartment, where pressure is lower (Fig. 29-1). The main features of the three common herniations—temporal lobe–tentorial, cerebellar–foramen magnum, and subfalcial—are summarized below:

Temporal lobe–tentorial herniation A mass in one cerebral hemisphere forces the medial part of the temporal lobe (usually the uncus) medially and downward through the tentorial opening. Thalamus and midbrain are displaced laterally and compressed against the contralateral margin of the tentorium. The cerebral peduncle opposite to the mass is creased; the aqueduct is narrowed; the perimesencephalic subarachnoid space is obliterated; the ipsilateral oculomotor nerve is compressed; one or both posterior cerebral arteries are intermittently occluded, with hemorrhagic infarction of one or both occipital lobes; and secondary (Duret) hemorrhages form in the midbrain and upper pons.

Cerebellum–foramen magnum herniation The medulla and inferior-mesial parts of the cerebellum are thrust downward into the cervical canal by a posterior fossa or central cerebral mass. Stiff neck may be an early sign, progressing to decerebrate posturing and coma. The medulla is pushed forward and compressed, with lethal effects (respiratory arrest).

Subfalcial herniation The medial part of one cerebral hemisphere, usually the cingulate gyrus, is pushed contralaterally under the falx. This herniation is more readily recognized by arteriography and MRI than by its clinical manifestations.

CLINICAL MANIFESTATIONS

In general, patients with brain tumors are likely to present clinically in one of three ways:

1. With mental impairment, convulsions, headaches, and focal neurologic signs, occurring singly or in various combinations.
2. With evidence of increased intracranial pressure.
3. With specific intracranial tumor syndromes.

The intracranial tumors that are most likely to cause each of these syndromes, along with their main clinical features, are summarized in Tables 29-2, 29-3, and 29-4. Special diagnostic procedures and treatment are considered separately.

Usual Diagnostic Tests

CT scanning and MRI visualize all intracranial tumors and should be the initial investigative procedures when symptoms or signs of increased ICP are present. Plain films of the chest should always be obtained to help rule out metastatic disease. Exceptionally, skull films in a particular plane will be needed to show an

TABLE 29-2 Tumors Presenting with Impairment of Mental Function, Headaches, Seizures, or Focal Neurologic Signs: Increased Intracranial Pressure a Late Development

Glioblastoma multiforme (anaplastic astrocytoma)	20% of all intracranial tumors, 55% of all gliomas; mainly cerebral but may affect all parts of brain and cord, widely infiltrative; survival about 12 months in most cases
Astrocytomas, grades 1 and 2	25–30% of cerebral gliomas; cerebral hemispheres common sites in adults, brainstem and cerebellum more often in children; slowly growing, tendency to form cysts; survival for many years
Oligodendroglioma	5–7% of intracranial gliomas; frontal lobes are most common site, slowly growing; survival many years if low grade
Ependymoma	Common sites: fourth ventricle (particularly in children), conus medullaris and filum terminale; survival depends on degree of anaplasia
Meningioma	15% of all primary intracranial tumors, highest incidence in seventh decade; more frequent in women; common sites: sylvian region, superior parasagittal surfaces, lesser wing of sphenoid, tuberculum sellae, cerebellopontine angle, spinal canal; very slow growing, with symptoms depending upon tumor site
Primary cerebral lymphoma	May arise in any part of the brain (monofocal or multifocal), usually in adult life; clinical course similar to glioblastoma; lymphocytes, mononuclear and tumor cells often found in CSF; immunosuppressed patients at risk; median survival less than 24 months
Metastatic carcinoma	Three main patterns: (1) to skull and dura from carcinoma of breast and prostate, and multiple myeloma; may involve cranial nerves and pituitary; (2) brain metastases from lung, breast, melanoma, rectocolon, kidney; (3) meningeal carcinomatosis or leukemic infiltration of leptomeninges and cranial and spinal nerve roots. Average survival 6 months; patients with bony metastases survive longer.

enlarged sella, optic foramen, or superior orbital fissure or skull-bone thickening with meningioma. The combination of CT-MR and arteriography may reveal enough of the characteristics of a glioma to make biopsy unnecessary.

TABLE 29-3 Tumors Causing Mainly Increased Intracranial Pressure and Hydrocephalus, Without Conspicuous Focal or Lateralizing Signs

Medulloblastoma and cystic astrocytoma of cerebellum	Mainly in children 4 to 8 years; begins with listlessness, vomiting, headaches; later, squint, stumbling gait, falling, and papilledema
Ependymoma and papilloma	Clinical syndrome similar to medulloblastoma but more protracted; two-thirds of patients present with increased ICP, others with vomiting, dysphagia, paresthesias of extremities, vertigo, head-tilt
Hemangioblastoma of cerebellum (von Hippel-Lindau disease)	Dominant inheritance; retinal angioma and polycythemia often conjoined; may develop multiple spinal cord lesions and syringomyelia
Pinealoma (includes germinoma and teratoma of pineal)	Onset in adolescence and adulthood; symptoms and signs of increased ICP, including paralysis of upward gaze and pupils fixed to light (Parinaud syndrome); precocious puberty in males with teratoma
Colloid (paraphysial) cyst of third ventricle	Signs of intermittent or persistent increased ICP and hydrocephalus
Craniopharyngioma	In children and adolescents, retardation of sexual maturation and growth, combined with visual loss from chiasmal-optic nerve lesions; in adults, signs of hydrocephalus, mild corticospinal and hypothalamic signs

Treatment

Surface tumors such as meningiomas and acoustic neuromas are amenable to complete surgical removal. Meningiomas of the base of the brain (sphenoid wing, olfactory groove, tuberculum sellae, and posterior fossa) may infiltrate bone and can be excised only partially. Radiation therapy is then given.

For gliomas, the common practice is biopsy with partial excision, radiation therapy up to 5000 rads over 3 to 4 weeks, and antitumor drug therapy. In the case of glioblastoma multiforme, this program prolongs useful life by several months. Dexamethasone is used to control cerebral edema.

Each of the special tumors that cause hydrocephalus or regional syndromes require special combinations of surgical and radiation therapy.

PARANEOPLASTIC DISORDERS

Designated by this term is a group of neurologic disorders that occur in patients with carcinoma or other types of neoplasia, even though the nervous system has not been invaded or compressed by the tumor. Presumably the tumors which induce

TABLE 29-4 Distinctive Tumor Syndromes: Local Signs Predominate and General Cerebral Deficits and Increased ICP Are Late or Absent

Acoustic neuroma (schwannoma)	Usually solitary; may be part of neurofibromatosis, either solitary (Type I) or bilateral (Type II, autosomal dominant); unilateral neurosensory deafness, loss of balance, facial weakness and loss of sensation, later ataxia of ipsilateral limbs and gait and raised intracranial pressure
Carotid body tumor	Painless mass at bifurcation of common carotid, below angle of jaw; grows slowly; compresses cranial nerves IX to XII and sympathetics; rarely familial and bilateral
Pituitary adenomas (with enlarged sella, rule out empty sella syndrome by CT-MRI)	
Prolactinomas (usually chromophobe, sometimes acidophilic adenoma)	Increased incidence with age; headache, bitemporal hemianopia or mixed optic nerve-chiasmal changes; sella turcica expands; hypothyroidism, hypoadrenalism; in females, amenorrhea, galactorrhea, serum prolactin increased (>100 ng/mL); in males, impotence
Acromegaly-gigantism (eosinophilic adenoma)	Oversecretion of growth hormone (GH); before puberty, gigantism; after puberty, acromegaly; sometimes prolactin also increased
Cushing disease (basophil or nonbasophil adenoma)	Oversecretion of ACTH; sella not enlarged; truncal obesity, striae, hirsutism; hypertension; glycosuria; amenorrhea; osteoporosis; muscle weakness; mental changes
Meningioma of sphenoid ridge	Mainly in women; average age 50 years; unilateral exophthalmos, slight temporal bulge, anosmia, ocular palsies, Tolosa-Hunt syndrome, monocular blindness
Meningioma of olfactory groove	Older adults; anosmia and frontal lobe signs; high CSF protein
Meningioma of tuberculum sellae	Older adults; mainly women; bitemporal hemianopia with normal sized sella
Glioma of brainstem	Onset mainly in childhood; progressive cranial nerve and long tract signs; increased ICP late; prognosis varies with degree of anaplasia
Glioma of optic nerve and chiasm	Mainly in children and adolescents, sometimes with neurofibromatosis; progressive loss of vision with optic atrophy or chiasmal field defect
Chordoma	Common sites, clivus and sacrococcygeal region; cauda equina syndrome or successive multiple cranial nerve signs, with conduction deafness, facial pain, and ataxia
Nasopharyngeal or sinus tumors	Multiple upper canial nerve abnormalities; nasopharyngeal mass; erosion base of skull
Tumors of foramen magnum	Pain in occiput and posterior neck; combination of lower cranial nerve, cervical cord, and cerebellar signs

these effects elaborate enzymes or antibodies capable of reacting with the nervous system. The most familiar of these remote effects and the chapters in which they are discussed are listed below:

1. Polyneuropathy (Chap. 44).
2. Polymyositis or dermatomyositis (Chap. 47).
3. Myasthenic-myopathic syndrome of Lambert-Eaton (Chap. 51).
4. Carcinomatous cerebellar degeneration (see the *Principles*, pp. 549–550).
5. Limbic encephalitis (see *Principles*, p. 550).
6. Progressive multifocal leukoencephalopathy (Chap. 31).
7. Necrotizing myelopathy (Chap. 34).

For a more detailed discussion of this topic, see Adams and Victor: *Principles of Neurology*, 4th ed, pp 516–553.

ADDITIONAL READING

Anderson NE, Cunningham JM, Posner JB: Autoimmune pathogenesis of paraneoplastic neurological syndromes. *CRC Crit Rev Neurobiol* 3:245, 1987.

Fishman RA: *Cerebrospinal Fluid in Diseases of the Nervous System*, Philadelphia, Saunders, 1980.

Henson RA, Urich H: *Cancer and the Nervous System*. Oxford, Blackwell, 1982.

Martuza RI: Genetics of neuro-oncology. *Clin Neurosurg* 21:417, 1984.

Posner JB: Primary lymphoma of the CNS. *Neurol Alert* 5:21, 1987.

Russell DS, Rubinstein LJ: *Pathology of Tumours of the Nervous System*, 5th ed. Baltimore, Williams & Wilkins, 1989.

Walker RW, Posner JB: Central nervous system neoplasms, in Appel SH (ed): *Current Neurology*, vol 5. New York, Wiley, 1984, chap 9, pp 285–322.

30 Nonviral Infections of the Nervous System

PYOGENIC INFECTIONS

The most important of the pyogenic infections in decreasing order of their frequency are bacterial meningitis (also called leptomeningitis), brain abscess, subdural empyema, dural sinus thrombophlebitis, and focal bacterial encephalitis. In all of these and other conditions, bacteria reach the brain in one of two ways: by hematogenous spread (i.e., septicemia or infected emboli) or by extension from infected cranial structures (ears, sinuses, osteomyelitic foci, or penetrating cranial injuries).

Bacterial Meningitis

Definition This consists essentially of a bacterial infection of the pia and arachnoid and the fluid that they enclose. Since the subarachnoid space is continuous around the brain, spinal cord, and optic nerves, an infective agent (or blood or tumor cells) gaining entry to any one part of the space spreads to all of it. Thus *meningitis is always cerebrospinal*. Infection also reaches the ventricles either directly from the choroid plexuses or by reflux from the subarachnoid space. All structures bathed by the CSF—ependyma, choroid plexuses, cranial and spinal nerves, and surface veins and arteries—are exposed to the meningeal infection.

Epidemiology *Streptococcus pneumoniae, Neisseria meningitidis, Hemophilus influenzae,* and *Listeria monocytogenes*—the most common bacteria causing meningitis—have a worldwide distribution. Mainly they occur in the fall, winter, and spring months. Each has a relatively constant seasonal incidence, although epidemics of meningococcal meningitis tend to occur in roughly 10-year cycles. This form of meningitis is most frequent in children and adolescents but occurs throughout adult life. *Hemophilus influenzae* meningitis affects mainly children between the ages of 2 months and 7 years but is now being reported in adults over 50 years of age. Pneumococcal meningitis predominates in the very young and old. *Escherichia coli, Staphylococcus aureus, group A streptococci, Klebsiella, Pro-*

teus, and *Listeria monocytogenes* are associated with immunodeficiency states, trauma, and neurosurgical procedures, including ventricular shunts.

Pathogenesis and pathology The usual route by which bacteria reach the meninges is the blood stream (septicemia). Other pathways are direct extension from ears and infected sinuses, surgical operations, and rarely from congenital neuroectodermal fistulae and skull fractures.

Once bacteria enter the CSF, they excite an acute inflammatory reaction, mainly in the vascular pia. Hyperemia, exudation of blood proteins, and migration of neutrophils occur within hours. This exudate continues to accumulate for the next few days. Thereafter lymphocytes and then plasma cells begin to appear in the pia as part of an immune response. Veins in the pia may thrombose and cause brain infarction. As the meningeal exudate blocks the subarachnoid space and the foramens of Luschka and Magendie, tension hydrocephalus develops. There is also an ependymitis, which may contribute to the obstruction of CSF flow. Cranial nerves as they pass through purulent exudate in the subarachnoid space may be involved. Although the brain is not invaded by bacteria, their toxins diffuse through the pia and along the Virchow-Robin spaces and excite a subpial reaction. The thin arachnoid, especially in infants, may be transgressed, with the development of a subdural inflammatory reaction and a hygroma. If the meningitis is not treated successfully, arteritis and thrombosis may result.

Clinical features Fever, severe headache, generalized convulsions, various degrees of drowsiness and confusion, and even coma are the usual manifestations in adults and older children. Signs of meningeal irritation—stiffness of the neck on forward flexion, with flexion of the knees and hips (Brudzinski sign) and inability to completely extend the legs (Kernig sign)—become evident. In infants and newborns, in whom meningitis is often lethal, the infection expresses itself by fever and bulging of the fontanels, vomiting, drowsiness, and in some instances, convulsions; stiff neck may not be evident.

Clinical clues as to the type of meningitis are as follows:

1. Petechial and purpuric rash and circulatory collapse—meningococcal meningitis with Waterhouse-Friderichsen syndrome.
2. Ventriculoatrial or peritoneal shunt—coagulase-negative *Staphylococcus*.
3. Complication of lumbar puncture or spinal anesthesia—*Pseudomonas*.
4. Upper respiratory and ear infections in children—*H. influenzae*.

5. Immunocompromised host—*Strep. pneumoniae, Listeria monocytogenes.*
6. Infection of ears, sinuses, lung, heart valves—*Strep. pneumoniae.*

Ancillary examinations The single most important laboratory procedure is lumbar puncture and examination of the spinal fluid. The CSF is usually under increased pressure (200 to 400 mmH_2O), is cloudy owing to the presence of cells (mainly polymorphonuclear, a few hundred to 10,000 mm^3), and contains bacteria seen on Gram stain, increased protein (100 to 500 mg/dL), and decreased glucose (<40 mg/dL) or <40 percent of the blood glucose, which should be measured simultaneously. The fluid needs to be cultured. CSF latex agglutination for bacterial antigens is especially useful for partially treated meningitis. Also, throat and blood cultures should be obtained. The white cells in the blood are increased with a shift to the left.

Films of sinuses and chest are indicated after treatment is underway as are CT scanning and MRI to exclude brain abscess and subdural empyema. Actually, brain abscess rarely complicates meningitis. In infants and children ultrasound is preferred because anesthesia is not required. Brain imaging is best performed before the LP.

Treatment Bacterial meningitis is a medical emergency. Every hour of delay in starting antibacterial therapy increases the risk of permanent cerebral damage. Treatment with broad spectrum antibiotics should be started while awaiting identification of the organism (ampicillin 12 g/day in adults or ampicillin 400 mg/kg and chloramphenicol 100 mg/kg per day in children).

In Table 30-1 are listed the recommended antibiotic drugs and their dosages for the different types of meningitis. Persistent and recurrent subdural hygromas usually respond to repeated aspiration or shunting.

Preventive measures should not be neglected. All household contacts of patients with meningitis, particularly children, should receive rifampin, 20 mg/kg daily PO for 4 days. Immunization against *Neisseria meningitidis* is effective and should be given during epidemics. Children at 24 months of age should be vaccinated against *H. influenzae.*

Bacterial Encephalitis

In acute and subacute bacterial endocarditis (SBE) the brain is seeded with bacteria-laden emboli. In SBE, the bacteria are characteristically of low virulence and do not produce brain abscesses. However, the emboli of acute bacterial endocarditis

TABLE 30-1 Treatment of Bacterial Meningitis

Type	Drug	Adult dose	Pediatric dose
Pneumococcal or meningococcal	Penicillin G*	12–15 million units/day IV divided every 3 h	300,000 units/kg per day IV divided every 2–6 h
H. influenzae	Chloramphenicol	6 g/day IV divided every 6 h	75–100 mg/kg per day IV, IM, or p.o. divided every 6 h
	Or ampicillin	12–14 g/day IV divided every 4 h	300–400 mg/kg per day IV divided every 4 h
	Or cefotaxime	6–12 g/day IV divided every 4 h	150 mg/kg per day IV divided every 6 h
Enterobacteriaceae	Ampicillin	As above	As above
	Or gentamicin	200 mg/day IV divided every 8 h; 5–10 mg/day intrathecal	3 mg/kg per day IM divided every 8 h; 5 mg day intrathecal
Pseudomonas	Cefotaxime	As above	As above
Staph. aureus	Nafcillin	6 g/day IV divided every 4 h	200–300 mg/kg per day IV divided every 6 h

* In adults with any one of the three major meningitides, who are allergic to the penicillins, chloramphenicol, 6 g/day IV, can be used.

do give rise to miliary abscesses, infarcts, small hemorrhages and bacterial meningitis; large abscesses are rare. SBE causes sterile meningeal reactions, infarcts, and rarely mycotic aneurysms and hemorrhage. Treatment is directed to the endocarditis and septicemia.

Legionnaire's disease, *Mycoplasma pneumoniae*, and *Listeria monocytogenes* infections may cause multiple foci of inflammation in the brain—strictly speaking a picture of bacterial encephalitis.

Subdural Empyema

This is a purulent infection of the subdural space, stemming usually from disease of the frontal or ethmoid sinuses or middle ears and mastoid cells. Pus accumulates over one cerebral hemisphere. The arachnoid prevents a sufficient number of organisms from entering the subarachnoid space and inducing a bacterial meningitis. There is, however, a polymorphonuclear pleocytosis (50 to 1000 per mm^3) and an elevated CSF protein; the glucose is normal. Meningeal veins that underly the empyema become thrombosed and give rise to cortical infarction, which is the cause of the cerebral symptoms.

Diagnosis is based on the presence of a known sinus or ear infection, generalized headache and fever, rapid accession of focal seizures, hemiparesis, hemisensory loss and aphasia, and a sterile CSF under increased pressure. CT scanning and MRI disclose the extracerebral accumulation of pus.

Treatment consists of administration of large doses of wide spectrum antibiotics (20 to 24 million units penicillin per day plus chloramphenicol, 2 to 4 g/day, modified according to bacteriologic findings) and surgical drainage.

Extradural Abscess

This is usually associated with osteomyelitis of a cranial bone. Local pain and tenderness, purulent discharge from an ear or sinus, affection of cranial nerves V and VI (Gradenigo syndrome), and a normal CSF (except for a few cells) are the usual manifestations. *Staphylococcus aureus* is the most common agent. Vigorous administration of antibiotics and, later, surgical removal of the infected bone are the recommended treatment.

Intracranial Thrombophlebitis and Aseptic Venous Thrombosis

The *lateral sinus* may become thrombosed in the course of an ear infection and block cerebral venous drainage sufficiently to cause a rise in CSF pressure. Facial and nasal infections may lead to thrombosis of the anterior part of the cavernous sinus on one or both sides, manifested by orbital edema and involvement of cranial nerves III, IV, and VI and ophthalmic division of V. Thrombosis of the superior longitudinal sinus and its draining veins gives rise to headache, seizures, and unilateral or bilateral paralysis, mainly of the legs.

The occurrence of these conditions should always be suspected in the presence of some other form of intracranial suppuration—meningitis, sinus or ear infection, subdural empyema, extradural or brain abscess—or some disease state that renders the blood hypercoagulable (e.g., polycythemia, congenital heart disease, postpartum and postoperative states, sickle cell anemia). Thrombosis of major venous sinuses can often be detected by MRI, and the diagnosis can be corroborated by direct jugular venography or by failure of the superior sagittal sinus to fill during the late phase of carotid arteriography. Treatment consists of large doses of antibiotics, after which surgery on the offending ear or sinus may be necessary.

Brain Abscess

The brain is resistant to abscess formation, but this will occur under conditions that cause necrosis of tissue with simultaneous bacterial infection. The disease states that are conducive to the formation of brain abscess are chronic pulmonary infections (peribronchial pneumonitis, bronchiectasis, lung abscess); chronic and recurrent sinusitis, otitis, or mastoiditis; congenital heart disease or pulmonary vascular malformation; distant infection of skin, bone, and kidney; and rarely acute bacterial endocarditis. In a considerable proportion of cases, the source of the abscess cannot be determined.

The abscess, as it forms over a period of several weeks, passes through several stages—from localized suppurative encephalitis to complete encapsulation. There may be one or several abscesses, depending on the cause. Those secondary to ear and sinus infection are single with one or more daughter abscesses and are localized in the part of the brain nearest the source. Thus, with frontal-ethmoidal sinusitis, the abscess tends to form in the frontal lobe; with sphenoid sinusitis, in the frontal or anterior temporal lobe; with otitis media, in the middle or posterior temporal lobe; and with mastoiditis, in the cerebellum.

Clinical manifestations Headache is the most frequent presenting symptom, followed by drowsiness, confusion, focal or generalized seizures, and focal motor, sensory, visual field, and language disorders. The focal signs may vary with the location of the abscess. With frontal abscess, frontal headache, hemiparesis, and unilateral contraversive seizures are the most prominent manifestations; with temporal lobe abscess, frontotemporal headache, upper homonymous quadrantanopia, dysnomia, and other aphasic symptoms if left-sided; and with cerebellar abscess, postauricular headache, ipsilateral ataxia, and paresis of gaze to the side of the lesion with gaze-paretic nystagmus.

In all types of abscess, the CSF pressure is elevated and there is usually a pleocytosis with elevated protein but normal glucose. The symptoms progress over a period of two or more weeks. CT scanning and MRI reveal the lesion(s).

Treatment Acute suppurative encephalitis requires the administration of 20 to 24 million units of penicillin G and 4 to 6 g chloramphenicol daily IV in divided doses. The initial elevation of ICP is managed by IV mannitol, followed by dexamethasone 6–12 mg every 6 h. Failure to respond to these measures requires aspiration of the abscess for precise bacteriologic diagnosis and open surgical drainage if the abscess is single and superficial. If the abscess is deep, aspiration and injection of antibiotics are the only treatment, which may have to be repeated. Multiple abscesses can be treated only by parenteral antibiotics (penicillin and chloramphenicol).

Tuberculous Meningitis

Once frequent, tuberculous meningitis is now rarely seen in the United States and western Europe, reflecting the decreasing incidence of pulmonary tuberculosis. However, the disease is still common in India and other underdeveloped countries and is being reported with increasing frequency in AIDS patients.

The *causal agent, Myobacterium tuberculosis*, usually reaches the brain via the blood stream, the bacteremia occurring intermittently with pulmonary tuberculosis. The meningitis may be a manifestation of miliary tuberculosis or occur in association with one or more tuberculomatous foci in the brain, which spread infection to the meninges. Otitic, renal, or other sources are rare.

The *pathologic reaction* differs from other meningitides in that the meningeal exudate is mainly basal and there are myriads of small tubercles (foci of caseation, epithelioid cells, and Langhans' giant cells) on the external surface of the brain and ependyma. Tension hydrocephalus is usually present. Brain infarction is frequent because of meningeal arteritis.

Clinical and laboratory features Fever, headache, confusion, and lethargy evolve less acutely than in other forms of bacterial meningitis, and cranial nerve palsies are prominent. Occasionally the disease presents by some focal cerebral sign or with signs of increased ICP.

The CSF formula is diagnostic: Increased pressure, pleocytosis (100 to 500 cells/mm^3, with lymphocytes predominating after a few days); protein increased to 100 to 200 mg/dL, and low glucose (<40 mg/dL). When this spectrum of changes is found in a febrile patient and fungal infections and meningeal carcinomatosis can be excluded, antituberculous therapy should be instituted at once. Tubercle bacilli are often difficult to find in smears of CSF, and cultures do not become positive for 3 to 4 weeks or longer.

Chest films may demonstrate the source of the infection, and CT scanning and MRI may reveal hydrocephalus, tuberculomas, or zones of infarction.

Treatment If unrecognized and untreated, tuberculous meningitis is invariably fatal. Treatment consists of administration of a combination of drugs: (1) isoniazid (5 mg/kg daily in adults and 10 mg/kg for children); (2) rifampin (600 mg daily for adults and 15 mg/kg for children); and (3) a third drug, which may be ethambutol (15 mg/kg per day), ethionamide (750 to 1000 mg daily in divided doses after meals), or pyrazinamide (30 to 50 mg/kg per day). The drugs need to be given for 18 to 24 months as a rule. Details of administration, adverse effects, etc., are discussed in the *Principles*.

Ventricular shunting may be needed for patients who remain stuporous with large ventricles.

Sarcoidosis

This disease involves the peripheral or central nervous system in about 5 percent of cases. It may present as a solitary granulomatous mass, especially in or around the pituitary stalk, or elsewhere. Single or multiple cranial or peripheral nerves may be implicated. A relatively common combination of abnormalities are chronic uveitis, parotitis, and facial nerve involvement (uveoparotid syndrome).

Diagnosis is based on the general medical findings (lesions of the uveal tract, skin, lungs, and bones); blood findings, including hyperglobulinemia and increased concentration of angiotensin-converting enzyme; and biopsy of a peripheral lesion (noncaseating granuloma). Contrast-enhanced CT scanning and MRI may show meningeal involvement and white matter lesions, respectively.

Recent onset of symptoms requires treatment with corticosteroids given over a period of many months. (See the *Principles*.)

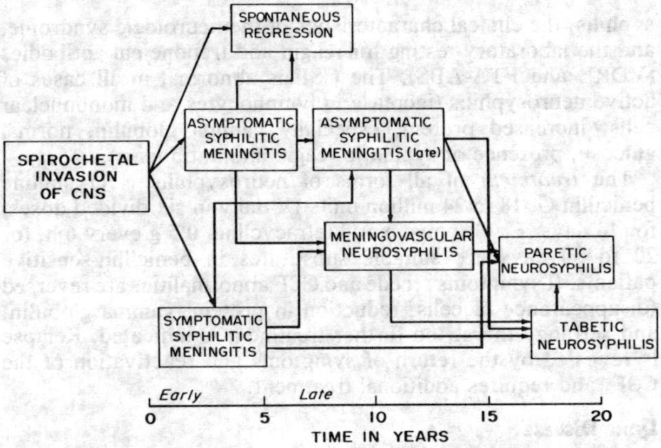

FIG. 30-1 Diagram of the evolution of neurosyphilis.

Neurosyphilis

Treponema pallidum is the recognized cause of a wide range of neurologic syndromes, which include acute syphilitic meningitis, meningovascular syphilis, syphilitic meningo-encephalitis (general paresis or paretic neurosyphilis), syphilitic lumbosacral radiculitis (tabes dorsalis), other forms of myelitis, and optic neuritis. The incidence of these late forms of syphilis has decreased dramatically during the past three to four decades.

As indicated in Fig. 30-1, all of these syndromes derive from a common, low-grade, often asymptomatic syphilitic meningitis. In fact, this is the most chronic of any known form of meningitis and may be active for 10 to 15 years. In its more subacute phase (within 2 years of infection) it may present with headache, drowsiness, and cranial nerve palsies (*meningeal syphilis*). After 2 to 10 years, arterial inflammation may result in a stroke (*meningovascular syphilis*). *General paresis* is a gradual dementing meningoencephalitis appearing 15 to 20 years after the onset of infection. *Tabes dorsalis* (literally a wasting of the dorsal funiculi of the spinal cord secondary to lumbosacral radiculitis) presents, after 15 to 20 years, with a chronic syndrome of lancinating pains in the legs, gastric crises of pain, deep sensory loss and ataxia, impotence, hypotonia of the bladder and urinary incontinence, Charcot joints, and Argyll Robertson pupils. *Optic neuritis* is often added; it consists of unilateral and later bilateral loss of vision and optic atrophy.

Diagnosis is based on a history of primary or secondary

syphilis, the clinical characteristics of the neurologic syndrome, and the laboratory testing for reagin and treponemal antibodies (VDRL and FTA-ABS). The CSF is abnormal in all cases of active neurosyphilis (increase in lymphocytes and mononuclear cells, increased protein, especially gamma globulin, normal glucose, presence of syphilitic reagin and antibodies).

The *treatment* of all forms of neurosyphilis is crystalline penicillin G, 18 to 24 million units IV daily in six divided doses, for 14 days. Erythromycin and tetracycline, 0.5 g every 6 h, for 20 to 30 days are suitable substitutes in penicillin-sensitive patients. If symptoms recede and CSF abnormalities are reversed (disappearance of cells, reduction in protein, gamma globulin, and serology titers), no further treatment is indicated. Relapse is revealed by the return of symptoms and reactivation of the CSF, and requires additional treatment.

Lyme Disease

This disease, known in Europe as *erythema chronicum migrans,* has been encountered with increasing frequency during the past decade. The infective agent is the spirochete *Borrelia burgdorferi,* and the vectors are the common ixodid ticks. The initial manifestation, at the site of the tick bite, is an enlarging erythematous lesion, sometimes surrounded by satellites. The skin lesion may be overlooked or disregarded but is followed, weeks to months later, by arthritis (two-thirds of cases), cardiac manifestations (15 percent), and neurologic complications (8 percent). The disease is not fatal but can lead to prolonged disability if not recognized and treated. The neurologic involvement most often takes the form of a fluctuating meningoencephalitis (headache, stiff neck, nausea and vomiting, chronic fatigue) with cranial or peripheral neuritis and sometimes a polymyositis. A myelitic syndrome is also documented. Meningeal symptoms are associated with a CSF lymphocytosis (up to 3000 per mm^3), an elevated protein content, but normal glucose.

Diagnostic laboratory tests are the indirect immunofluorescence assay and the enzyme-linked immunosorbent assay (ELISA). The use of oral penicillin, tetracycline, or erythromycin in the initial stage of the disease will prevent the cardiac, arthritic, and neurologic manifestations. The onset of meningeal symptoms requires high doses of antibiotics—penicillin, 20 million units daily IV for 10 days, or tetracycline, 500 mg qid for 30 days. Concomitant administration of prednisone is said to be helpful.

Fungal Infections of the CNS

These are much less common than bacterial infections. Cryptococcosis, candidiasis, aspergillosis, mucormycosis, coccidioidomycosis, blastomycosis, and actinomycosis have all been identified, but only the first three occur with any degree of regularity. These infections may arise without obvious predisposing cause, but more often they complicate some other disease process, such as malignancy or one that suppresses the body's immune responses (*opportunistic infections*).

Cryptococcosis (formerly called torulosis) is the fungal infection seen most often in eastern United States. It gives rise to a subacutely evolving meningitis and meningoencephalitis, the symptoms of which are much the same as tuberculous meningitis. The CSF findings are also similar. *Specific diagnosis* depends upon identifying *Cryptococcus neoformans* in Gram stains of the CSF, culturing the organism on Sabouraud glucose agar, and a positive latex agglutination test for the cryptococcal polysaccharide antigen in the CSF. *Treatment* consists of IV administration of amphotericin B. After a test dose of 5 mg, the drug is given in a dosage of 1.0 mg/kg every second day to a total of 2 to 3 g. The addition of flucytosine (150 mg/kg per day) results in fewer failures and decreased nephrotoxicity, but the mortality is still about 40 percent.

Infections Caused by Protozoa and Worms

Of the protozoal infections, only *toxoplasmosis* is observed with any frequency in the United States and Europe. Immunocompromised adults, notably those with AIDS, are particularly vulnerable. In healthy adults, the infection is usually asymptomatic, but an infected mother may transmit the disease to her unborn fetus. The disease takes the form of a multifocal encephalitis with inflammatory necrotic foci, large enough to be seen by CT scanning and MRI. Diagnosis is established by finding the organisms in the CSF sediment and by a positive Sabin-Feldman test. Treatment with sulfadiazine (2 to 6 g daily) and pyrimethamine (25 mg daily) should be continued for at least 4 weeks, and lifelong in patients with AIDS.

Cysticercosis and *schistosomiasis* are major infections in certain parts of the world, and involvement of the nervous system greatly worsens the outcome. Cysticercosis (the larval or intermediate stage of infection with the pork tapeworm *Taenia solium*) causes focal inflammatory lesions in the brain, which become encysted and calcified and often epileptogenic. Large intraventricular cysts may cause hydrocephalus. The calcified lesions are readily seen on CT scans.

Rarely, the ova of trematodes (schistosomiasis) cause necrotizing foci in the brain or spinal cord. *Treatment* of both cysticercosis and schistosomiasis has been greatly enhanced by the use of the antihelminthic agent praziquantel.

Trichinosis presents essentially as a self-limiting polymyositis, involving cranial muscles and heart. Rarely, cerebral emboli complicate the mycocarditis (see *Principles*).

For a more detailed discussion of this topic, see Adams and Victor: *Principles of Neurology*, 4th ed, pp 554–589.

ADDITIONAL READING

Coonrod JD, Dans PE: Subdural empyema. *Am J Med* 53:85, 1972.

Finkel M: Lyme disease and its neurologic complications. *Arch Neurol* 45:99, 1988.

Kroll JS, Moxon ER: Acute bacterial meningitis, in Kennedy PGE, Johnson RT (eds): *Infections of the Nervous System*. Boston, Butterworth, 1987, chap 2, pp 2–22.

Leys, D, Destee A, Petit H, Warot P: Management of subdural intracranial empyemas should not always require surgery. *J Neurol Neurosurg Psychiatry* 49:635, 1986.

Reik L: Spirochetal infections of the nervous system, in Kennedy PGE, Johnson RT (eds): *Infections of the Nervous System*. Boston, Butterworth, 1987, chap 4, pp 43–75.

Swartz, MN: "Chronic meningitis"—many causes to consider. *N Engl J Med* 317:957, 1987.

Walsh, TJ, Hier DB, Caplan LR: Fungal infections of the central nervous system: Comparative analysis of risk factors and clinical signs in 57 patients. *Neurology* 35:1654, 1985.

31 Viral Infections of the Nervous System

Viruses enter the body in many ways—via the respiratory passages (mumps, measles, varicella), the oral-intestinal route (enteroviruses) or the genital-mucosal route (herpes), by inoculation (arboviruses, AIDS), or transplacentally (rubella, cytomegalus virus). Another pathway is along peripheral nerves (herpes, rabies). Once the nervous system is invaded, the virus multiplies in selective regions of the brain or spinal cord or in the choroid plexuses and meninges. Six syndromes are thus induced, occurring with such regularity that if recognized they not only stamp the infection as viral but also indicate the identity of the virus. These syndromes are as follows:

1. Acute anterior poliomyelitis
2. Herpes zoster ganglionitis
3. Acute aseptic (nonsuppurative) meningitis
4. Acute encephalitis or meningoencephalitis
5. Chronic infections due to "slow viruses" and unconventional agents
6. Acquired immunodeficiency syndrome (AIDS)

SYNDROME OF ACUTE ANTERIOR POLIOMYELITIS

In the past, this syndrome was almost invariably due to one of the three types of poliovirus. Antipoliomyelitic vaccines have practically eliminated the disease, but occasional cases still occur in unvaccinated children and in adults exposed to a vaccinated child. A similar, though generally benign, syndrome can be caused by other enteroviruses, such as Coxsackie viruses A and B and echoviruses.

Clinical features Fever, malaise, headache, nausea and vomiting, and stiffness and aching of muscles are followed, in three to four days, by pain in the back and neck and signs of mild meningeal irritation and then weakness or paralysis of muscles.

In most cases the disease arrests in the preparalytic phase and cannot be distinguished from other viral diseases that give rise to aseptic meningitis. The latter are considered further on.

Paralysis, when it develops, usually attains its maximum severity in 48 hours or less, rarely longer. The distribution of paralysis is quite variable. Weakness of one or both legs or an arm and both legs are the most common forms. Trunk muscles may be severely affected, or paralysis may be purely bulbar, with fatal respiratory failure. Tendon reflexes are lost. Paresthesias and muscle pain are frequent complaints, but sensory loss cannot be demonstrated. Bladder and smooth muscles are usually spared. The CSF shows a modest increase in cells, mainly mononuclear, and in protein, but the glucose is normal.

The final outcome is an atrophic, areflexive paralysis, always less severe than the acute paralysis. A gradual increase in weakness may occur 20 to 30 or more years after the acute paralytic illness.

Pathologic changes Destruction of anterior horn cells with phagocytosis of cell remnants by microgliacytes, gliosis, and perivascular meningeal infiltrates of lymphocytes and monocytes comprise the principal changes. Nerve cells in the bulbar motor nuclei, dentate nuclei, and motor cortex are also involved.

Treatment Prevention is the essence. The Sabin vaccine, which consists of attenuated live virus, is administered orally to infants in two doses 8 weeks apart, with boosters at 1 year and 4 years of age. Poliomyelitis may follow vaccination (0.02 to 0.04 cases per million doses).

Treatment of paralytic poliomyelitis is purely supportive, utilizing respiratory assistance and physical therapy.

SYNDROME OF HERPES ZOSTER

This well-known disorder (also called zona or "shingles") is caused by the varicella-zoster virus. It has an overall incidence of three to five cases per thousand per year and is considerably more frequent in the elderly and in those with malignancies, particularly lymphoma and Hodgkin disease. Herpes zoster probably represents a reactivation of varicella virus infection which has been latent in sensory ganglia following the primary infection with chicken pox.

Clinical features The characteristic manifestations are radicular pain, a vesicular cutaneous eruption spread over two or three dermatomes on one side of the body, and in some cases sensory and motor impairment in the segments bearing the skin lesions. The vesicular eruption is preceded for 3 to 4 days (or as long as 7 days) by dysesthesias in the involved dermatomes; or there may be severe localized pain suggestive of pleurisy or an acute abdominal condition.

Any part of the body may be affected, but thoracic lesions are the most frequent. When cranial ganglia are affected, two special syndromes with prominent paralytic features appear: (1) *ophthalmic herpes*, with pain and eruption in the distribution of the first division of the trigeminal nerve, ophthalmoplegia, and risk of corneal ulceration; and (2) so-called *geniculate herpes* (Ramsay Hunt syndrome), with facial paralysis, otic-palatal vesiculation, vertigo, and deafness. *Herpes occipitocollaris*, with involvement of palate, pharynx, neck, and retroauricular region, depends upon herpetic infection of the ganglia of cranial nerves IX and X and upper cervical roots. The CSF may contain 10 to 100 cells and a slightly increased amount of protein.

Pain and dysesthesia last for 1 to 4 weeks in most cases, but in as many as one-third of patients, pain persists for months or even years and creates a difficult therapeutic problem.

Pathologically there is an intense inflammation in two or three dorsal root or cranial nerve ganglia and in corresponding posterior and anterior roots, adjacent meninges, and gray matter of the spinal cord on one side. The latter lesion is a veritable poliomyelitis, but the neuronal destruction is more in the posterior than in the anterior horn. Myelitis and encephalitis are rare complications.

Treatment A course of acyclovir (800 mg five times daily for 7 days), if begun within 48 h after the appearance of the rash, shortens the period of acute pain and hastens the healing of the vesicles. It does not prevent the occurrence of postherpetic neuralgia, however. In nonimmunosuppressed patients, prednisone (45 to 60 mg/day for 7 days, then tapered) decreases the incidence of postherpetic neuralgia. The latter disorder is best treated by a combination of carbamazepine and amitriptyline, beginning with small doses that are gradually increased to 400 to 800 and 75 to 150 mg/day, respectively.

THE SYNDROME OF ASEPTIC MENINGITIS

The term *aseptic meningitis* designates a common clinical syndrome consisting of fever, headache, and other signs of meningeal irritation and a predominantly lymphocytic pleocytosis with normal CSF glucose. Photophobia and pain on movement of the eyes are other common complaints. Sometimes drowsiness and confusion are added, making it difficult to distinguish a pure meningitis from a meningoencephalitis. The CSF reaction is the same in both—pleocytosis, mainly lymphocytes, up to 1000 per mm^3, increase in protein, but normal glucose. Very rarely, the glucose level is reduced.

Most cases of aseptic meningitis are due to viral infections, but there are important nonviral causes as well.

Viral Causes of Meningitis

1. Enteroviral infections: Echovirus, Coxsackie, and nonparalytic poliomyelitis. Peak incidence in August and September. These viruses account for 80 percent of cases of established viral etiology.
2. Mumps: Highest incidence is in late winter and spring. Male-to-female ratio is 3 : 1.
3. Herpes simplex, type 2 (rarely type 1), and Epstein-Barr (EB) virus.
4. Lymphocytic choriomeningitis: Lymphocyte count in CSF may be 1000 per mm^3 or higher. Infection is acquired by contact with infected hamsters and mice, mainly in late fall and winter.
5. Adenovirus infections.
6. HIV (AIDS) may cause an acute, self-limited aseptic meningitis with a clinical picture like that of infectious mononucleosis (EB virus).

Most of these conditions are benign. Diagnosis is by viral isolation and serologic tests performed during the acute and convalescent phases of the illness. A specific cause cannot be established in one-quarter or more of cases of presumed viral origin, despite careful cultures and neurologic studies.

Nonviral Causes of Aseptic Meningitis

1. Spirochetal infections: Syphilitic meningitis and Lyme disease, described in Chap. 30. Leptospirosis, with a peak incidence in August, is acquired by contact with contaminated urine of rats, dogs, swine, and cattle.
2. *Mycoplasma pneumoniae:* Cold agglutinins in the serum toward the end of the first week of illness are diagnostic.
3. Bacterial infections lying adjacent to the meninges.
4. Neoplastic invasion of meninges by lymphoma or carcinoma.
5. Recurrent inflammatory meningitides of obscure origin—Vogt-Koyanagi-Harada syndrome (iridocyclitis, depigmentation of skin, deafness); meningitis with serum sickness and connective tissue disease such as lupus erythematosus; Behçet disease (relapsing meningitis, iridocyclitis, ulcers of mouth and genitalia).

In the diagnosis of aseptic meningitis, it is important to rule out tuberculosis, cryptococcosis, Lyme disease, syphilis, and inadequately treated bacterial meningitis, all of which require urgent treatment.

SYNDROME OF ACUTE ENCEPHALITIS

In this class of viral diseases, a febrile illness is expressed by meningitis, to which are added the following neurologic abnormalities in various combinations: impairment of consciousness (confusion, stupor, and coma); seizures; mutism or aphasia; hemiparesis, with asymmetry of reflexes and Babinski signs; involuntary movements, cerebellar ataxia, and polymyoclonia; and cranial nerve palsies. With the exception of herpes simplex encephalitis, the viral encephalitides are seasonal and occur in epidemic form. Diagnosis in other circumstances usually proves to be incorrect. In other words, viral encephalitis is in effect a *meningoencephalitis*, and mild forms of encephalitis, in which the meningeal symptoms and CSF abnormalities predominate, cannot be distinguished from viral (aseptic) meningitis, as mentioned in the preceding section.

Causation

The causes of acute viral meningoencephalitis in their approximate order of frequency are as follows:

1. Mumps virus
2. Arboviruses (Eastern, Western, and Venezuelan equine, St. Louis, California, and Colorado tick fever viruses)
3. Herpes simplex and EB viruses
4. Lymphocytic choriomeningitis virus
5. Enteroviruses (Coxsackie and echoviruses)
6. Cytomegalovirus
7. Adenoviruses
8. Rabies virus

Herpes Simplex Encephalitis

This, the most serious of the viral encephalitides, occurs sporadically throughout the year, in patients of all ages and in all parts of the world. It is caused by type 1 herpes simplex virus, very rarely by type 2 (genital herpes).

The symptoms, consisting of fever, headache, confusion, stupor, and coma, evolve over a period of several days. Additional symptoms in some patients include olfactory and gustatory hallucinations, temporal lobe seizures, changes in personality and behavior, and aphasia. The latter symptoms betray the localization of the disease process in the inferior and medial parts of the temporal lobes and orbital parts of the frontal lobes. The lesions are characterized by intense inflammation, often hemorrhagic, and pannecrosis of nearly all tissue elements.

Intranuclear eosinophilic inclusions are found in neurons and glial cells.

The lesions can be seen by CT scanning and MRI. The CSF findings are like those of other encephalitides (predominantly mononuclear pleocytosis, elevated protein, normal glucose), except that there may be as many as several thousand red cells. Certain EEG findings (periodic high-voltage sharp waves in the temporal leads and slow wave complexes at 2- to 3-second intervals) should suggest the diagnosis. If the diagnosis is reasonably certain, it is preferable to proceed at once with treatment. Brain biopsy carries a greater risk than the inappropriate use of antiviral agents.

About half the patients with this disease do not survive, and many of those who do are left with a severe amnesic state and seizures.

Treatment consists of the administration of *acyclovir* (30 mg/kg per day for 14 days). Initiation of treatment early in the illness (before the onset of stupor and coma) significantly reduces mortality and the severity of the residual neurologic deficits.

Nonviral Forms of Encephalitis

Numerous bacterial, fungal, parasitic, and noninfectious diseases may simulate the viral encephalitides and need to be distinguished from them. These nonviral diseases, many of which require urgent therapeutic intervention, are listed in Table 31-1.

CHRONIC INFECTIONS DUE TO "SLOW VIRUSES" AND UNCONVENTIONAL AGENTS

Subacute sclerosing panencephalitis This is a slowly evolving inflammatory disease appearing in children and adolescents several years after an attack of measles. It is characterized by a dementia, focal or generalized seizures, ataxia of gait, and myoclonus. The EEG is typical—periodic bursts of high-voltage slow waves followed by a flat pattern. Gamma globulin and measles antibodies are greatly elevated in the CSF. Since measles vaccine became widely used, the neurologic disease has virtually disappeared.

A subacute progressive panencephalitis occurring many years after congenital rubella has also been identified.

Progressive multifocal leukoencephalopathy (PML) This disease is usually associated with Hodgkin disease, lymphoma, or chronic leukemia and less often with tuberculosis, sarcoid, AIDS, or other states of immunosuppression. It develops over a 3- to 6-month period, with focal cerebral, brainstem, and cerebellar

TABLE 31-1 Diseases Simulating Viral Encephalitis

- Rickettsial
  - Rocky Mountain spotted fever
  - Typhus
- Bacterial
  - *Mycoplasma pneumoniae*
  - Leptospirosis
  - Lyme disease
  - Syphilis (secondary or meningovascular)
  - Listeriosis
  - Brucellosis (particularly *Brucella melitensis*)
  - Tuberculosis
  - Typhoid fever
  - Parameningeal infections (epidural, petrositis)
  - Partially treated bacterial meningitis
  - Subacute bacterial endocarditis
  - Brain abscess
- Fungal
  - Cryptococcosis
  - Coccidioidomycosis
  - Histoplasmosis
  - North American blastomycosis
  - Candidiasis
- Parasitic
  - Toxoplasmosis
  - Cysticercosis
  - Echinococcosis
  - Trypanosomiasis
  - *Plasmodium falciparum*
  - Amebiasis (*Naegleria* and *Acanthamoeba*)
- Neoplastic
  - Carcinomatous meningitis
  - Gliomatosis cerebri
- Vascular
  - Granulomatous angiitis
  - Systemic lupus erythematosus
- Others
  - Sarcoid
  - Behcet syndrome
  - Oculocephalic syndromes

signs. The lesions are demyelinative in nature. Inclusion bodies are seen in oligodendrocytes, and astrocytes are gigantic and show tumor-like mitoses. A polyoma virus—designated JC virus—has been isolated from the lesions. There is no effective treatment.

Subacute spongiform encephalopathy (SSE) This disease, also referred to as *Creutzfeldt-Jakob disease*, is characterized by a rapidly progressive dementia in association with cerebellar ataxia, heightened startle reaction, and diffuse myoclonic jerks. The CSF is normal. In many cases, the EEG is diagnostic—high-voltage slow and sharp waves on an increasingly flat background ("burst suppression"). As the disease advances, the patient becomes totally unresponsive and the outcome is invariably fatal, usually in less than a year.

The disease affects principally the cerebral and cerebellar cortices, where there is a diffuse loss of neurons, gliosis, and a striking vacuolation of the tissues. Inflammatory changes are absent, and no inclusion bodies have been observed. The disease is due to an unconventional virus-like agent, which can be transmitted to chimpanzees, with an incubation period of more than a year. Pathologically and epidemiologically SSE resembles a disease first recognized among natives of New Guinea and known as kuru.

There is no known treatment. Precautions need to be taken in the medical care of these patients, like those recommended for patients with hepatitis B (see *Harrison's Principles of Internal Medicine*).

THE ACQUIRED IMMUNODEFICIENCY SYNDROME (AIDS)

This new viral syndrome is characterized by an acquired and unusually profound depression of cell-mediated immunity (cutaneous anergy, lymphopenia, reversal of T-helper/T-suppressor cell ratios, and depressed in vitro lymphoproliferative response to various antigens and mitogens). The causative virus, originally called human T-cell lymphotropic virus (HTLV), is now generally referred to as human immunodeficiency virus (HIV or HIV-1). The diseases it induces, due to the effects of the virus itself and a wide array of opportunistic infections and neoplasms, are grouped under the name acquired immunodeficiency syndrome (AIDS).

Epidemiology AIDS is mainly a disease of homosexual or bisexual men (72 percent) and of male and female drug users (17 percent). A smaller group at risk are hemophiliacs (and other patients who receive transfusions or injections of blood products) and infants born of mothers with AIDS. There is a small group of heterosexual men who appear to have been infected by prostitutes. Four-fifths of the patients in the United States reside in New York, California, New Jersey, and Florida.

Clinical manifestations These range from the asymptomatic seroconversion state to widespread lymphadenopathy, diarrhea, and weight loss (AIDS-related complex, or ARC) to full-blown AIDS, comprising all of the complications listed in Table 31-2. In approximately one-third of patients, the CNS or PNS has been

TABLE 31-2 Neurologic Complications in HIV-1 Infected Patients

- Brain
  - Predominantly nonfocal
    - AIDS dementia complex (subacute-chronic HIV encephalitis)
    - Acute HIV-related encephalitis
    - Cytomegalovirus encephalitis
    - Herpes simplex virus encephalitis
    - Metabolic encephalopathies
  - Predominantly focal
    - Cerebral toxoplasmosis
    - Progressive multifocal leukoencephalopathy
    - Cryptococcosis
    - Varicella-zoster virus encephalitis
    - Tuberculous brain abscess/tuberculoma
    - Neurosyphilis (meningovascular)
    - Vascular disorders—notably nonbacterial endocarditis and cerebral hemorrhages associated with thrombocytopenia
    - Primary CNS lymphoma
- Spinal cord
  - Vacuolar myelopathy
  - Herpes simplex or zoster myelitis
- Meninges
  - Aseptic meningitis (HIV)
  - Cryptococcal meningitis
  - Tuberculous meningitis
  - Syphilitic meningitis
  - Metastatic lymphomatous meningitis
- Peripheral nerve and root
  - Infectious
    - Herpes zoster
    - Cytomegalovirus polyradiculopathy
  - Virus or immune related
    - Acute and chronic inflammatory HIV polyneuritis
    - Mononeuritis multiplex
    - Sensorimotor demyelinating polyneuropathy
    - Distal painful sensory polyneuritis
  - Muscle
    - Polymyositis and other myopathies

Source: Brew et al.

clinically involved by the time of death, and at postmortem nearly all patients prove to have CNS lesions.

The neurologic manifestations are too numerous and varied to describe in detail. They are listed in Table 31-2 and are described in the references at the end of this chapter.

Laboratory tests Many screening tests are now available, all of them based on an enzyme-linked immunoassay (ELISA). While highly sensitive, there is a high incidence of false positives. The

Western blot test, which identifies antibodies to viral proteins, is more specific and is being used to confirm a positive screening test.

Treatment There is as yet no satisfactory treatment for the primary HIV infection. Azidothymidine (AZT) has been helpful in controlling *Pneumocystis carinii* infections and possibly HIV infection. There is some recent evidence that low-dosage AZT taken over a long period of time may prevent seroconversion individuals from developing AIDS.

The opportunistic infections and the lymphomas should be treated individually.

For a more detailed discussion of this topic, see Adams and Victor: *Principles of Neurology*, 4th ed, pp 590–616.

ADDITIONAL READING

Brew B, Sidtis J, Petito CK, Price RW: The neurologic complications of AIDS and immunodeficiency virus infection, in Plum F (ed): *Advances in Contempoary Neurology*. Philadelphia, FA Davis, 1988, chap 1.

Johnson RT: *Viral Infections of the Nervous System*. New York, Raven, 1982.

Leehey M, Gilden D: Neurologic disorders associated with the HIV and HIV-1 viruses, in Appel SH (ed): *Current Neurology*, vol 10. St. Louis, Mosby/Year Book Publishers, 1990.

Matthews WB: Slow infections, in Kennedy PGE, Johnson RT (ed): *Infections of the Nervous System*. London, Butterworth, 1987, pp 227–247.

Richardson EP Jr: Progressive multifocal leukoencephalopathy. *N Engl J Med* 265:815, 1961.

Rosenblum ML, Levy RM, Bredesen DE (eds): *AIDS and the Nervous System*. New York, Raven, 1988.

Whitley RJ: The frustrations of treating herpes simplex virus infections of the central nervous system. *JAMA* 259:1067, 1988.

Whitley RJ: Viral encephalitis. *N Engl J Med* 323:242, 1990.

32 | Cerebrovascular Diseases

Cerebrovascular disease follows heart disease and cancer as the most frequent cause of death in the western world. And at least one-half of all neurologic patients in general has some type of cerebrovascular disease.

The term *cerebrovascular disease* denotes any abnormality of the brain resulting from a pathologic process of blood vessels. The pathologic change in the vessels takes the form of occlusion by thrombus or embolus, or of rupture, and the resulting parenchymal changes in the brain are of two types: ischemia, with and without infarction, and hemorrhage. Rarer forms of cerebrovascular disease are those due to altered permeability of the vascular wall and increased viscosity or other changes in the quality of blood. These changes underlie the strokes that complicate diseases such as sickle-cell anemia and polycythemia and account for the headache, brain edema, and convulsions of hypertensive encephalopathy. There are many more types of cerebrovascular disease; these are listed in Table 32-1, and their relative frequency is indicated in Table 32-2.

The stroke syndrome The distinctive mode of presentation of cerebral vascular disease is the stroke, defined as any sudden or acute nonconvulsive focal neurologic deficit. In its most severe form the patient becomes hemiplegic or falls senseless, an event so dramatic that it is given its own name—apoplexy, cerebrovascular accident, stroke, or shock. If death does not follow within hours or days, there is nearly always some degree of recovery of function. This temporal profile of neurologic events, whether condensed into several hours or days, is diagnostic. Variations in the temporal profile reflect the type of vascular lesion. Embolic strokes characteristically begin with absolute suddenness, and they may at times recede rapidly or they may last. Thrombotic strokes may have a similarly abrupt onset, but often they are somewhat slower in evolution, over a period of minutes to hours or even days. Cerebral hemorrhage from its onset causes a deficit that is steadily progressive for hours or longer.

TABLE 32-1 Causes of Cerebral Vascular Disease

1. Atherosclerotic thrombosis
2. Transient ischemic attacks
3. Embolism
4. Ruptured or unruptured saccular aneurysm or AVM
5. Arteritis
   a. Meningovascular syphilis, arteritis secondary to pyogenic and tuberculous meningitis, rare infective types (typhus, schistosomiasis, malaria, trichinosis, mucormycosis, etc.)
   b. Connective tissue diseases (polyarteritis nodosa, lupus erythematosus), necrotizing arteritis, Wegener arteritis, temporal arteritis, Takayasu disease, granulomatous or giant cell arteritis of the aorta, and giant cell granulomatous angiitis of cerebral arteries
6. Cerebral thrombophlebitis: secondary to infection of ear, paranasal sinus, face, etc.; with meningitis and subdural empyema; debilitating states, postpartum, postoperative, cardiac failure, hematologic disease (polycythemia, sickle-cell disease), and of undetermined cause
7. Hematologic disorders: polycythemia, sickle-cell disease, thrombotic thrombocytopenic purpura, thrombocytosis, etc.
8. Trauma to carotid artery
9. Dissecting aortic aneurysm
10. Systemic hypotension with arterial stenoses: "simple faint," acute blood loss, myocardial infarction, Stokes-Adams syndrome, traumatic and surgical shock, sensitive carotid sinus, severe postural hypotension
11. Complications of arteriography
12. Neurologic migraine with persistent deficit
13. With tentorial, foramen magnum, and subfalcial herniations
14. Miscellaneous types: fibromuscular dysplasia, excessive x-irradiation, unexplained middle cerebral artery territory infarction in closed head injury, pressure of unruptured saccular aneurysm, local dissection of carotid, middle cerebral, or vertebral-basilar arteries, complication of oral contraceptives
15. Undetermined cause as in children and young adults: moyamoya; multiple, progressive intracranial arterial occlusions (Taveras).

The major neurovascular thrombotic and embolic syndromes—their symptoms and signs, and the corresponding regions of cerebral damage—are shown in Figs. 32-1 to 32-7.

Atherosclerotic-Thrombotic Infarction

The large intracranial arteries, like the aorta and coronary arteries, are predisposed to atherosclerotic changes. Favored sites are the common and internal carotid, the vertebral and basilar, and the stems of the major cerebral arteries. Factors enhancing this predilection are hypertension, diabetes mellitus, and hyperlipidemia, both genetic and dietary.

TABLE 32-2 Major Types of Cerebrovascular Diseases and Their Frequency

	Harvard stroke series (756 successive cases)*	BCH autopsy series (179 cases)†
Atherosclerotic thrombosis	244 (32%)	21 (12%)
Lacunes	129 (18%)	34 (18.5%)
Embolism	244 (32%)	57 (32%)
Hypertensive hemorrhage	84 (11%)	28 (15.5%)
Ruptured aneurysms and vascular malformations	55 (7%)	8 (4.5%)
Indeterminate		17 (9.5%)
Other‡		14 (8%)

* Compiled by J Mohr, L Caplan, D Pessin, P Kistler, and G Duncan at Massachusetts General Hospital and Beth Israel Hospital, Boston.
† Compiled by CM Fisher and RD Adams in an examination of 780 brains during the year 1949 at Mallory Institute of Pathology, Boston City Hospital.
‡ Hypertensive encephalopathy, cerebral vein thrombosis, meningovascular syphilis, and polyarteritis nodosa.

More than one-half of patients who develop a thrombotic stroke have one or more brief warning episodes, called transient ischemic attacks (TIAs), the diagnosis and treatment of which may prevent an oncoming stroke (see further on). The thrombotic stroke, whether or not it is preceded by warning attacks, develops in one of the following ways: Most often there is an abrupt onset of the neurologic deficit, evolving over a few minutes to a few hours; or there may be a stuttering onset with intermittent progression over several hours or a day or longer; or symptoms may regress for hours and then advance again. More perplexing still is the rare stroke in which the deficit advances in a series of steps over a period of weeks. Often the onset is during sleep; the patient awakens paralyzed.

The pattern of the neurologic deficit is determined by the site of arterial occlusion and the available anastomotic arrangements.

Ancillary examinations Noninvasive blood flow procedures, such as carotid Doppler studies, may reveal a stenotic or occluded artery. This can be verified by angiography, but this procedure carries a small risk of worsening the neurologic deficit. Digital subtraction angiography (DSA), preferably by the arterial route, more safely but less clearly visualizes the aorta and its main cranial branches. One can see by these several techniques both stenotic segments or occlusion of arteries and sometimes mural thrombi that may become embolic (artery-to-artery embolism).

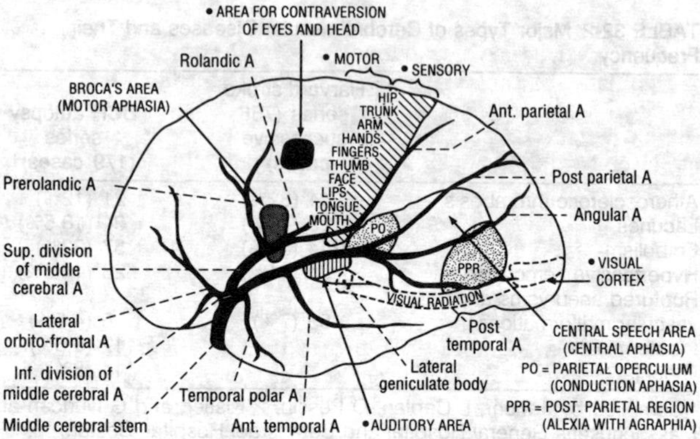

FIG. 32-1 Diagram of a cerebral hemisphere, lateral aspect, showing the branches and distribution of the middle cerebral artery and the principal regions of cerebral localization. Following is a list of the clinical manifestations of infarction in the territory of this artery and the corresponding regions of cerebal damage.

Signs and symptoms	*Structures involved*
Paralysis of the contralateral face, arm, and leg	Somatic motor area for face and arm and the fibers descending from the leg area to enter the corona radiata
Sensory impairment over the contralateral face, arm, and leg (pinprick, cotton touch, vibration, position, two-point discrimination, stereognosis, tactile localization, barognosis, cutaneographia)	Somatic sensory area for face and arm and thalamoparietal projections
Motor speech disorder	Broca's area and frontal operculum of the dominant hemisphere
"Central" aphasia, word deafness, anomia, jargon speech, alexia, agraphia, acalculia, finger agnosia, right-left confusion (the last four comprise the Gerstmann syndrome)	Central language area and parieto-occipital cortex of the dominant hemisphere
Apractagnosia (amorphosynthesis), anosognosia, hemiasomatognosia, unilateral neglect, agnosia for the left half of external space, "dressing apraxia," "constructional apraxia," distortion of visual coordinates, inaccurate localization in the half field, impaired ability to judge distance, upside-down reading, visual illusions	Usually nondominant parietal lobe. Loss of topographic memory is usually due to a nondominant lesion, occasionally to a dominant one

FIG. 32-1 (*continued*)

Signs and symptoms	*Structures involved*
Homonymous hemianopia (often superior homonymous quadrantanopia)	Optic radiation deep to second temporal convolution
Paralysis of conjugate gaze to the opposite side	Frontal contraversive field or fibers projecting therefrom
Avoidance reaction of opposite limbs	Parietal lobe
Miscellaneous:	
Ataxia of contralateral limbs(s)	Parietal lobe
So-called Bruns ataxia or apraxia of gait	Frontal lobes (bilateral)
Loss or impairment of optokinetic nystagmus	Supramarginal or angular gyrus
Limb-kinetic apraxia	Premotor or parietal cortical damage
Mirror movements	Precise location of responsible lesions not known
Cheyne-Stokes respiration, contralateral hyperhidrosis, mydriasis (occasionally)	Precise location of responsible lesions not known
Pure motor hemiplegia	Upper portion of the posterior limb of the internal capsule and the adjacent corona radiata

Treatment Opinion is divided as to whether the administration of IV heparin and oral coumadin, begun as early as possible, are capable of arresting a propagating thrombotic process. Surgical revascularization of an accessible neck vessel may be effective if done within a few hours, but this is feasible in only a tiny proportion of stroke victims. Tissue plasminogen activators are too new to evaluate; so far they have not lived up to their promise. Vasodilators may do more harm than good because they may draw blood away from the marginal zones of the infarct (penumbra). Steroids are indicated only to control the swelling of massive infarcts and threatened herniation.

The long-term therapy of individuals with completed thrombotic infarcts is equally uncertain. Physiotherapy prevents frozen joints and assists the patient in coping with his disabilities but does not hasten the return of function. The prevention of further strokes or heart attacks by long-term anticoagulant or "antiplatelet" drugs have their advocates but are only of minimal value at best.

Prognosis When seen at the onset, prediction of the outcome is difficult, since it depends on whether the stroke is still progressing or has been completed. The mortality rate is high in comatose

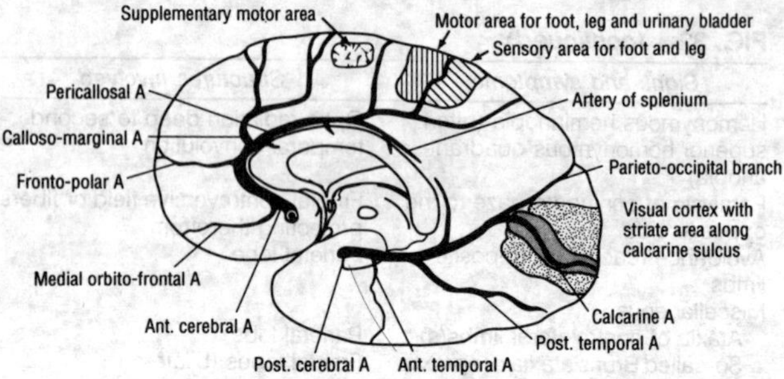

FIG. 32-2 Diagram of a cerebral hemisphere, medial aspect, showing the branches and distribution of the anterior cerebral artery and the principal regions of cerebral localization. Following is a list of the clinical manifestations of infarction in the territory of this artery and the corresponding regions of cerebral damage.

Signs and symptoms	*Structures involved*
Paralysis of opposite foot and leg	Motor leg area
Paresis of opposite arm	Involvement of arm area of cortex or fibers descending therefrom to corona radiata
"Cortical" sensory loss over toes, foot, and leg	Sensory area for foot and leg
Urinary incontinence	Posteromedial part of superior frontal gyrus (bilateral)
Contralateral grasp reflex, sucking reflex, gegenhalten (paratonic rigidity), (all rare)	Premotor cortex (area 6 and supplementary motor area of 8)
Abulia (akinetic mutism), slowness, delay, lack of spontaneity, whispering, motor inaction, reflex distraction to sights and sounds	Uncertain localization—probably deep medial-orbital (usually bilateral)
Impairment of gait and stance (gait "apraxia")	Inferomedial frontal–striatal (?)
Mental impairment (perseveration and amnesia)	Localization unknown
Miscellaneous:	
Dyspraxia of left limbs	Corpus callosum
Tactile aphasia in left limbs	Corpus callosum
Cerebral paraplegia	Motor leg area bilaterally (due to bilateral occlusion of anterior cerebral arteries)

Note: Hemianopia does not occur; transcortical aphasia occurs rarely (p. 189).

patients. In every group of stroke patients there is, over a period of years, a rising mortality from coronary thrombosis, and this is as much of a hazard as recurrent cerebral thrombosis.

Transient Ischemic Attacks (TIAs)

These are defined as transitory neurologic deficits due to ischemia in the territory of a given artery, lasting for minutes to hours and followed by complete restoration of function. There is a demonstrable temporary arrest in local blood flow. Literally hundreds of attacks may occur or only a few. As remarked above, such attacks may anticipate an oncoming thrombotic stroke.

Carotid branch TIAs take the form of monocular blindness (amaurosis fugax), hemiparesis, hemisensory syndromes, aphasia, dyscalculia, and confusion. Vertebral-basilar branch attacks consist of blindness, hemianopia, diplopia, dizziness, dysarthria, dysphagia, facial weakness or numbness, hemiplegia or quadriplegia, and sensory syndromes, all in various combinations.

TIAs that are long-lasting (several hours to a day) or of diverse pattern are nearly always embolic. Some declare that all TIAs are embolic, others that they represent transient changes in local flow due to altered viscosity of the blood, hypotension, or other mechanism.

Management Patients who present with TIAs should be investigated with noninvasive Doppler flow studies, DSA, and arteriography. If the symptoms are those of carotid TIAs and the lesion is localized to the carotid artery in the neck (high-grade stenosis or an ulcerated plaque), endarterectomy may halt the symptomatic progress. If the disease is most apparent in the intracranial portion of the carotid artery or in the vertebral-basilar system, one resorts to long-term coumadin or aspirin therapy.

Embolic Infarction

Cerebral embolism is the single most frequent cause of stroke. If one adds the strokes of indeterminate origin (most of which are probably embolic) to those of proven embolism, then 40 percent of all strokes will be embolic, compared to 32 percent of thrombotic ones (see Table 32-2).

Most cerebral emboli arise in the heart (auricular fibrillation, myocardial infarction with mural thrombi, endocarditis). Others come from the lungs, aorta, or large cranial arteries. Unlike a thrombus, which adheres to the vessel wall, the embolic particle is friable and migratory. The embolus may disintegrate before tissue necrosis can occur, or if the tissue is infarcted, it becomes hemorrhagic as circulation is restored.

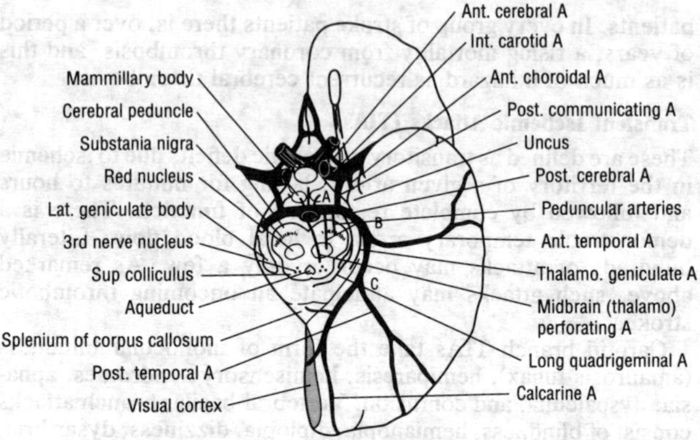

FIG. 32-3 Inferior aspect of the brain showing the branches and distribution of the posterior cerebral artery and the principal anatomic structures supplied. Listed below are the clinical manifestations produced by infarction in its territory and the corresponding regions of damage.

Signs and symptoms	*Structures involved*
	Peripheral territory
Homonymous hemianopia	Calcarine cortex or optic radiation; hemiachromatopsia may be present. Macular or central vision is preserved if striate area is spared.
Bilateral homonymous hemianopia, cortical blindness, unawareness or denial of blindness; achromatopsia; inability to perceive and touch objects not centrally located; apraxia of ocular movements.	Bilateral occipital lobe possibly with involvement of parieto-occipital region
Dyslexia without agraphia, color anomia	Dominant calcarine cortex and posterior part of corpus callosum
Memory defect	Inferomedial portions of temporal lobe bilaterally
Topographic disorientation and prosopagnosia	Calcarine and lingual gyri, usually bilateral
Simultanagnosia	Dominant visual cortex, sometimes bilateral
Unformed visual hallucinations, metamorphopsia, teleopsia, illusory visual spread, palinopsia, distortion of outlines, photophobia	Calcarine cortex

FIG. 32-3 (*continued*)

Signs and symptoms	*Structures involved*
Central territory	
Thalamic syndrome: sensory loss (all modalities), spontaneous pain and dysesthesias, choreoathetosis, intention tremor, mild hemiparesis	Ventral posterolateral nucleus of thalamus in territory of thalamogeniculate artery. Involvement of the adjacent subthalamic nucleus or its pallidal connections results in hemilballismus and choreoathetosis.
Thalamoperforate syndrome: (1) superior, crossed cerebellar ataxia; (2) inferior, crossed cerebellar ataxia with ipsilateral third nerve palsy (Claude syndrome)	Dentatothalamic tract and issuing third nerve
Weber snydrome—third nerve palsy and contralateral hemiplegia	Issuing third nerve and cerebral peduncle
Contralateral hemiplegia	Cerebral peduncle
Paralysis or paresis of vertical eye movements, skew deviation, sluggish pupillary responses to light, slight miosis and ptosis (retraction nystagmus and "tucked-in" eyelids may be associated)	Supranuclear structures in high midbrain tegmentum ventral to superior colliculi (interstitial nucleus of medial longitudinal fasciculus, and posterior commissure)
Contralateral ataxic or postural tremor	Dentatothalamic tract (?) after decussation. Precise site of lesion unknown.
Decerebrate attacks	Damage to motor tracts between red and vestibular nuclei

Note: Tremor in repose has been omitted because of the uncertainty of its occurrence in the posterior cerebral artery syndrome. Peduncular hallucinosis has been associated with bilateral lesions of the pars reticulata of the substantia nigra (McKee et al).

Clinical manifestations Of all ischemic strokes the embolic type develops most rapidly, literally within several seconds or a minute. While the brain is the most frequent site of cardiac embolism, other parts (spleen, kidney, gastrointestinal tract, legs) may also be involved. Again, the stroke pattern accords with the neurovascular syndromes displayed in Figs. 32-1 to 32-7. Branches of the middle cerebral arteries are the most frequently involved. About one-third of embolic infarcts become hemorrhagic, a phenomenon that can be exposed by serial CT scans.

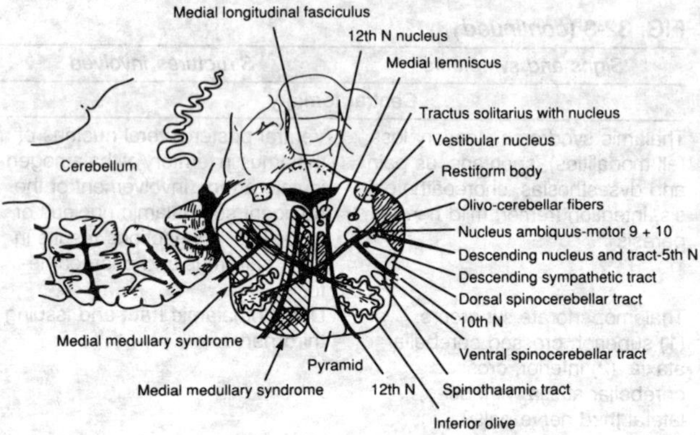

FIG. 32-4

Signs and symptoms	*Structures involved*
1. Medial medullary syndrome (occlusion of vertebral artery or branch of vertebral or lower basilar artery)	
a. On side of lesion: paralysis with atrophy of half the tongue	Issuing twelfth nerve
b. On side opposite lesion	
(1) Paralysis of arm and leg sparing face	Pyramidal tract
(2) Impaired tactile and proprioceptive sense over half the body	Medial lemniscus
2. Lateral medullary syndrome (occlusion of any of five vessels—vertebral, posterior inferior cerebellar, or superior, middle, or inferior lateral medullary arteries)	
a. On side of lesion	
(1) Pain, numbness, impaired sensation over half the face	Descending tract and nucleus of fifth nerve
(2) Ataxia of limbs, falling to side of lesion	Uncertain—restiform body, cerebellar hemisphere, olivocerebellar fibers, spinocerebellar tract (?)
(3) Vertigo, nausea, vomiting	Vestibular nuclei and connections
(4) Nystagmus, diplopia, oscillopsia	Vestibular nuclei and connections
(5) Horner syndrome (miosis, ptosis, decreased sweating)	Descending sympathetic tract

FIG. 32-4 (*continued*)

Signs and symptoms	*Structures involved*
(6) Dysphagia, hoarseness, paralysis of vocal cord, diminished gag reflex	Issuing fibers ninth and tenth nerves
(7) Loss of taste (rare)	Nucleus and tractus solitarius
(8) Numbness of ipsilateral arm, trunk, or leg	Cuneate and gracile nuclei
(9) Hiccup	Uncertain
b. On side opposite lesion: impaired pain and thermal sense over half the body, sometimes face	Spinothalamic tract
3. Total unilateral medullary syndrome (occlusion of vertebral artery); combination of medial and lateral syndromes	
4. Lateral pontomedullary syndrome (occlusion of vertebral artery); combination of medial and lateral syndromes	
5. Basilar artery syndrome (the syndrome of the lone vertebral artery is equivalent); a combination of the various brainstem syndromes plus those arising in the posterior cerebral artery distribution. The clinical picture comprises bilateral long-tract signs (sensory and motor) with cerebellar and cranial nerve abnormalities.	
a. Paralysis or weakness of all extremities, plus all bulbar musculature	Corticobulbar and corticospinal tracts bilaterally
b. Diplopia, paralysis of conjugate lateral and/or vertical gaze, internuclear ophthalmoplegia, horizontal and/or vertical nystagmus	Ocular motor nervers, apparatus for conjugate gaze, medial longitudinal fasciculus, vestibular apparatus
c. Blindness, impaired vision, various visual field defects	Visual cortex
d. Bilateral cerebellar ataxia	Cerebellar peduncles and the cerebellar hemispheres
e. Coma	Tegmentum of midbrain, thalami
f. Sensation may be strikingly intact in the presence of almost total paralysis. Sensory loss may be syringomyelic or the reverse or involve all modalities	Medial lemniscus, spinothalamic tracts or thalamic nuclei

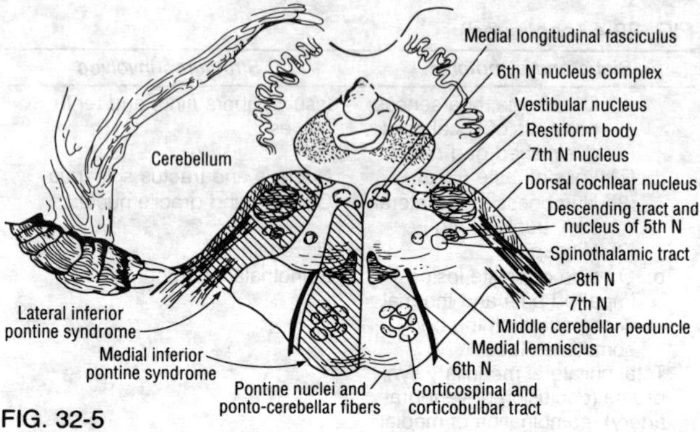

FIG. 32-5

Signs and symptoms	*Structures involved*
1. Medial inferior pontine syndrome (occlusion of paramedian branch of basilar artery)	
a. On side of lesion	
(1) Paralysis of conjugate gaze to side of lesion (preservation of convergence)	Pontine "center" for lateral gaze (PPRF)
(2) Nystagmus	Vestibular nuclei and connections
(3) Ataxia of limbs and gait	Middle cerebellar peduncle (?)
(4) Diplopia on lateral gaze	Abducens nerve or nucleus
b. On side opposite lesion	
(1) Paralysis of face, arm, and leg	Corticobulbar and corticospinal tracts in lower pons
(2) Impaired tactile and proprioceptive sense over half of the body	Medial lemniscus
2. Lateral inferior pontine syndrome (occlusion of anterior inferior cerebellar artery)	
a. On side of lesion	
(1) Horizontal and vertical nystagmus, vertigo, nausea, vomiting, oscillopsia	Vestibular nerve or nucleus
(2) Facial paralysis	Seventh nerve or nucleus
(3) Paralysis of conjugate gaze to side of lesion	Pontine "center" for lateral gaze (PPRF)
(4) Deafness, tinnitus	Auditory nerve or cochlear nucleus
(5) Ataxia	Middle cerebellar peduncle and cerebellar hemisphere
(6) Impaired sensation over face	Descending tract and nucleus fifth nerve

FIG. 32-5 (*continued*)

Signs and symptoms	*Structures involved*
b. On side opposite lesion: impaired pain and thermal sense over half the body (may include face)	Spinothalamic tract
3. Total unilateral inferior pontine syndrome (occlusion of anterior inferior cerebellar artery); lateral and medial syndromes combined	

The *immediate prognosis* for a patient with embolic infarction is much the same as for a patient with thrombotic infarction, except that recession of the neurologic deficit tends to be more rapid in the former. Always there is a threat of recurrent embolism.

Treatment Nothing really can be done about an infarct that has already occurred, and treatment is directed to the prevention of recurrent embolism. Of all strokes, the embolic ones are the most amenable to long-term anticoagulation with coumadin and antiplatelet drugs. However, early heparinization of a potentially hemorrhagic infarct, particularly if the infarct is large and the patient is hypertensive, carries a risk of increased bleeding. Hemorrhage occurs in approximately 30 percent of all embolic cerebral infarcts and may require 3 to 4 days to become apparent. For this reason we perform a CT scan and an LP 3 to 4 days following embolism. If there is no evidence of hemorrhage we proceed with IV heparin, introduced gradually, followed by coumadin.

INTRACRANIAL HEMORRHAGE

The many causes of intracranial hemorrhage are listed in Table 32-3. The most important of these are primary intracerebral hemorrhage, ruptured saccular aneurysm and arteriovenous malformation (AVM), and trauma, including epidural and subdural hematomas.

Primary Intracerebral Hemorrhage

Also called hypertensive because most cases occur in patients with an elevated blood pressure, the occurrence of primary cerebral hemorrhage does not necessarily correlate with the presence or degree of hypertension. In an unknown proportion of cases amyloidosis of arteries is an important factor.

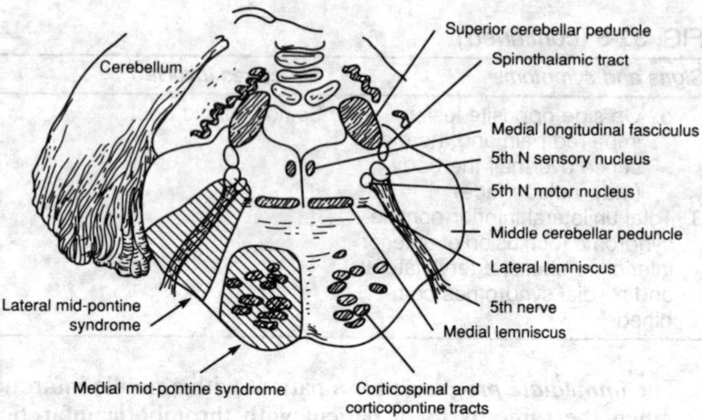

FIG. 32-6

Signs and symptoms	*Structures involved*
1. Medial midpontine syndrome (paramedian branch of mid-basilar artery)	
a. On side of lesion: ataxia of limbs and gait (more prominent in bilateral involvement)	Middle cerebellar peduncle
b. On side opposite lesion	
(1) Paralysis of face, arm, and leg	Corticobulbar and corticospinal tracts
(2) Deviation of eyes	
(3) Variably impaired touch and proprioception when lesion extends posteriorly. Usually the syndrome is purely motor.	Medial lemniscus
2. Lateral midpontine syndrome (short circumferential artery): on side of lesion	
a. Ataxia of limbs	Middle cerebellar peduncle
b. Paralysis of muscles of mastication	Motor fibers or nucleus of fifth nerve
c. Impaired sensation over side of face	Sensory fibers or nucleus of fifth nerve

Of all the cerebrovascular diseases, this is the most dramatic and most deserving of the name apoplexy. The patient is literally felled in his tracks or is seized with a headache and rapidly sinks into coma. Death follows in hours or days. At autopsy, a massive hemispheral clot swells the brain and bloodies the ventricular and subarachnoid fluid.

A lesser magnitude of hemorrhage is also possible. In 20 to 30 percent of cases, the headache is trivial, and a focal neurologic deficit may occur without loss of consciousness and be indistinguishable clinically from an infarct. Only with CT scanning is a discrete hemorrhage recognized. All gradations between large and small hemorrhages may be observed.

The common sites of brain hemorrhage in order of their frequency are (1) putaminal-capsular (50 percent), (2) lobar, (3) thalamic, (4) cerebellar, and (5) pontine.

With large *putaminal hemorrhages*, patients quickly lapse into stupor and coma with hemiplegia. The onset may be with headache, and hemiplegia may evolve over a period of 5 to 30 min, with deviation of the eyes to the side of the lesion, followed by progressive confusion, stupor, coma, and signs of upper brainstem compression. As indicated above, a small putaminal-capsular hemorrhage may behave clinically like an embolic or thrombotic ischemic stroke, and its true nature is disclosed by CT scan.

The clinical picture of *lobar hemorrhage* will of course depend on its location: occipital (pain around ipsilateral eye and homonymous hemianopia), temporal (pain in or anterior to ear, partial hemianopia, fluent aphasia), frontal (contralateral hemiplegia and frontal headache), or parietal (anterior temporal headache and contralateral hemisensory defect). The occurrence of one of these syndromes in conjunction with rapidly progressive headache, vomiting, and stupor is diagnostic and CT scanning is corroborative. The taking of anticoagulants and the presence of an underlying arteriovenous malformation (AVM) or metastatic tumor are other causes that need always to be considered.

In *thalamic hemorrhage*, the sensory defect is more prominent than hemiparesis or hemianopia. Aphasia may be present with dominant lesions and amorphosynthesis with nondominant ones. Ocular abnormalities are frequent, particularly downward deviation of the eyes and small, nonreactive pupils. The prognosis relates closely to the size of the hemorrhage.

Pontine hemorrhage is characterized by the rapid evolution of coma and total paralysis, decerebrate rigidity, and small but reactive pupils. Survival is possible with small hemorrhages (±1 cm).

With *cerebellar hemorrhage*, loss of consciousness at the onset is unusual. Vomiting, occipital headache, vertigo, gross ataxia, inability to stand or sit, and forced deviation of the eyes to the side opposite the lesion are the usual manifestations.

Prognosis Approximately two-thirds of patients with primary intracerebral hemorrhage and nearly all comatose ones succumb.

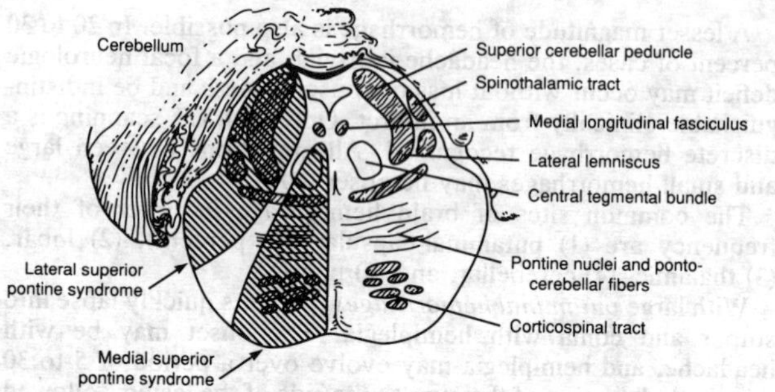

FIG. 32-7

Signs and symptoms	*Structures involved*
1. Medial superior pontine syndrome (paramedian branches of upper basilar artery)	
a. On side of lesion	
(1) Cerebellar ataxia	Superior and/or middle cerebellar peduncle
(2) Internuclear ophthalmoplegia	Medial longitudinal fasciculus
(3) Rhythmic myoclonus of palate, pharynx, vocal cords, respiratory apparatus, face, oculomotor apparatus	Central tegmental tract
b. On side opposite lesion	
(1) Paralysis of face, arm, and leg	Corticobulbar and corticospinal tracts
(2) Rarely touch, vibration, and position senses are affected	Medial lemniscus
2. Lateral superior pontine syndrome (syndrome of superior cerebellar artery)	
a. On side of lesion	
(1) Ataxia of limbs and gait, falling to side of lesion	Middle and superior cerebellar peduncles, superior surface of cerebellum, dentate nucleus
(2) Dizziness, nausea, vomiting, horizontal nystagmus	Vestibular nuclei
(3) Paresis of conjugate gaze (ipsilateral)	Uncertain
(4) Loss of optokinetic nystagmus	Uncertain artery
(5) Skew deviation	Uncertain
(6) Miosis, ptosis, decreased sweating over face (Horner syndrome)	Descending sympathetic fibers

FIG. 32-7 (*continued*)

Signs and symptoms	*Structures involved*
b. On side opposite lesion	
(1) Impaired pain and thermal sense on face, limbs, and trunk	Spinothalamic tract
(2) Impaired touch, vibration, and position sense, more in leg than arm	Medial lemniscus (lateral portion)

Surgical removal of the clot is seldom successful in saving life, though a few patients with a lobar or cerebellar hemorrhage may be salvaged.

Patients with small hemorrhages usually survive, sometimes for years, and with striking regression of focal signs. In the acute stage, control of intracranial pressure, by measures outlined in Chap. 28, should be undertaken.

Ruptured Saccular Aneurysm

This is the fourth most frequent cerebrovascular disease. The aneurysm consists of a small (2 mm to 2 cm, average 8 to 10 mm), berry-shaped dilatation of a surface artery. Mostly they lie in the crotch of a bifurcating artery on or near the circle of Willis. In most instances they are small and clinically silent until the age of 35 to 65 years, when they rupture and give rise to a subarachnoid hemorrhage.

There may be one or several aneurysms, but with subarachnoid hemorrhage only one will be found to have bled. Why the aneurysm forms in the first place is not certain. A congenital defect of the internal elastic lamina and media of the vessel wall is the most widely accepted theory. The frequent concurrence of such aneurysms with AVMs supports a theory of congenital origin.

Clinical manifestations Occasionally, the aneurysm may, by a process of oozing and accretion of surface clots, reach a large size (3 to 4 cm) and press on cranial nerves or other structures, but most are recognized when they rupture and cause a subarachnoid hemorrhage. This produces severe headache of acute onset, nausea, vomiting, and signs of meningeal irritation. The occurrence of these symptoms in an adult who is not febrile and has no focal or lateralizing neurologic signs is virtually diagnostic of a ruptured saccular aneurysm. However, some cases of aneurysmal hemorrhage are accompanied by focal neurologic signs. An aneurysm at the junction of the internal carotid and posterior communicating arteries may damage the adjacent oculomotor nerve; one at the anterior–middle cerebral junction,

TABLE 32-3 Causes of Intracranial Hemorrhage (Including Intracerebral, Subarachnoid, Ventricular, and Subdural)

1. Primary (hypertensive) intracerebral hemorrhage
2. Ruptured saccular aneurysm
3. Ruptured AVM
4. Undetermined cause (normal blood pressure, no aneurysm or AVM)
5. Trauma including postraumatic delayed apoplexy
6. Hemorrhagic disorders: leukemia, aplastic anemia, thrombocytopenic purpura, liver disease, complication of anticoagulant therapy, hyperfibrinolysis, hypofibrinogenemia, hemophilia, Christmas disease, etc.
7. Hemorrhage into primary and secondary brain tumors
8. Septic embolism, mycotic aneurysm
9. With hemorrhagic infarction, arterial or venous
10. With inflammatory disease of the arteries and veins
11. With arterial amyloidosis
12. Miscellaneous rare types: after vasopressor drugs, upon exertion, during arteriography, during painful urologic examination, as a late complication of early-life carotid occlusion, complication of carotid-cavernous AV fistula, with anoxemia, migraine, teratomatous malformations. Herpes simplex encephalitis and acute necrotizing hemorrhagic encephalopathy may be associated with up to 2000 red blood cells or more per cubic millimeter in the CSF; tularemia, anthrax, and *Pseudomonas meningitis* and snake venom poisoning may cause bloody CSF.

the nearby optic nerve; and one at the first bifurcation of the middle cerebral artery may bleed into the brain and cause hemiplegia.

A large subarachnoid hemorrhage may be immediately fatal, the only form of cerebrovascular disease that results in sudden death. Or there may be a generalized convulsion. Most patients reach the hospital in a conscious state. The diagnosis is established by CT scanning and an LP. Angiography visualizes the aneurysm in 95 percent of cases.

Approximately 40 percent of untreated bleeding aneurysms rerupture within 2 months (most of them in the second or third week), and the majority of these prove fatal. The second major complication of ruptured aneurysm is vascular spasm and cerebral infarction, occurring in the territory of the artery harboring the aneurysm and most often during the second week. Hydrocephalus, due to blockage of the CSF pathways by blood, may develop 2 to 4 weeks following rupture. Cerebral salt wasting and SIADH may also be observed.

Treatment and prognosis Early diagnosis, direct surgical exposure of the aneurysm, and its obliteration by a clip placed on its neck is the only sure treatment. However, if the patient is in deep stupor or coma, the surgical mortality is so high as to be unacceptable. The preference then is to sedate the patient, control the blood pressure, and prevent convulsions until consciousness is regained. The antifibrinolytic agents aminocaproic acid (1 to 1.5 g/h IV) or tranexamic acid (6 to 12 mg/day) impede lysis of the clot, but this effect is largely offset by an increased incidence of vascular spasm and infarction. There is no certain method of preventing the latter; intravascular volume expansion may do so, but this measure can only be used safely in the postoperative period. Evidence in recent years indicates that the use of calcium channel blockers (nimodipine, 60 mg every 4 h for 21 days) may be helpful in preventing vasospasm and infarction.

Lumbar puncture is necessary to confirm the presence of an inconclusive meningeal syndrome, but repeated taps for the removal of bloody CSF is no longer practiced. In some cases, the aneurysm cannot be seen angiographically, even when the procedure is repeated after the vascular spasm has subsided. In such cases, the outlook for survival is better than that of patients with an untreated demonstrable aneurysm.

Arteriovenous Malformation (AVM)

These hamartomatous malformations are about one-third as frequent as saccular aneurysms. They may be only 1 cm or even less in size or so large as to occupy the major portion of a lobe of the cerebrum or of the brainstem or cerebellum. They consist of a mass of small vessels fed by large arteries and drained by large veins. In most instances they are asymptomatic until they bleed into the subarachnoid space, brain, or ventricle. A small proportion are manifested by a progressive neurologic deficit due to gradual enlargement or to shunting of blood through enlarged vascular channels ("intracerebral steal"). In a significant number of cases there are focal seizures or a migraine syndrome, for which one should initiate a search for the AVM by an enhanced CT scan or MRI. Hemorrhage, the feared complication, may be recurrent and fatal, but the risk of death is less than with bleeding from ruptured aneurysm.

A separate group of vascular malformations is made up of a cluster of enlarged veins (cavernous VM). Often these are angiographically negative but can be seen by MRI. They bleed frequently. In some cases they are multiple and familial.

If small and accessible in a "quiet zone" of the brain, AVMs can be extirpated with an acceptably low mortality and morbidity. With large and complicated AVMs, preoperative embolization of large feeding vessels with Silastic pellets is a valuable adjuvant procedure. If inoperable, focused gamma or proton radiation will obliterate small lesions in 80 to 90 percent of cases and probably help the large ones as well.

APPROACH TO THE STROKE PATIENT

The physician may be confronted by a number of stroke problems, each of which needs to be managed in particular ways, depending upon the clinical status of the patient and the underlying disease.

For the comatose stroke patient (massive hypertensive or subarachnoid hemorrhage, or massive cerebral or brainstem infarction), one attempts diagnosis and provides symptomatic care. CT scanning or MRI are the only needed diagnostic procedures. As a rule, no specific therapy is possible. In rare cases surgical aspiration of clot is helpful, providing the patient is not yet comatose.

A recently completed or an evolving stroke in a noncomatose patient is the most frequent clinical problem. The type of stroke should be determined by clinical and laboratory methods and the patients treated according to the plan outlined above. Since the patient will probably survive, long-term plans need to be made for rehabilitation and the prevention of further strokes.

Strokes inobvious to the general physician should be kept in mind—a small subarachnoid hemorrhage from a leaking aneurysm; a posterior cerebral artery occlusion with only a homonymous visual field defect (found by testing visual fields); a cerebellar hemorrhage not evident unless the patient is made to sit up, stand, or walk; a mild paraphasic difficulty, which may be misinterpreted as a confusional state or a psychosis.

Finally, there is the patient who gives a history of a stroke in the past but has since fully recovered. Here a premium attaches to accurate diagnosis of the type of stroke and the application of measures that reduce the risk of further strokes.

For a more detailed discussion of this topic, see Adams and Victor: *Principles of Neurology*, 4th ed, pp 617–692.

ADDITIONAL READING

Barnett HJM: The EC/IC bypass study group. Failure of extracranial-intracranial arterial bypass to reduce the risk of ischemic stroke. Results of an international randomized trial. *N Engl J Med* 313:1191, 1985.

Barnett HJM, Mohr JP, Stein BM, Yatsu FM (eds): *Stroke. Pathophysiology, Diagnosis and Management*. New York, Churchill Livingstone, 1986.

Caplan LR: "Top of the basilar" syndrome. *Neurology* 30:72, 1980.

Chester EM, Agamanolis DP, Banker BQ, Victor M: Hypertensive encephalopathy: A clinicopathologic study of 20 cases. *Neurology* 28:298, 1978.

Crawford PM, West CR, Chadwick DW, et al: Arteriovenous malformations of the brain; natural history in unoperated patients. *J Neurol Neurosurg Psychiatry* 49:1, 1986.

Fisher CM: Lacunar strokes and infarcts: A review. *Neurology* 32:871, 1982.

Heyman A, Wilkinson WE, Heyden S, et al: Risk of stroke in asymptomatic persons with cervical arterial bruits. *N Engl J Med* 302:838, 1980.

Kubik CS, Adams RD: Occlusion of the basilar artery—a clinical and pathological study. *Brain* 69:73, 1946.

McKee AC, Levine DN, Kowall NW, Richardson EP Jr: Peduncular hallucinosis associated with isolated infarction of the substantia nigra pars reticulata. *Ann Neurol* 27:500, 1990.

Shields RW Jr, Laureno R, Lachman T, Victor M: Anicoagulant-related hemorrhage in acute cerebral embolism. *Stroke* 15:426, 1984.

Toole V: *Cerebrovascular Disorders*, 4th ed. New York, Raven, 1990.

Toole JF, Yuson CP, Janeway R: Transient ischemic attacks: A study of 225 patients. *Neurology* 28:746, 1978.

Weisberg LA: Thalamic hemorrhage: Clinical CT correlations. *Neurology* 36:1382, 1986.

33 | Craniocerebral Trauma

Head injury is such a commonplace event that at any one time as much as 1 percent of the population is suffering from its effects as a result of road injuries and other accidents. The basic problem is both simple and complex—simple because there is usually no question as to etiology and complex because of the abstruse mechanisms of a number of secondary and delayed effects.

Severe head injuries often require the care of a neurosurgeon, but even a neurosurgeon can often do no more than clean the scalp wound or open the skull in order to aspirate a clot. For the great majority of head-injured patients, the management is medical and the neurologist is as competent to manage these cases as the neurosurgeon. The neurologist must therefore be versed in diagnosis of the types of head injury and their treatment.

DEFINITIONS

Most head injuries in civilian life are nonpenetrating or "blunt." The term *concussion* implies a violent agitation of the brain from a blow to the head, resulting in a transient loss of neurologic function. The word *contusion* refers to a bruising of the brain, beneath the point struck ("coup" injury) or on the opposite side ("contrecoup" injury). However, contusional injury comprises a wide spectrum of pathologic changes, such as local edema, hemorrhage, shattering of nerve fibers, and brain herniation. For this complex of changes we will use the term "*contusion-plus*."

Concerning the mechanisms of concussion and contusion-plus, two points deserve emphasis:

1. The brain is capable of motion separate from the skull, owing to the fact that it is virtually floating in CSF. With a brisk blow that sets the head in motion (acceleration injury), movement of the brain lags. Or if a moving head strikes an immovable object (deceleration injury), motion of the head is arrested but not that of the brain. Moreover, the brainstem is anchored in the posterior fossa, beneath the tentorium, and does not move. As a result, there occurs a torque or rotational movement of the cerebral hemispheres, with maximum stress

on the high brainstem reticular formation. This is the most plausible explanation of the fact that concussion occurs only if the head is mobile when struck.

2. As the cerebral hemispheres undergo torsion, the surface convolutions are flung against bony prominences of the inner skull surface and folds of dura, causing both the coup and contrecoup bruises and hemorrhages. Thus contusion is a kind of epiphenomenon of the same mechanism that produces concussion. The rotational changes are believed by some neuropathologists to shear or rupture axons of nerve fibers in the white matter, quite apart from surface bruising. The skull may or may not be fractured.

Skull Fractures

The severity of cerebral injury correlates only roughly with skull fracture. A seemingly slight injury may fracture a temporal bone (and at the same time lacerate a meningeal artery, producing an epidural hemorrhage); conversely, there may be severe concussion and contusion without skull fracture. The fractures themselves, especially basilar ones, acquire significance because they may injure the optic or other cranial nerves and sometimes allow ingress or air (pneumocele) or bacteria or egress of CSF from paranasal sinuses or ears (rhinorrhea, otorrhea). A fracture through the sphenoid bone or sella may tear a carotid artery or branch thereof, producing a carotid-cavernous fistula or the pituitary stalk may be torn, with development of a hypothalamic-pituitary syndrome.

Concussion and Contusion-Plus

A blunt injury in which the head accelerates or decelerates at a critical velocity change of 27 to 30 ft/s (for a macaque) results in an instantaneous loss of consciousness, which may last seconds, minutes, or hours. The longer the duration of unconsciousness, the greater the likelihood that some combination of contusion, laceration, hemorrhage, and localized edema has been added. The latter changes are responsible for hemiparesis, aphasia, and other focal signs as well as for the signs of shift of central structures and temporal lobe–tentorial herniation. Pupillary and ocular-motor damage indicate primary or secondary brainstem injury.

In the first hours of severe injury, vital signs may fail, and brain death results. More frequently, patients are conscious or rapidly regaining consciousness when first seen (minor head injury). With purely concussive injury, the patient passes quickly through a state of drowsiness and confusion to one of full recovery (with the qualifications noted further on). When the effects of contusion-plus are added, the period of initial unconsciousness is more prolonged, and recovery is of varying degrees of completeness. The sequelae of the various forms of head injury are considered below.

Acute Epidural Hemorrhage

This is caused by bleeding from a meningeal artery, occasionally a vein, torn by a temporal or parietal fracture. The patient may or may not have been concussed and may have regained consciousness; but then as the clot expands over a period of hours, the patient becomes hemiplegic and comatose. The CT scan is diagnostic. Early recognition is essential. Unless the clot is removed and the torn vessel ligated, death is invariable.

Acute and Chronic Subdural Hematomas

With the contusion-plus type of injury, there is nearly always some degree of subarachnoid hemorrhage and, not infrequently, subdural hemorrhage as well. The latter is readily detected by CT scanning and MRI. All but the smallest subdural clots need to be removed surgically and the bleeding controlled.

Chronic subdural hematomas pose an entirely different problem. The head injury, particularly in the elderly and in those taking anticoagulant drugs, may have been trivial and even forgotten. A bridging vein, as it passes from the pia-arachnoid to a dural sinus, is torn, and this permits blood to accumulate under low pressure in the subdural space. The usual site is over one cerebral hemisphere (sometimes bilateral) and occasionally interhemispheric or subcerebellar. The clot excites membrane formation from the dura; the membranes enclose the clot and attach it to the dura. As the blood disintegrates over 2 to 3 months, the fluid mass enlarges, compressing and displacing the underlying brain. Headache, drowsiness, confusion, hemiparesis, and dysphasia follow. The hematoma and its compressive effects are visible by MRI and CT scanning. If the symptoms are severe and progressive, surgical drainage is life-saving and recovery can be complete. Small hematomas regress naturally.

Penetrating Injuries

These are mainly due to gunshot wounds of the head, and if vital centers are struck, death is instantaneous. Many patients reach the emergency ward where the physician's primary objective is to assure respiratory and cardiovascular stability. The wound needs to be cleaned and debrided. CT scanning or MRI will indicate whether shell fragments or an expanding intracranial hemorrhage is an immediate threat to survival. The problem is mainly surgical, and the clinical status of the patient determines the timing of planned operative intervention.

SEQUELAE OF HEAD INJURY

Concussion invariably leaves the patient with a permanent gap in memory, extending from a point before the injury occurred until the time he can form consecutive memories. The duration of the retrograde and anterograde amnesia, particularly the latter, is the most reliable index of the severity of the concussive injury.

Concussion and even more trivial injuries (in which there is no concussion) may also leave the patient with persistent headache, fatigue, irritability, giddiness, difficulty in concentration, disturbed sleep, anxiety, and depression. This syndrome is common and has been given many names—postconcussion syndrome, traumatic neurasthenia, and *posttraumatic nervous instability*, which is the one we prefer. These symptoms may persist for weeks, months, or a year or more. The syndrome is more frequent and prolonged when compensation or litigation is an issue. Settlement of the legal problem, reassurance, and appropriate use of antianxiety and antidepression medication are essential steps in the rehabilitation program.

In respect to patients with contusion-plus, all gradations in the severity of neurologic sequelae can be observed. Some patients, following a protracted period of coma, may open their eyes and appear to be awake but betray no signs of cognition or responsiveness (*persistent vegetative state*, see Chap. 16). Other patients, in whom the symptoms fall just short of those of the persistent vegetative state, remain severely and permanently "brain-damaged."

In the majority of patients with contusion-plus, the consequences of brain damage recede, usually in the first 6 months and often to a surprising degree. Nevertheless, many patients are left with troublesome symptoms. Delayed onset of seizures is to be expected in 25 to 40 percent of contused patients (but not in those with pure concussion). Focal deficits—hemiparesis, dysphasia, frontal lobe disorder—may persist in mild form in patients with hemispheral injuries and cerebellar ataxia and various upper brainstem abnormalities in those who have had temporal lobe–tentorial herniations. Mental and personality changes may develop and cause serious problems in social adjustment; these demand expert neuropsychiatric care.

ADDENDUM

Limitations of space preclude a full account of many problems based on head injury. We have omitted discussion of posttraumatic syncope; immediate traumatic epilepsy; particular cranial nerve injuries with skull fractures; traumatic meningitis, subarachnoid hemorrhage, and hydrocephalus; acute contusional swelling of the brain; traumatic dissecting aneurysm of the carotid artery; traumatic migraine; delayed traumatic cerebral hemorrhage; CSF rhinorrhea; dementia-pugilistica (the "punch-drunk" syndrome); and the predictors of outcome of head injury (e.g., the Glasgow coma scale). The reader will find a discussion of these topics in the *Principles* and other references in the suggested reading list.

Spinal cord trauma is described in the following chapter.

For a more detailed discussion of this topic, see Adams and Victor: *Principles of Neurology*, 4th ed, pp 693–717.

ADDITIONAL READING

Adams JH, Graham DI, Murray LS, Scott G: Diffuse axonal injury due to nonmissile head injury in humans: An analysis of 45 cases. *Ann Neurol* 12:557, 1982.

British Medical Journal: A Group of Neurosurgeons: Guidelines for initial management after head injury in adults. *Br Med J* 288:983, 1984.

Corsellis JAN, Bruton CJ, Freeman-Browne D: The aftermath of boxing. *Psychol Med* 3:270, 1973.

Gennarelli TA, Thibault LE, Adams JH, et al: Diffuse axonal injury and traumatic coma in the primate. *Ann Neurol* 12:564, 1982.

Jennett B, Teasdale G: *Management of Head Injuries: Contemporary Neurology*, no. 20. Philadelphia, Davis, 1981.

Ommaya AK, Grubb RL, Naumann RA: Coup and contrecoup injury: Observations on the mechanisms of visible brain injuries in the rhesus monkey. *J Neurosurg* 35:503, 1971.

Ropper AH, Kennedy SK (eds): *Neurological and Neurosurgical Intensive Care*, 2nd ed. Rockville, MD, Aspen, 1988.

Symonds CP: Concussion and contusion of the brain and their sequelae, in Feiring EH (ed): *Brock's Injuries of the Brain and Spinal Cord and Their Coverings*, 5th ed. New York, Springer, 1974, chap 4, pp 100–161.

34 | Diseases of the Spinal Cord

Many disease processes affect the spinal cord predominantly or exclusively and produce a number of distinctive syndromes. The latter relate to the special anatomic features of the cord: great length compared to width; predominance of conductive tracts over central segmental gray matter; tight enclosure by pia-arachnoid, which renders the cord intolerant to acute edematous lesions; apposition to the spine and predilection to diseases thereof; and precarious vascular arrangements.

The most commonly observed and important disorders of the spinal cord can be grouped into the following clinical syndromes:

1. Paraplegia or quadriplegia due to complete transverse lesions of the spinal cord
2. The syndrome of subacute or chronic spinal paraparesis with or without sensory changes and ataxia
3. The syndrome of segmental sensory dissociation with brachial amyotrophy (syringomyelic syndrome)

PARAPLEGIA OR QUADRIPLEGIA DUE TO COMPLETE TRANSVERSE LESIONS

Spinal Cord Trauma

This is the most widely studied example of complete spinal cord transection and the prototype of other acute transverse lesions (vascular, demyelinative, compressive) giving rise to paraplegia or quadriplegia. Penetration of the spinal canal by a missile is the common cause in wartime. In civilian life the usual mechanism is a vertical compression of the spinal column, to which is added the immediate effect of antero- or retrohyperflexion. The resultant tearing of spinal ligaments, permits the dislocation of an upper vertebra anteriorly on the one below, often with fracture. The spinal cord is literally crushed. In cases of cervical spondylosis an abrupt, forceful extension of the neck can also severely damage the cervical cord.

Clinical effects The immediate effect of spinal cord transection is a loss of all motor, sensory, autonomic, and sphincteric function below the level of the lesion. Or, if at first the loss of function is not complete, edema makes it so in a few hours. If the lesion is above the C4 level, respiration is paralyzed as well.

The subsequent effects are divided into two stages: the stage of *spinal shock* and the stage of *heightened reflex activity*. Spinal shock is expressed by a loss of all reflex activity below the level of the lesion, an atonic bladder with overflow incontinence, atonic bowel (paraytic ileus), gastric dilatation, and loss of genital reflexes and vasomotor control. After a period of 1 to 2 weeks, sometimes longer, spinal flexor reflexes (Babinski signs, flexor spasms) and then tendon reflexes begin to appear. Simultaneously, bladder tone and gastric and bowel function begin to recover. Gradually the tendon reflexes become hyperactive, and the bladder becomes spastic (frequency and urgency of urination, small capacity of bladder with automatic emptying). Also, autonomic functions (vasomotor and sweating reactions) become hyperactive. The paralyzed legs remain in flexion or in extension if the cord lesion is not complete. In the latter case, there may be some return of motor and sensory function below the lesion. The gray matter over two or three spinal segments is destroyed, and paralyzed arm or hand muscles become atrophic and areflexic; when this effect predominates over tract injury, it is referred to as a *central cord syndrome*.

Crush injuries of the lowermost thoracic and upper lumbar spine are in position to damage the spinal cord, cauda equina, or both.

The *treatment* of spine fracture and dislocation are mainly orthopedic—to reduce subluxation, assure fixation of the spine, and reduce spinal cord edema by administration of corticosteroids. Whether or not laminectomy and cord decompression are helpful is still a matter of controversy. In patients with complete spinal cord lesions the prevailing opinion is against laminectomy.

An acute, complete or nearly complete transverse cord lesion in the *absence of trauma* should lead to a consideration of the following:

1. Ischemic infarction of the cord, due to occlusion of a major segmental artery arising from a vertebral artery (supplying the cervical cord) or the aorta (supplying the thoracic and lumbar cord). Dissecting aortic aneurysm, arteritis, and atherosclerosis of the collateral arterial vessels are the usual causes. Rarely, there is thrombosis of the anterior spinal artery itself.
2. Hemorrhage into the spinal cord (hematomyelia) from an arteriovenous malformation, or epidural or subdural hemorrhage, e.g., from anticoagulant drugs.

3. Acute necrotizing or demyelinative myelopathy. These lesions are more often subacute in evolution (see below), but they may strike with such suddeness as to suggest spinal cord apoplexy.
4. Epidural abscess. Again this lesion is more often subacute in evolution.

SYNDROME OF SUBACUTE OR CHRONIC SPINAL PARAPARESIS WITH OR WITHOUT ATAXIA

This is the mode of presentation of a number of important spinal cord diseases of diverse type.

Cervical Spondylosis with Myelopathy

This is perhaps the most frequently observed myelopathy in general hospitals. It is essentially a degenerative disease of the lower cervical vertebrae in which some combination of degenerating and bulging disc(s), vertebral exostoses, and thickened ligamentum flavum are often engrafted on a congenitally narrow spinal canal; it compromises the cervical cord and roots by compression and possibly by reduction of the blood supply along radicular arteries.

Clinically, the syndrome consists of a triad of (1) painful, stiff neck with limitation of the range of movement; (2) radicular pain and numbness and reduced reflexes in an arm; and (3) symmetric or asymmetric spastic paraparesis and ataxia with signs of lateral and posterior column affection.

The condition is chronic and diagnosis is made by MRI or by myelography combined with CT scanning and by the exclusion of other spinal cord diseases.

In the early stages of the disease, the use of a soft collar may be sufficient to relieve the stiffness and pain in the neck and brachialgia. With progressive myelopathy a posterior decompressive laminectomy or an anterior approach (depending on the sites of osteophytic overgrowth) halts the progression of the disease and may lead to some improvement.

Demyelinative Myelopathy

Among young adults in northern climates, multiple sclerosis is the most frequent cause of an asymmetric paraparesis with hyperreflexia and sensory ataxia. About one-third of patients with multiple sclerosis exhibit this essentially spinal form of the disease. This and other forms of demyelinative disease—postinfectious and postvaccinal myelitis and acute necrotizing myelitis—are discussed in the following chapter.

Spinal Cord Tumors

Conventionally, these are divided into three groups: (1) tumors that lie within the spinal cord (*intramedullary*), (2) others lying on the surface of the cord and arising from the meninges or a spinal root (extramedullary-intradural), and (3) still others in the epidural space (*extradural*) but in a position to compress the spinal cord. Intrinsic cord tumors are usually astrocytomas or ependymomas of various degrees of malignancy. Extramedullary intradural tumors are most often neurofibromas or meningiomas. Extradural tumors usually prove to be manifestations of multifocal systemic neoplasia, i.e., metastatic carcinomas, lymphomas, plasmacytomas, or chordomas. Nonneoplastic extramedullary tissue masses also occur—hematopoiesis, lipomas, and epidural lipomatosis (complicating prolonged steroid therapy).

Radicular pain in combination with asymmetric or symmetric sensory and motor tract involvement and variable sphincteric dysfunction, evolving over weeks or months, constitute the prototypic syndrome. The pace of the disease varies with the type of tumor. Some of the ependymomas progress slowly over months or years, whereas the time course of epidural lymphomas and metastatic carcinomas is measured in days or weeks. Radicular symptoms are prominent with neurofibromas but may occur also with meningiomas and other tumors. Infrequently, an intramedullary tumor induces a frank central or syringomyelic syndrome (see further on).

The treatment of most spinal tumors, even the intramedullary ones, is surgical excision with radiation therapy. Epidural carcinomas and lymphomas are exceptions to this rule; they respond as well or better to radiation and chemotherapy as to surgery. Some lymphomas are so sensitive to radiation that a few exposures, supplemented by steroid therapy, will adequately relieve the cord compression.

Spinal Arachnoiditis

This is a relatively rare disorder characterized by thickening of the arachnoidal membranes and the formation of adhesions between arachnoid and dura, the result of connective tissue proliferation. Arachnoiditis of the thoracic cord presents clinically by a combination of root and spinal cord symptoms, mimicking spinal cord tumor. Some cases can be traced to syphilis or to some other therapeutically resistant chronic meningitis. Others follow the injection of certain substances, such as penicillin or Pantopaque (see Chap. 2) into the subarachnoid space. Increasingly frequent is the occurrence of a circumscribed lumbar arachnoiditis complicating repeated surgery for lumbar discs. In some cases no preceding event can be recognized.

Epidural Abscess

Skin infection in the region of the back or a bacteremia may permit seeding of the epidural space or a vertebral body, which in turn gives rise to an osteomyelitis with extension to the epidural space. Rarely, infection is introduced by a lumbar puncture needle or laminectomy. Fever and local pain and tenderness in the back is followed within a few days by radicular pain and a rapidly progressive paraparesis and sensory loss in the lower parts of the body, with sphincteric paralysis. Lumbar puncture shows a modest pleocytosis and high protein content, with normal glucose, but more importantly, a dynamic block (positive Queckenstedt test).

These CSF and clinical findings call for immediate investigation with MRI and myelography, followed by laminectomy and drainage, and the administration of appropriate antibiotics. Osteomyelitis, if present, can be dealt with subsequently. Laminectomy must be performed before paralysis becomes established if permanent damage to the cord is to be avoided.

Subacute Combined Degeneration (SCD) of the Cord

This is the name applied to the spinal cord disease resulting from a deficiency of cobalamin (vitamin B_{12}). It begins with symptoms and signs of posterior column disorder, affecting both legs more or less simultaneously and followed after some weeks by a symmetric paraparesis with either increased or decreased tendon reflexes and Babinski signs. The spinal cord lesion may precede the megaloblastic anemia by months or a year or more, particularly in patients taking folic acid.

Multiple sclerosis, tropical spastic paraparesis, syphilitic meningomyelitis, and combined system disease of nonpernicious anemia type may also cause ataxic paraparesis and must be differentiated from SCD. The diagnosis and treatment of SCD are discussed further in Chap. 37. If treated at its onset, or soon thereafter, striking improvement may be obtained by cobalamin therapy; hence the overriding importance of early diagnosis.

Radiation Myelopathy

This iatrogenic disease appears many months (12 to 15 months in most cases) after radiation therapy to the region of the spine. Clinically it takes the form of a transverse myelopathy that develops insidiously and progresses irregularly for several weeks or months. Pathologically there is coagulation necrosis of both gray and white matter, extending over several segments of the cord and corresponding with the level of the irradiated zone. In most cases this complication can be avoided if the total dose of a given course of radiation is kept below 5000 rads and is given over a period of 30 to 70 days.

Myelopathies Due to Viral Diseases

A vacuolar myelopathy, clinically and pathologically similar to that of vitamin B_{12} deficiency, may complicate AIDS. Another retrovirus (HTLV-1) has been implicated in the etiology of an endemic spastic paraparesis observed in tropical and subtropical climates. These and other viral myelitides (poliomyelitis, herpes zoster, etc.) are discussed in Chap. 31.

Friedreich Ataxia and Familial Spastic Paraparesis

These hereditary forms of myelopathy are described in Chap. 41.

Lathyrism and Tropical Spastic Paraparesis

Lathyrism, common in some parts of India and Africa, takes the form of a chronic spastic paraparesis, with variable degrees of sensory loss and sphincteric disturbances. It is probably due to a neurotoxic amino acid (BOAA) contained in chickling peas, which are consumed in large amounts during periods of famine.

Tropical spastic paraparesis comprises a syndrome of progressive spastic weakness of the legs, impaired function of bladder and bowel and variable low back pain and sensory impairment. It develops over many years in adults residing in the tropics and has been traced to HTLV-1 retrovirus infection.

SYNDROME OF SEGMENTAL SENSORY DISSOCIATION WITH BRACHIAL AMYOTROPHY (SYRINGOMYELIC SYNDROME)

This syndrome is usually due to syringomyelia, i.e., central cavitation of the spinal cord, predominantly cervical, of undetermined cause. Rarely, it is associated with spinal cord tumor (especially hemangioblastoma) or occurs as a late complication of spinal cord trauma. Clinically, syringomyelia is distinguished by segmental weakness and atrophy of the hands and arms with loss of reflexes and a segmental loss of sensation of dissociated type (i.e., loss of pain and temperature sense and preservation of the sense of touch and pressure) in a "cape" distribution over the neck, shoulders, and arms. Later in the illness there is weakness and ataxia of the legs from involvement of corticospinal tracts and posterior columns. Pain in the neck and arms, kyphoscoliosis, and lower brainstem signs (syringobulbia) are frequently associated.

There are two main types of syringomyelia: (1) an idiopathic type, which has its onset in early adult life and is unassociated with obstruction at the foramen magnum, and (2) a type that is associated with a Chiari malformation and signs of obstruction at the foramen magnum. Both types are readily visualized by MRI. Traumatic necrosis and arachnoiditis may contribute to the formation of a spinal cord syrinx.

The treatment of syringomyelia is far from satisfactory. If a Chiari malformation contributes to the clinical picture, unroofing the upper cervical canal up to and including the foramen magnum is advisable. The shunting of the syrinx into the peritoneal cavity or venous system has given unpredictable results.

CONCLUSIONS

In approaching the multitude of diseases that affect the spinal cord, one's primary concern is not to overlook those for which treatment is possible. These are spinal cord tumors and epidural abscess, subacute combined degeneration due to vitamin B_{12} deficiency, chronic spinal meningitis (syphilitic, tuberculous, parasitic), cervical spondylosis, some vascular malformations, and some types of demyelinative myelitis (see Chap. 35). As for the others, diagnosis is advantageous but not crucial, since it does not lead to definitive therapy.

For a more detailed discussion of this topic, see Adams and Victor: *Principles of Neurology*, 4th ed, pp 718–754.

ADDITIONAL READING

Barnett HJM, Foster JB, Hudgson P: *Syringomyelia*. Philadelphia, Saunders, 1973.

Greenberg HS, Kim JH, Posner JB: Epidural spinal cord compression from metastatic tumor. *Ann Neurol* 8:361, 1980.

Herrick M, Mills PE Jr: Infarction of spinal cord. *Arch Neurol* 24:228, 1971.

Petito CK, Navia BA, Cho ES, et al: Vacuolar myelopathy pathologically resembling subacute combined degeneration in patients with AIDS. *N Engl J Med* 312:374, 1985.

Rossier AB, Foo D, Shillito J: Post-traumatic cervical syringomyelia. *Brain* 108:439, 1985.

Shaw MDM, Russell JA, Grossart KW: The changing pattern of arachnoiditis. *J Neurol Neurosurg Psychiatry* 41:97, 1978.

Sloof JH, Kernohan JW, MacCarty CS: *Primary Intramedullary Tumors of the Spinal Cord and Filum Terminale*. Philadelphia, Saunders, 1964.

Wilkinson M: *Cervical Spondylosis*, 2nd ed. Philadelphia, Saunders, 1971.

35 Multiple Sclerosis and Related Demyelinative Diseases

In speaking of disease, the term *demyelinative*, as a defining adjective, is used in two ways. One, which is incorrect in our opinion, is to specify any disease that involves the white matter (myelin, axis cylinders, oligodendrocytes), whether tumor, infarct, or whatever. The other and more correct usage is to denote a disease that affects mainly the myelin sheaths of nerve fibers, leaving axons and their cells of origin intact. Other attributes of a truly demyelinative process are a lack of secondary or wallerian degeneration (because of sparing of axis cylinders) and a perivenous pattern of distribution.

The diseases that are listed in Table 35-1 conform to this latter definition, and all of them share another attribute, that of being idiopathic. Omitted from this tabulation are a number of demyelinative disorders such as subacute combined degeneration due to vitamin B_{12} deficiency, progressive multifocal leukoencephalopathy, and the cortical demyelination of hypoxic encephalopathy—in each of which the causative factor is known.

MULTIPLE SCLEROSIS

Definition

Multiple sclerosis (MS) is a disease of the CNS, beginning most often in late adolescence and early adult life and expressing itself by discrete and recurrent attacks of spinal cord, brainstem, cerebellar, optic nerve, and cerebral dysfunction, the result of foci of destruction of myelinated fibers. The attacks are subacute in onset but may be acute and are often followed by recession of symptoms and even recovery.

Epidemiology

The geography of the disease is noteworthy. In the northern United States and Canada, Great Britain, and northern Europe, the prevalence is high—30 to 80 per 100,000 population. In the southern parts of Europe and the United States the prevalence falls to 6 to 14 per 100,000, and in equatorial regions, to less than 1 per 100,000. Persons who migrate from a high- to a low-risk

TABLE 35-1 Classification of the Demyelinative Diseases

I. Multiple sclerosis (disseminated or insular sclerosis)
   A. Chronic relapsing encephalomyelopathic form
   B. Acute multiple sclerosis
   C. Neuromyelitis optica
II. Diffuse cerebral sclerosis (encephalitis periaxalis diffusa) of Schilder and concentric sclerosis of Baló
III. Acute disseminated encephalomyelitis
   A. Following measles, chickenpox, smallpox, and rarely mumps, rubella, and influenza
   B. Following rabies or smallpox vaccination
IV. Acute and subacute necrotizing hemorrhagic encephalitis
   A. Acute encephalopathic form (hemorrhagic leukoencephalitis of Hurst)
   B. Subacute necrotic myelopathy?

area (or vice versa) after the age of about 15 years retain the risk of their place of origin. Before that age, they acquire the risk of the place to which they migrate. Familial incidence is low. Certain histocompatibility (HLA) antigens are more frequent in the MS population (HLA-DR2, -DR3, -B7, and -A3). The occurrence of MS is low in children. Adult females are more susceptible than males (1.7 : 1.0) and whites more than blacks.

Clinical Manifestations

The disease may occur in asymptomatic form, the lesions being found at autopsy in "silent regions" of the CNS. The first attack comes without warning and may be mono- or polysymptomatic. In one-fifth of the cases, the onset is acute, i.e., the deficit attains its maximum severity in minutes or hours. Weakness or numbness of a limb, monocular visual loss, diplopia, vertigo, facial weakness or numbness, ataxia, and nystagmus are the most common presenting symptoms, and they occur in various combinations. Remission after the first attack is to be expected. Recurrences represent a recrudescence of earlier lesions plus the effects of new ones, predominantly the former. Over a variable period, usually measured in years, the patient becomes increasingly handicapped, with an asymmetric paraparesis and obvious signs of corticospinal tract disease, sensory and cerebellar ataxia, urinary incontinence, optic atrophy, nystagmus, internuclear ophthalmoparesis, and dysarthria. Seizures occur in 3 to 4 percent of patients. Mental changes are variable, depending on whether spinal or cerebral lesions predominate and whether the latter are numerous. The late established stage may not be reached until 20 or 25 years have elapsed. Once the advanced stage is attained, deterioration may be so slow as to suggest the presence of a degenerative disease. Other patients fail rapidly, within 3 to 4 years, and in rare instances, the patient succumbs within months of onset (acute MS).

There are no systemic signs other than fatigue.

Pathology

Multiple discrete lesions of myelin destruction, called plaques, range in size from a few millimeters to several centimeters. The regions around the lateral ventricles are common sites, and the perivenous relationship of the lesions is most evident in this location, but the lesions can be anywhere in the CNS. The lesions vary also in appearance; fresh ones filled with macrophages are ivory or cream colored and old gliotic ones are gray. Perivascular cuffs of lymphocytes and mononuclear cells are more frequent in recent lesions. The neurons and most but not all the axis cylinders are spared. Cavitation of one or more old lesions may occur.

Pathogenesis

There is much evidence to favor an early life viral infection as the initial event in the pathogenesis of MS. However, all attempts to isolate a virus have failed. Whatever the initial event, an autoimmune, cell-mediated inflammatory process focused on CNS myelin or some component thereof appears to be the basis of the recurrent attacks and plaque formation.

Diagnosis

Once there is evidence of multiple CNS lesions that have produced remitting symptoms over a period of time—without evidence of syphilis or other infections, metastatic tumor, or cerebral arteritis (Behçet disease, lupus erythematosus)—the diagnosis becomes certain with a high degree of accuracy. A single lesion causing recurrent symptoms must be regarded with suspicion. While it may be due to MS, certain solitary lesions of other type (vascular malformation of the brainstem, Chiari malformation, or a tumor of the foramen magnum, clivus, or cerebellopontine angle) may produce a clinical picture that closely mimics MS.

Laboratory Findings

In about 80 percent of established cases, the CSF is abnormal. There may be a mild mononuclear pleocytosis and a modest increase in total protein, but the gamma globulin fraction is greatly increased (greater than 10 percent of the total protein).

Even more sensitive indices of MS are the increase in the IgG index and the electrophoretic demonstration of oligoclonal IgG bands. Lesions that are not clinically manifest may be revealed by visual, auditory, and somatosensory evoked potential studies and by MRI; this provides proof that the disease is truly multiple.

Treatment

The administration of ACTH or prednisone, given over a period of weeks, appears to hasten the resolution of nascent lesions. ACTH is given IV, 80 units in 500 mL dextrose and water daily for 3 days, then 40 units of gel IM bid for 7 days. The dose is then decreased by 10 units every 3 days, but if symptoms recur, 20 to 40 units every other day may be required for several weeks or months. IV methylprednisolone (500 mg for 3 to 5 days) or comparable doses of oral prednisone are probably as effective as ACTH. These drugs have not prevented or reduced the incidence of recurrences, nor do they halt the disease in the late deteriorative stage.

Immunosuppression therapy with drugs such as azathiaprine or cyclophosphamide, given over a period of years, has its advocates.

DIFFUSE CEREBRAL SCLEROSIS (SCHILDER DISEASE)

The sporadic case of massive cerebral demyelination in one or several foci proves usually to be an example of cerebral multiple sclerosis. This form of the disease, referred to as Schilder disease, differs from the usual form in being more frequent in childhood and adolescence and in the rapidity with which it may progress to a state of severe disability (weeks or months).

The *clinical manifestations* indicate that the lesions involve tracts of myelinated fibers (optic nerves, geniculocalcarine tracts, corticospinal tracts, posterior or lateral columns of spinal cord, lemnisci of brainstem, and cerebellar peduncles), i.e., are truly leukoencephalopathic. The characteristic lesion is a large, sharply outlined demyelinative focus involving an entire lobe or hemisphere and extending to the opposite hemisphere across the corpus callosum, but careful examination usually discloses additional lesions of MS in the brainstem, optic nerves, or spinal cord. Some degree of remission and relapse under these circumstances and the laboratory findings mentioned above support the diagnosis of MS.

Differential Diagnosis

To be distinguished from Schilder disease are a number of other white matter diseases, not strictly demyelinative; they are called *leukodystrophies*. The known forms of leukodystrophy, distinguished by their pathology, are metachromatic leukodystrophy, globoid-body leukodystrophy (Krabbe disease), sudanophilic leukodystrophy, and adrenoleukodystrophy. These diseases are familial. Usually they begin in infancy and childhood, but each has been observed to have its onset in adult life, particularly adrenoleukodystrophy. The latter is essentially a male (sex-linked) disease diagnosed by finding evidence of adrenal insufficiency and very long chain fatty acids in cultured fibroblasts.

Progressive multifocal leukoencephalopathy is another disease that figures in the differential diagnosis of cerebral MS. However, most of the patients are elderly. The disease takes the form of a focal cerebral lesion, developing over a period of weeks, usually on a background of known lymphatic leukemia, Hodgkin disease, or other lymphoma and less often with other types of neoplasia or AIDS. Regional multifocality is demonstrated by CT scan and MRI. The CSF is usually normal (see Chap. 31).

ACUTE DISSEMINATED ENCEPHALOMYELITIS (Postinfectious, Postexanthem, Postvaccinal Encephalomyelitis; Acute Perivascular Myelinoclasis)

All of these terms refer to a distinctive form of demyelinative disease, which evolves over a period of several hours or days in the setting of a viral exanthematous disease (measles, rubella, chickenpox), after smallpox or rabies vaccination, and rarely with mumps or influenza. Cerebral, cerebellar, or spinal cases appear acutely, along with a pleocytosis. In cerebral cases, death may occur within days. With survival, there is often a gratifying recovery of function. The lesions are microscopic and consist of perivenous zones of demyelination with perivascular cuffing of lymphocytes and mononuclear cells. The changes are quite different from those of a viral infection, and a virus has never been obtained from the cerebral tissue. An autoimmune reaction is postulated. Steroid therapy is of uncertain benefit. The widespread use of measles vaccine, the discontinuation of smallpox vaccination, and the introduction of new tissue culture vaccines for rabies have greatly reduced the incidence of this disease process.

ACUTE NECROTIZING HEMORRHAGIC ENCEPHALOMYELITIS (Leukoencephalitis of Hurst)

This is the most fulminant of the acute demyelinative processes, affecting mainly adults who have had a recent respiratory infection, sometimes due to *Mycoplasma pneumoniae*. Within hours there may be seizures, a massive hemiplegia or quadriplegia, and a polymorphonuclear pleocytosis up to 3000 per mm^3, with increased CSF protein but normal glucose. No bacteria are seen or isolated by culture. In one of our cases, brain swelling and herniation ended life within 6 h. A slower form of the disease, developing over 1 to 2 weeks and with slight pleocytosis, has been seen.

The lesions combine intense perivascular inflammation and demyelination with many small hemorrhages and meningeal inflammation. Only the white matter is affected. No virus has been isolated. Corticosteroid therapy (IV dexamethasone, 6 to 10 mg every 6 h) has been beneficial in some of our cases.

A similar lesion may affect only the spinal cord (acute necrotizing myelitis) or the spinal cord and optic nerves (one type of neuromyelitis optica).

For a more detailed discussion of this topic, see Adams and Victor: *Principles of Neurology*, 4th ed, pp 755–774.

ADDITIONAL READING

Adams RD, Kubik CS: The morbid anatomy of the demyelinative diseases. *Am J Med* 12:510, 1952.

Ebers GC: Optic neuritis and multiple sclerosis. *Arch Neurol* 42:702, 1985.

Ebers GC, Bulman DE, Sadovnick AD: A population-based study of multiple sclerosis in twins. *N Engl J Med* 315:1638, 1986.

Jacobs L, Kinkel PR, Kinkel WR: Silent brain lesions in patients with isolated idiopathic optic neuritis. *Arch Neurol* 43:452, 1986.

Johnson RT, Griffin DE, Hirsch RL, et al: Measles encephalomyelitis—clinical and immunologic studies. *N Engl J Med* 310:137, 1984.

McDonald WI: The mystery of the origin of multiple sclerosis. *J Neurol Neurosurg Psychiatry* 49:113, 1986.

Mathews WB, Acheson ED, Batchelor JR, Weller RO (eds): *McAlpine's Multiple Sclerosis*. New York, Churchill Livingstone, 1985.

Ormerod IEC, McDonald WI, DuBoulay GH, et al: Disseminated lesions at presentation in patients with optic neuritis. *J Neurol Neurosurg Psychiatry* 49:124, 1986.

Paty DW, Asbury AK, Herndon RM, et al: Use of magnetic resonance imaging in the diagnosis of multiple sclerosis: Policy statement. *Neurology* 36:1575, 1986.

Poser CM, Goutiers F, Carpentier M: Schilder's myelinoclastic diffuse sclerosis. *Pediatrics* 77:107, 1986.

Weiner HL, Hafler DA: Immunotherapy of multiple sclerosis. *Ann Neurol* 23:211, 1988.

36 The Inherited Metabolic Diseases of the Nervous System

Advances in biochemistry have made possible the discovery of more than a hundred new diseases of the nervous system; conversely, the study of many of these diseases has opened new fields in neurochemistry. The diseases that fall into this category are too numerous to describe individually. Because they vary as to the time of life when they become clinically manifest, a logical way of grouping them is by the age period in which they are most likely to appear, viz., in the neonatal period, in infancy, in early and late childhood, and so forth. Because of restrictions of space, it will be possible to present only a few illustrative examples from each of these age periods. Information about the rest of them can be found in the *Principles* and in the monographs of Scriver et al and of Adams and Lyon, listed in the references.

In general terms, the diseases being considered here are hereditary, and the ones appearing early are almost always transmitted as autosomal recessive traits. In other words, the mother bears the abnormal gene but does not herself suffer from the disease clinically; during intrauterine life, her normal metabolism protects the fetus, which is then normal for a variable period postnatally. This fact is important because it offers the prospect of prevention. Indeed, biochemical screening of large populations at birth has identified those at risk for several inherited metabolic diseases, and in some instances the effects of these diseases have been prevented.

METABOLIC DISEASES IN THE NEONATAL PERIOD

As indicated above, the infant is normal at birth; only after several days or weeks do these diseases begin to express themselves. The clinical syndrome that ensues is relatively nonspecific for the reason that the immature nervous system has only a limited number of ways of expressing disorders of function. The usual clinical manifestations are reduced alertness and responsivity, lack of normal support reactions of the body and neck, loss of the Moro and startle responses, quivering of the face and limbs, hyper- or hypotonia, disturbances of ocular control (oscillations, nystagmus, loss of vestibulo-ocular reflexes), poor feeding, unstable temperature and respiratory control, and seizures.

The most frequently inherited metabolic diseases of the neonatal period are galactosemia, maple-syrup urine disease; one of the hyperammonemic syndromes; sulfite oxidase deficiency; and ketotic and nonketotic hyperglycinemia.

Galactosemia is a typical example. The onset of symptoms is in the first days of life, after the ingestion of milk. Vomiting and diarrhea are followed by a failure to thrive, drowsiness, inattentiveness, hypotonia, and diminished vigor of the normal neonatal automatisms. There is enlargement of the liver and spleen, jaundice, and anemia. Impaired psychomotor development, cataracts, visual impairment, and cirrhosis become manifest in survivors. The biochemical abnormality is a defect in galactose-1-phosphate uridyl transferase (G-1-PUT). The diagnostic laboratory findings are an elevated blood galactose level, low glucose, galactosuria, and a deficiency of G-1-PUT in red and white blood cells. The treatment is dietary, using milk substitutes.

Differential diagnosis The other common inherited metabolic disease of this period is *phenylketonuria*. Also, *cretinism* is sometimes hereditary. Statewide screening tests of neonates and the introduction of dietary control measures and early thyroid replacement have significantly modified the effects of these two diseases.

Nonhereditary metabolic disorders, notably *hypoglycemia* and *hypocalcemia,* need to be distinguished from hereditary ones. The former are readily recognized by simple biochemical tests and respond well to correction with glucose or calcium.

Parturitional *anoxic-ischemic encephalopathy* and *developmental anomalies,* the other major categories of disease at this time of life, can usually be distinguished by their earlier postnatal onset and other findings.

HEREDITARY METABOLIC DISEASES OF EARLY INFANCY

Beyond the neonatal period diagnosis becomes easier, because then there is evident psychosensorimotor regression after a period of normal development—the hallmark of hereditary metabolic disease. The common clinical manifestations are a loss of vision, head control, interest in the surroundings, and hand-eye coordination; a failure to walk, stand, and sit; and the occurrence of seizures.

The most important members of this group are the *lysosomal storage diseases,* in which there is a genetic deficiency of enzymes necessary for the degradation of specific glycosides or peptides. As a result, the intracytoplasmic lysosomes become engorged with undegraded material, with eventual damage to nerve cells. Often the cells of other organs are similarly affected.

The lysosomal storage diseases are listed in Table 36-1. In addition to the sphingolipidoses, which are the ones most likely to occur in infancy, the table includes the storage diseases of childhood and adolescence, to be considered further on.

G_{M2} gangliosidosis (Tay-Sachs disease) is the best known lysosomal storage disease of infancy. Mainly it affects Jewish infants of eastern European (Ashkenazi) background. The onset is usually by the fourth month of life, with an abnormal startle to acoustic stimuli, listlessness and irritability, and delay in psychomotor development (or regression if onset is at 4 to 6 months). These are followed by hypotonia and then spasticity of the axial musculature, visual failure, cherry-red spots in the retina, seizures, enlarging head (due to an enlarging brain), and death within a few years.

The abnormality here is a deficiency of hexosaminidase A, with accumulation of ganglioside in neurons and retinal ganglion cells. The enzyme defect can be found in serum, white blood cells, and cultured fibroblasts from amniotic fluid, permitting the detection of an affected fetus or a heterozygote carrier of the disease. The disease has been practically eradicated by screening of the ethnic group in which it occurs for the recessive enzyme defect.

INHERITED METABOLIC DISEASES OF LATE INFANCY AND EARLY CHILDHOOD

The following are the hereditary metabolic diseases that appear most often in this age period (1 to 4 years):

1. Many of the milder disorders of amino acid metabolism
2. Metachromatic, globoid-body, and sudanophilic leukodystrophies
3. Late infantile G_{M1} gangliosidosis
4. Late infantile Gaucher disease and Niemann-Pick disease
5. Neuroaxonal dystrophy
6. The mucopolysaccharidoses
7. The mucolipidoses
8. Fucosidosis
9. The mannosidoses
10. Aspartylglycosaminuria
11. Jansky-Bielschowsky ceroid lipofuscinosis
12. Cockayne syndrome

In this group, most attention has been given to the aminoacidurias, for which large-scale screening programs have been instituted in most parts of the Western world. Phenylketonuria is the most familiar example.

The usual type of *phenylketonuria* (there are several milder variants) is transmitted as an autosomal recessive trait. Again, the baby is normal at birth and during the first year but then begins to lag in psychomotor development. By 5 to 6 years the IQ has fallen to less than 50 and often to less than 20. Hyperactivity, aggressivity, clumsy gait, fine tremors of the hands and body, poor coordination, odd posturing, digital mannerisms, and rhythmias are the usual clinical manifestations. Many patients have a light complexion, and seizures occur in 25 percent. High serum levels of phenylalanine (15 mg/dL) are diagnostic. The disease is due to a deficiency of the hepatic enzyme phenylalanine hydroxylase. A low phenylalanine diet instituted at birth and continued for the first 5 to 10 years of life prevents the psychomotor decline. Severe mental retardation as a result of this disease has become a rarity. However, a normal treated homozygous mother, if untreated during pregnancy, will invariably give birth to an affected baby.

Diagnosis In general terms, in distinguishing among the diseases of this group, it is useful to determine whether a particular syndrome is primarily one of white matter (oligodendrocytes and myelin) or gray matter (neurons). This approach narrows the list of possible diseases and facilitates diagnosis. Indicative of the former (*leukodystrophies*) are early onset of spastic paralysis with or without ataxia, loss of tendon reflexes, and visual impairment with optic atrophy but normal retinas. Seizures and mental deterioration are late events. Gray matter diseases (*poliodystrophies*) are characterized by the early occurrence of seizures, myoclonus, blindness with retinal changes, and mental regression; spastic paralysis and signs of sensorimotor tract involvement occur later. The neuronal storage diseases, described in the earlier section, as well as neuroaxonal dystrophy and the lipofuscinoses conform to the pattern of gray matter disease. Metachromatic, globoid-body, and sudanophilic leukodystrophies exemplify the white matter diseases.

INHERITED METABOLIC DISEASES OF LATE CHILDHOOD AND ADOLESCENCE

By this time of life the hereditary metabolic diseases tend to be more selective in their effects on the nervous system and more chronic. Also, the maturation processes of the CNS are nearing completion, so that it has nearly the same capacity for clinical expression as that of the adult. Therefore, the predominant syndrome often provides a clue as to diagnosis.

TABLE 36-1 Lysosomal Storage Diseases

	Enzyme deficiency	Accumulated metabolite
	Sphingolipidoses	
G_{M1} gangliosidosis	G_{M1} ganglioside β-galactosidase	G_{M1} ganglioside, galactose-containing oligosaccharides
Type 1—infantile, generalized		
Type 2—juvenile		
G_{M2} gangliosidosis		
Tay-Sachs disease	Hexosaminidase A	G_{M2} ganglioside
Sandhoff disease	Hexosaminidases A and B	G_{M2} ganglioside, globoside
AB variant	G_{M2} activator factor	G_{M2} ganglioside
Sulfatidoses		
Metachromatic leukodystrophy	Aryl sulfatase A	Sulfatide
Activator factor deficiency	Cerebroside sulfate sulfatase activator factor	Sulfatide
Mucosulfatidosis (multiple sulfatase deficiency)	Aryl sulfatases A, B, C; steroid sulfatase; iduronate sulfatase, heparan *N*-sulfatase	Sulfatide, steroid sulfate, heparan sulfate, dermatan sulfate
Krabbe disease	Galactocerebrosidase	Galactocerebroside
Fabry disease	α-Galactosidase A	Ceramide trihexoside
Gaucher disease		
Infantile form	β-Glucosidase	Glucocerebroside
Adult form	β-Glucosidase	Glucocerebroside
Niemann-Pick disease	Sphingomyelinase	Sphingomyelin
Farber disease	Ceramidase	Ceramide
	Mucopolysaccharidoses	
Hurler-Scheie syndrome	α-Iduronidase	Dermatan sulfate, heparan sulfate
Hunter disease	Iduronate sulfatase	Dermatan sulfate, heparan sulfate

Sanfilippo disease		
Type A	Heparan *N*-sulfatase	Heparan sulfate
Type B	α-*N*-Acetylglucosaminidase	Heparan sulfate
Type C	Heparan-*N*-acetyltransferase	Heparan sulfate
Type D	α-*N*-Glucosamine-6-sulfatase	Heparan sulfate
Morquio disease		
Type A	*N*-Acetylgalactosamine-6-sulfate sulfatase	Keratan sulfate
Type B	β-Galactosidase	Keratan sulfate
Maroteaux-Lamy disease	Arylsulfatase B	Dermatan sulfate
β-Glucuronidase deficiency (Sly disease)	β-Glucuronidase	Dermatan and heparan sulfate
	Mucolipidoses	
Type I	α-*N*-Acetylneuraminidase	Sialyloligosaccharides
Type II (I-cell disease)	Cellular deficiency of many lysosomal	Mucopolysaccharide, glycolipid
Type III (pseudo-Hurler polydystrophy)	enzymes; increased levels of same enzymes extracellular	
Type IV	Unknown	Mucopolysaccharide, ganglioside
	Oligosaccharidoses	
Fucosidosis	α-*L*-Fucosidase	Fucosyl-sphingolipids, oligosaccharides, and glycopeptides
Mannosidosis	α-Mannosidase	Mannosyl-oligosaccharides
Aspartylglucosaminuria	Aspartylglucosamine amide hydrolase	Aspartyl-2-deoxy-2-acetamidoglucosylamine
	Glycogenosis	
Pompe disease	α-Glucosidase	Glycogen
	Other lysosomal storage diseases	
Wolman disease	Acid lipase	Cholesterol esters, triglycerides
Acid phosphatase deficiency	Lysosomal acid phosphatase	Phosphate esters

Progressive Cerebellar Ataxias

The gradual development of cerebellar or sensory ataxia should raise the possibility of Friedreich ataxia, ataxia-telangiectasia, Bassen-Kornzweig acanthocytosis, prolonged vitamin E deficiency, Refsum disease (with polyneuropathy), Unverricht-Lundborg (Baltic) myoclonus, and the Cockayne syndrome. These can be differentiated by clinical and laboratory tests, as described in the *Principles*.

Parkinson Syndrome

The best-known disease that presents with this syndrome is the *hepatolenticular degeneration of Wilson*. This is an autosomal recessive disease of liver and brain that presents between 10 and 30 years of age, with a syndrome of tremor, extrapyramidal rigidity, dysarthria, and dysphagia and, in some cases, with cerebellar ataxia and dementia. Kayser-Fleischer (KF) rings of copper pigment gradually form in the deep layers of the corneas and are pathognomonic of the disease. Altered liver function is an invariable feature but is prominent in only some of the childhood cases.

Diagnostic findings in Wilson disease are KF rings by slit lamp examination, low serum ceruloplasmin and copper, high copper content in liver biopsy, and abnormal CT scan of the basal ganglia. Early diagnosis and control of copper levels (low dietary copper, D-penicillamine, 1 to 2 g/day orally, or zinc acetate or trientine) will prevent the neurologic symptoms or cause them to regress.

Other diseases inducing an extrapyramidal syndrome are Hallervorden-Spatz disease, childhood Huntington chorea, Leigh subacute encephalomyelopathy, Chediak-Higashi disease, and the juvenile type of Niemann-Pick disease.

Syndrome of Dystonia, Chorea, and Athetosis

This syndrome has been described in Chap. 4. Diseases that are most likely to express themselves by this syndrome are Lesch-Nyhan disease, familial calcification of the basal ganglia and cerebellum, lipofuscinosis, torsion dystonia (chemistry and pathologic basis unknown), and late-onset Niemann-Pick disease.

Familial Polymyoclonias

In late childhood and adolescence, a diffuse, arrhythmic jerking of the limbs, often in conjunction with seizures and cerebellar ataxia, is characteristic of the following conditions: (1) Lafora-body polymyoclonus; (2) juvenile cerebroretinal (ceroid) degeneration; (3) the cherry-red spot–myoclonus syndrome (sialidosis or neuraminidosis); (4) the rare, juvenile onset form of G_{M2} gangliosidosis; (5) late-onset Gaucher disease; and (6) mitochondrial encephalopathy. A benign degenerative form is also known (dyssynergia cerebellaris myoclonica of Ramsay Hunt).

Polymyoclonus as a symptom was described in Chap. 5.

Bilateral Hemiplegia, Cerebral Blindness and Deafness, and Other Manifestations of Decerebration

Most of the hereditary leukodystrophies with onset during late childhood and adolescence present with this syndrome. The most familiar are sudanophilic leukodystrophy with bronzing of the skin and adrenal atrophy (adrenoleukodystrophy) and late-onset metachromatic leukodystrophy.

Two of the hereditary metabolic diseases—homocystinuria and Fabry disease—may cause strokes in the juvenile period of life.

Personality, Behavioral, and Cognitive Disorders

Disorders of these types, beginning in late childhood and adolescence, may sometimes be an early expression of hereditary metabolic disease. Although rare, diagnosis is possible if one keeps in mind that behavioral and personality disorders in these circumstances are usually accompanied by some decline in memory and intellectual function. In this respect, the psychiatric disturbances of the hereditary metabolic diseases differ from those of schizophrenia and manic-depressive psychosis. Also, sooner or later, other neurologic abnormalities (ataxia, rigidity, choreoathetosis, polyneuropathy, seizures) begin to appear. Diagnosis is made more difficult if the patient is addicted to opiates or if psychotropic drugs had been given for schizophrenia or manic-depressive disease, producing extrapyramidal symptoms.

Of the many hereditary metabolic diseases in this age period, the following are the most likely to demonstrate early regression of cognitive function in association with alterations of personality and behavior:

1. Wilson disease
2. Hallervorden-Spatz pigmentary degeneration
3. Lafora-body myoclonic epilepsy
4. Late-onset neuronal ceroid–lipofuscinosis (Kufs form)
5. Juvenile Gaucher disease (type III)
6. Some of the mucopolysaccharidoses
7. Adolescent Schilder disease, with or without adrenal atrophy (sudanophilic leukodystrophy)
8. Metachromatic leukodystrophy

9. Adult G_{M2} gangliosidosis
10. Mucolipidosis I (type I sialidosis)
11. Non-wilsonian copper disorder with dementia, spasticity, and paralysis of vertical eye movements
12. Childhood Huntington chorea

ADULT FORMS OF INHERITED METABOLIC DISEASE

Exceptionally, one of the diseases mentioned above assumes a relatively mild and chronic form or the disease may first appear in adult life. The hereditary metabolic diseases that we have observed in adults are listed below:

1. Metachromatic leukoencephalopathy
2. Adrenoleukodystrophy
3. Krabbe globoid body leukodystrophy
4. Kufs form of lipid storage disease
5. G_{M2} gangliosidosis
6. Wilson disease
7. Leigh disease
8. Gaucher disease
9. Niemann-Pick disease
10. Polysaccharide encephalopathy
11. Mucolipidosis, type I
12. Polyneuropathies (Andrade disease, porphyria, Refsum disease)

ADDENDUM

The reader must appreciate that the classification used in this chapter is somewhat arbitrary. Nearly every disease assigned to one age period may extend into another as a milder or more severe variant. Nearly every disease that usually presents with one dominant manifestation may at times present with some other neurologic abnormality. The plan adopted here—of categorizing these diseases by age period and syndromic relationship—is intended merely to facilitate diagnosis.

For a more detailed discussion of this topic, see Adams and Victor: *Principles of Neurology*, 4th ed, pp 775–819.

ADDITIONAL READING

Adams RD, Lyon G: *Neurology of Hereditary Metabolic Diseases of Children*. New York, Hemisphere, 1982.

Menkes JH: *Textbook of Child Neurology*, 4th ed. Philadelphia, Lea & Febiger, 1990, pp 28–138.

Scriver CR, Beaudet Al, Sly WS, Valle D (eds): *The Metabolic Basis of Inherited Disease*. New York, McGraw-Hill, 1989.

37 Diseases of the Nervous System Due to Nutritional Deficiency

Included here are those diseases in which the nervous system suffers injury from the lack of an essential nutrient in the diet or from some conditioning factor, which increases the need for such nutrients. The vitamins, and more particularly the B vitamins—thiamine, nicotinic acid, pyridoxine, pantothenic acid, folic acid, and cobalamin (vitamin B_{12})—are the most important. With the exception of pernicious anemia, which is due solely to vitamin B_{12} deficiency, most deficiency states are associated with a lack of multiple vitamins. In Western society, alcoholism is the condition that most often leads to dietary B vitamin deficiency. Starvation itself is usually not responsible, except in some infants and children who suffer the harmful effects of calorie-protein deprivation.

Nutritional deficiencies give rise to the following disorders of the nervous system:

1. The Wernicke-Korsakoff syndrome
2. Polyneuropathy (neuropathic beriberi)
3. Optic neuropathy
4. Pellagra
5. Syndrome of amblyopia, painful neuropathy, and orogenital dermatitis (Strachan syndrome)
6. Subacute combined degeneration (vitamin B_{12} deficiency)
7. Neurologic disorders due to a deficiency of pyridoxine and other B vitamins (pantothenic acid, folic acid)
8. Vitamin E deficiency
9. "Alcoholic" cerebellar degeneration

Wernicke-Korsakoff Syndrome

This syndrome, a combination of two clinically recognized diseases (one described by Wernicke and the other by Korsakoff) is a chronic thiamine deficiency associated most often but not exclusively with chronic alcoholism. The symptoms and signs of nutritional polyneuropathy are frequently added. The main symptomatology is some combination of diplopia and strabismus (bilateral abducens, horizontal and vertical gaze palsies), nystagmus that is both vertical and horizontal, vestibular and cerebellar ataxia, and a confusional psychosis. The latter is often transformed into a relatively restricted Korsakoff amnesic state. Some degree of weakness, distal and symmetric sensory loss, and areflexia of the legs are present in most cases. If untreated or if the patient is given IV glucose without the addition of thiamine, death may occur from an associated nutritional cardiomyopathy or from some other undefined effect of carbohydrate loading.

The *lesions* are those of a polioencephalopathy restricted to bilaterally symmetric regions of the medial thalamus, hypothalamus, periaqueductal gray matter, and structures in the floor of the fourth ventricle.

Treatment consists of the administration of thiamine chloride (50 mg IV and 50 mg IM daily, until the patient is consuming a full diet), instituted immediately upon recognition (or suspicion) of the disease. Such treatment arrests the disease, but because of residual damage, a horizontal gaze-evoked nystagmus, ataxia of gait ("alcoholic" cerebellar degeneration), and an amnesic (Korsakoff) state may persist.

Nutritional Polyneuropathy

This takes the form of a symmetric loss or impairment of motor, sensory, and reflex function, affecting feet and legs more than hands and arms and the distal parts of the limbs more than the proximal ones. As stated above, this type of neuropathy often accompanies the Wernicke-Korsakoff syndrome, but it also occurs alone, particularly in its most severe form (neuropathic beriberi). Special variants of alcoholic-nutritional polyneuropathies are extremely painful with burning and sweating of the feet and sometimes of the hands as well. The CSF protein is normal or only slightly elevated.

The nerve lesion involves axons as well as myelin sheaths, the degenerative process being most pronounced in the distal parts of the longest and largest myelinated fibers ("dying-back" neuropathy). Once the legs become paralyzed, recovery can occur only after axonal regeneration, a process that may require many months to a year or more. In time, the paralyzed muscles atrophy but nerve conduction is only moderately slowed.

The deficiency can be corrected by oral vitamin therapy or merely a balanced diet adequate in vitamins and is prevented by the same measures.

Deficiency Amblyopia

This is a relatively rare syndrome of subacute central visual loss with gradually developing pallor of the optic discs (optic atrophy). In the past alcohol and tobacco were thought to be causative ("tobacco-alcohol" amblyopia), but the disease is now known to be due to B vitamin deficiency. It overlaps the *Strachan syndrome* in which the amblyopia is associated with a painful and predominantly sensory polyneuropathy and orogenital dermatitis.

Subacute Combined Degeneration (SCD) and Pernicious Anemia (see also Chap. 34)

Long-standing deficiency of cobalamin (vitamin B_{12}) has two major effects; (1) a macrocytic megaloblastic anemia and (2) a separate spinal cord (and sometimes brain and peripheral nerve) degeneration, which may precede the hematologic effects. The neurologic disease has been traced to a failure of a cobalamin-dependent enzyme—methylmalonic CoA mutase, which is essential for the maintenance of myelinated fibers.

Clinical findings Distressing and persistent paresthesias of the feet and hands are usually the initial symptoms, followed by signs of posterior column involvement and then by weakness and signs of corticospinal disease. Rarely visual impairment is an early manifestation of B_{12} deficiency; more often the signs of affection of the optic and peripheral nerves occur late in the disease. Disorders of cerebral function (irritability, drowsiness, emotional instability, and confusion) occur early in the course of cobalamin deficiency. Rarely, with advanced disease, there may be a dementia, due to lesions of the cerebral white matter, similar to those of the spinal cord.

Diagnosis and treatment The chief obstacle to early diagnosis of SCD is the lack of parallelism between the hematologic and neurologic signs. Patients who receive folic acid and some who do not may maintain a normal hematocrit and mean corpuscular volume (MCV) for an indefinite period, while the neurologic signs worsen. In such patients one must search the blood smear for hypersegmented neutrophils and the marrow smear for megaloblasts. Serum cobalamin levels of less than 100 pg/mL are usually associated with neurologic symptoms and signs of SCD. Levels below 200 pg/mg, unassociated with symptoms, call for further investigation of cobalamin deficiency. The two-stage Schilling test is a reliable but not absolute indicator of cobalamin deficiency. The recently developed assays for serum methylmalonic acid and homocysteine appear to be the most sensitive means of detecting cobalamin deficiency (Allen et al, Lindenbaum et al).

A high index of suspicion and early recognition of SCD is essential, since the extent of neurologic improvement is governed by the duration of symptoms before treatment is instituted. Saturation of tissues depleted of vitamin B_{12} requires that large doses be given initially—1000 μg IM daily during hospitalization. This dosage of B_{12} is then given weekly for a month and then monthly for the rest of the patient's life.

Occasionally, folic acid deficiency has been reported to cause lesions identical to those of vitamin B_{12} deficiency.

Pellagra

This is a chronic deficiency state stemming from a lack of nicotinic acid or its amino acid precursor, tryptophan, and usually other B vitamins as well. In the Western world pellagra is observed only rarely, probably because of the widespread practice of fortifying breads and cereals with nicotinic acid. In developing countries, the disease is still common. The fully developed disease is characterized by dermatitis of areas exposed to sunlight, gastrointestinal disturbances (diarrhea), anemia, and neurologic disorder. The latter consists of insomnia, irritability, feelings of anxiety and depression, fatigability, and inattentiveness, progressing to mental dullness, apathy, and forgetfulness. Spinal cord signs and those of polyneuropathy are variably present.

The pathologic changes consist of swelling and central chromatolysis of cortical neurons and a symmetric degeneration of the dorsal columns and to a lesser extent of the corticospinal tracts. The peripheral nerve changes are indistinguishable from those of neuropathic beriberi.

Pyridoxine (Vitamin B_6) Deficiency

There are two types of vitamin B_6 deficiency encephalopathy. One is related to an inherited deficiency of the enzyme glutamic acid decarboxylase, of which vitamin B_6 is a cofactor; this disorder presents as prenatal and postnatal convulsions. The other is an acquired deficiency of the vitamin, either from simple dietary lack or from the therapeutic use of isoniazid or hydralazine, which form hydrazone complexes and make pyridoxal unavailable to the tissues. The latter type is a cause of anemia and polyneuropathy in patients being treated for tuberculosis and hypertension.

Paradoxically, excessive dosage of vitamin B_6, taken orally, may induce a sensory polyneuropathy.

Pantothenic acid deficiency also produces a sensory polyneuropathy, said to be of painful type.

Vitamin E Deficiency

A spinocerebellar ataxia, associated with a polyneuropathy and pigmentary retinopathy, has been traced to a deficiency of vitamin E. It is corrected by administration of the vitamin. A number of underlying diseases may lead to such a deficiency—nontropical sprue, extensive intestinal resections, chronic cholestatic hepatobiliary disease, fibrocystic disease, and other malabsorptive states. All of the reported cases have been in children.

Alcoholic Cerebellar Degeneration

This term refers to a common disorder in alcoholics characterized by a wide-based stance and gait, instability of the trunk, and ataxia of the legs. Arms are affected to a lesser extent, and dysarthria and nystagmus are distinctly uncommon. The pathologic changes consist of a degeneration of the neurocellular elements of the cerebellar cortex, particularly the Purkinje cells, restricted to the anterior-superior vermis and, in advanced cases, to the anterior parts of the anterior lobes.

These changes are similar in type and distribution to those found in the Wernicke-Korsakoff syndrome, and the same syndrome has been observed, albeit rarely, in states of malnutrition unassociated with alcoholism. Adequate diet arrests the process and may be attended by improvement.

Central pontine myelinolysis and *Marchiafava-Bignami disease* (degeneration of the corpus callosum) are rare disorders that are observed most often in alcoholics but are not confined to them. A nutritional etiology has been suggested but not established. They are considered in the next chapter, with the acquired metabolic diseases of the nervous system.

For a more detailed discussion of this topic, see Adams and Victor: *Principles of Neurology*, 4th ed, pp 820–845.

ADDITIONAL READING

Allen RH, Stabler SP, Savage DG, Lindenbaum J: Diagnosis of cobalamin deficiency. I. Usefulness of serum methylmalonic acid and total homocysteine concentrations. *Am J Hematol* 34:90, 1990.

Beck WS: Cobalamin and the nervous system. *N Engl J Med* 318:1752, 1988.

Ishii N, Nishihara Y: Pellagra among chronic alcoholics: Clinical and pathological study of 20 necropsy cases. *J Neurol Neurosurg Psychiatry*. 44:209, 1981.

Lindenbaum J, Healton EB, Savage DG, et al: Neuropsychiatric disorders caused by cobalamin deficiency in the absence of anemia or macrocytosis. *N Engl J Med* 318:1720, 1988.

Victor M: Polyneuropathy due to nutritional deficiency and alcoholism, in Dyck PJ, Thomas PK, Lambert EH, Bunge R (eds): *Peripheral Neuropathy*, 2nd ed. Philadelphia, Saunders, 1984, pp 1899–1940.

Victor M, Adams RD, Collins GH: *The Wernicke-Korsakoff Syndrome and Related Neurologic Disorders Due to Alcoholism and Malnutrition*. Philadelphia, Davis, 1989.

Victor M, Adams RD, Mancall EL: A restricted form of cerebellar degeneration occurring in alcoholic patients. *Arch Neurol* 1:577, 1959.

Victor M, Mancall EL, Dreyfus PM: Deficiency amblyopia in the alcoholic patient: A clinicopathologic study. *Arch Ophthalmol* 64:1, 1960.

38 Acquired Metabolic Diseases of the Nervous System

The nervous system is regularly affected by diseases that cause failure of the heart, lungs, liver, kidneys, pancreas, and endocrine organs. This aspect of neurology obviously touches every branch of internal medicine, and the resulting syndromes must be familiar to internists and neurologists alike. In fact, recognition of the neurologic syndrome often leads to the diagnosis of the underlying disease.

Table 38-1 classifies the acquired metabolic disorders of the nervous system according to the syndrome by which they present.

SYNDROME OF CONFUSION, STUPOR, AND COMA

Here the most common disorder is a lack of oxygenation of the brain, caused by failure of the heart and circulation or of the lungs and respiration. The most frequent circumstances are suffocation (drowning, strangulation, and tracheal obstruction by a foreign body, blood, or vomitus); carbon monoxide poisoning; respiratory failure from cranial trauma and paralytic diseases (Guillain-Barré, poliomyelitis); and various forms of circulatory collapse (myocardial infarction, infective and traumatic shock). In all of these conditions, the mechanism can be reduced to insufficient oxygenation of the brain; and since cerebral neurons have no capacity to store oxygen, they are destroyed when their oxygen supply is cut off (within 5 min if the anoxia is complete).

Mild degrees of hypoxia induce only inattentiveness, impairment of judgment, and motor incoordination, and there are essentially no lasting effects. Severe hypoxia causes coma, which, if not promptly reversed, usually results in permanent injury. In its most severe form, the comatose patient lapses rapidly into a state known as *brain death*, which is manifested by a complete lack of awareness of and responsivity to all manner of stimuli and abolition of all brainstem reflex activity, including respiration. The EEG is isoelectric. Only cardiac action and blood pressure are maintained, but nearly always, in these circumstances, circulatory failure follows within a few days. If the patient survives, as happens when brainstem structures are

TABLE 38-1 Classification of the Acquired Metabolic Disorders of the Nervous System

I. Metabolic diseases presenting as a syndrome of episodic confusion, stupor, or coma
   A. Hypoxic-hypotensive encephalopathy
   B. Hypercapnia
   C. Hypoglycemia
   D. Hyperglycemia
   E. Hepatic failure and Eck fistula
   F. Reye syndrome
   G. Uremia
   H. Other metabolic encephalopathies: acidosis due to diabetes mellitus or renal failure (see also inherited forms of acidosis in Chap. 36); Addison disease; bismuth subgallate intoxication
II. Disturbances of sodium and potassium: changes in osmolality
III. Metabolic diseases presenting as a progressive extrapyramidal syndrome
   A. Acquired hepatocerebral degeneration
   B. Hyperbilirubinemia and kernicterus
   C. Hypoparathyroidism
IV. Metabolic diseases presenting as cerebellar ataxia
   A. Hypothyroidism
   B. Hyperthermia and hypothermia
   C. Hyperthyroidism
V. Metabolic diseases causing psychosis or dementia
   A. Cushing disease and steroid encephalopathy
   B. Thyroid psychoses
   C. Hyperparathyroidism
   D. Pancreatic encephalopathy (?)
   E. Whipple disease

preserved, he or she may live on in a persistent vegetative state (see Chap. 16).

Often the period or degree of anoxia is difficult to measure. Although the patient may be pulseless or with blood pressure too low to measure, there may still be some circulation to the brain. Cerebral function may then be restored after a much longer period of apparent anoxia than 5 min. The attending physician, lacking these essential data, must therefore be prepared to institute resuscitative measures (clear airway, artificial respiration, cardiovascular support) as quickly as possible.

Hypercapnia (and Hypoxia) in Pulmonary Disease (Hypercarbia)

Chronic parenchymal lung disease, inadequacy of the respiratory centers, or severe weakness of the muscles of respiration causes a chronic respiratory acidosis with elevation of P_{CO_2}. Secondary polycythemia and heart failure (cor pulmonale) may accompany these disorders of ventilation, and there may be an added factor of pulmonary infection.

The neurologic syndrome comprises headache, papilledema, drowsiness, mental dullness, confusion, tremor, abrupt lapses in sustained muscle contraction (asterixis), and coma. In the fully developed state, the CSF is under increased pressure, and arterial P_{CO_2} may exceed 75 mmHg. The pH of blood and CSF are lowered to 7.15 to 7.25. In this setting, the administration of O_2 may be harmful because the low arterial O_2 may be the only stimulus to the respiratory center, the latter having become insensitive to CO_2.

Forced ventilation, to reduce CO_2 retention, using an intermittent positive pressure device and room air (or oxygen if hypoxia is severe); administration of digitalis and diuretics; venesection to reduce viscosity of the blood; and antibiotics for pulmonary infection are the usual therapeutic procedures. Opioids should be avoided because of their depressant effects upon the respiratory centers.

Hypoglycemic Encephalopathy

Since the brain is largely dependent upon glucose for its metabolism and has only a limited glucose reserve (1 to 2 g or 30 μmol/100 g of tissue), hypoglycemia cannot be tolerated for longer than about 90 min. In conditions such as insulin overdose, islet cell tumor, depletion of liver glycogen, acute nonicteric hepatoencephalopathy (Reye syndrome), glycogen storage disease, or an idiopathic state in infants, the blood glucose may fall to a critical degree. When it reaches a level of 30 mg/dL, hunger, sweating, headache, nervousness, and trembling develop; with a further drop in blood glucose, forced sucking, grasping, muscular spasms, and decerebrate rigidity appear, and in some patients, myoclonic twitching and seizures as well. At levels of 10 mg/dL or below, the patient becomes comatose, with dilated pupils, pale skin, shallow respiration, slow pulse, and hypotonicity of the limb musculature. Exceptionally, a relatively mild but persistent hypoglycemia, as occurs with islet cell tumors, may cause symptoms such as ataxia, chorea, rigidity, combativeness, drowsiness, and lethargy.

Infants tolerate marked reduction of blood glucose for a longer time than adults because of higher glucose reserves.

The administration of intravenous glucose restores brain function completely if given before or at the very onset of coma. If coma is prolonged, some degree of permanent damage results, and the patient then remains mentally impaired or shows other neurologic residua, like the ones that follow severe anoxia.

Hyperglycemia

Diabetic coma with hyperglycemia and ketoacidosis is correctible by proper medical measures. Usually in this condition the blood glucose is more than 400 mg/dL, the blood pH is less than 7.2, and P_{CO_2} is 10 meq/L or less. In *nonketotic hyperglycemia* the blood glucose may reach extremely high levels, in the range of 1000 mg/dL, and be associated with seizures and focal cerebral signs (hemiparesis, aphasia, visual field defect), as well as stupor and coma, because of the extreme hyperosmolality. Cautious administration of isotonic solutions and insulin may result in full recovery, but the mortality in the elderly diabetic is distressingly high.

Hepatic Encephalopathy

This is a generic term for the several cerebral disorders consequent upon impaired liver function. An *acute encephalopathy* may complicate fulminant hepatitis; an acute nonicteric form is associated with fatty infiltration of the liver and other organs (*Reye syndrome*). More common is the subacute encephalopathy that complicates all varieties of chronic liver disease; this is the type usually referred to as *hepatic stupor or coma*. Repeated attacks of the latter may result in permanent structural damage to the brain. There are in addition several hereditary hyperammonemic syndromes of infancy that cause episodic coma and seizures.

Probably all forms of hepatic encephalopathy have their basis in a disorder of nitrogen metabolism. Ammonia (NH_3) is formed in the bowel by the action of urease-containing organisms on dietary protein and is carried to the liver in the portal circulation. However, the NH_3 fails to be converted to urea, because of either hepatocellular disease or portal-systemic shunting of blood, or both. As a result, excessive amounts of NH_3 reach the systemic circulation and interfere with cerebral metabolism in a way that is not fully understood (see references to Zieve and to Cooper and Plum).

The *clinical syndrome of hepatic coma* consists essentially of a disorder of consciousness, ranging from confusion to stupor and coma, accompanied by a characteristic movement disorder and EEG abnormality. The disorder of movement, loosely referred to as a "flapping tremor," is in reality an intermittency of sustained muscle contraction (asterixis). The EEG changes occur early in the evolution of the syndrome and take the form of synchronous bursts of slow (delta) waves, which replace all normal activity as coma deepens. A fluctuating rigidity of the limbs, reflex sucking and grasping, and sometimes Babinski signs and focal or generalized seizures round out the clinical picture. The blood NH_3 levels usually exceed 200 μg/dL and may be much higher.

Hepatic coma is most often precipitated by high protein intake and gastrointestinal hemorrhage. Hypoxia, hypokalemia, electrolyte depletion, and excessive diuresis are contributory factors. Measures that lower blood NH_3 levels—low-protein diet, oral neomycin and neomycin enemas (to reduce urease-producing bacteria in the gastrointestinal tract), and the use of lactulose (which acidifies the bowel contents)—are of therapeutic benefit and lend support to the ammonia intoxication hypothesis.

In the *Reye syndrome of children*, an acute viral infection (varicella, influenza B, and others) precipitates the rapid development of fever, vomiting, an enlarging fatty liver, convulsions, stupor and coma, with decorticate or decerebrate rigidity, loss of brainstem reflexes, and death, all within a few days. The CSF is under high pressure but is acellular. NH_3 levels may exceed 500 μg/dL. SGOT levels are also high (several thousand units).

At autopsy the liver cells are filled with fine droplets of fat, which are also present in renal tubules, myocardium, and skeletal muscle fibers. The brain is swollen with cerebral and cerebellar herniations and only secondary hypoxic changes.

Control of fever, ventilation, osmolality of blood, electrolyte balance, and blood NH_3 before coma develops has resulted in a significant reduction in mortality. In children, salicylates given for a respiratory infection are believed to be capable of precipitating this syndrome. Knowledge of this effect is probably responsible for the striking decrease in the incidence of the Reye syndrome in recent years.

Uremic Encephalopathy

Several types of encephalopathy may develop in the course of renal failure and dialysis:

1. *Hypertensive encephalopathy:* This is a rapidly evolving syndrome in which severe hypertension (diastolic above 130 mmHg) is associated with headache, nausea and vomiting, visual disturbances due to retinal hemorrhages, exudates, and papilledema, convulsions, confusion, stupor, and coma. The BUN may be only modestly increased. In children and in women with eclampsia, which is probably a variety of hypertensive encephalopathy, the syndrome may develop with a lesser degree of hypertension. Cautious lowering of blood pressure, anticonvulsant medication, and immediate delivery of the infant in the eclamptic are the essential elements in treatment.

2. *Uremic twitch—convulsive syndrome:* A variety of motor phenomena—twitching, tremor, myoclonus, convulsions—may be associated with renal failure, sometimes when the patient is still mentally clear and the blood pressure is normal. The BUN is extremely high. Acidosis, hypocalcemia, and hypomagnesemia are added factors. Dialysis is the only effective treatment. Convulsions, which occur in about one-third of cases, respond to relatively low plasma concentrations of phenytoin and valproic acid.
3. *"Disequilibrium syndrome":* This term refers to a group of symptoms—headache, muscle cramps, agitation, drowsiness and convulsions—that have been observed in uremic patients during the third and fourth hours of hemodialysis or peritoneal dialysis. Sometimes the symptoms occur after completion of dialysis. Water intoxication and inappropriate ADH secretion are believed to cause a shift of H_2O into the brain and brain swelling.
4. *Dialysis dementia:* This syndrome complicates chronic hemodialysis. It begins as a hesitant stuttering dysarthria and incoordination of the speech musculature, followed by facial and generalized myoclonus and seizures and intellectual decline. Intermittent at first, occurring during or just after dialysis, the symptoms later become more persistent and eventually permanent, terminating life in 1 to 2 years.

   This encephalopathy probably represents a form of aluminum intoxication and has been practically eliminated by the universal practice of purifying the water used in dialysis.

CENTRAL PONTINE MYELINOLYSIS (CPM)

In this disease, the center of the basis pontis and other parts of the brain undergo a more or less symmetric noninflammatory demyelination. If the lesion is large, the patient becomes quadriplegic and pseudobulbar (pseudocoma or "locked-in" syndrome). About one-half of the cases occur in alcoholics, the remainder in association with a wide spectrum of serious systemic diseases, with severe and extensive burns, and following kidney and liver transplantation. CT scanning and particularly MRI have greatly enhanced our ability to make a premortem diagnosis, although the lesion may not be visualized for several days or for a week or more after the onset of symptoms.

The factor common to most cases of CPM is severe hyponatremia (95 to 120 meq/L). Although hyponatremia itself may cause severe CNS dysfunction (seizures, stupor, coma, and respiratory arrest), it does not cause CPM; the latter appears (but not in all cases) only after rapid correction or overcorrection of hyponatremia. Evidence from severely burned patients suggests that the production of hyperosmolality, rather than hypernatremia per se, is the critical factor in the pathogenesis of CPM. The optimum method for the correction of severe hyponatremia remains to be determined, but the best evidence to date, in animals and in man, indicates that this must be done cautiously, at a rate not exceeding 12 meq in the first 24 h and not exceeding 20 meq in the first 48 h.

See the *Principles* for descriptions of other acquired metabolic encephalopathies produced by electrolyte imbalance.

ACQUIRED METABOLIC DISEASES PRESENTING WITH PROMINENT EXTRAPYRAMIDAL AND CEREBELLAR SIGNS

Chronic acquired hepatocerebral degeneration and *hypoparathyroidism* with basal ganglia and cerebellar calcification are the best known examples. *Kernicterus* is another, a complication of *erythroblastosis fetalis*. Chorea has been reported in *hyperthyroidism*.

A patient with any type of cirrhosis, with or without preceding attacks of hepatic coma, may present with a slowly progressive syndrome of dysarthria, choreoathetosis, cerebellar ataxia, and mental deterioration. The neurologic abnormality correlates best with chronic hyperammonemia and may improve to some extent when it is corrected (see above).

In *hypoparathyroidism*, both choreoathetosis and ataxia, unilateral or bilateral, and symptoms of parkinsonism have followed long after the early hypocalcemic manifestations of tetany and convulsions. The late neurologic effects appear to be related to basal ganglionic and cerebellar deposits of calcium, which are readily visible by CT scan and MRI.

Myxedema is said to produce a cerebellar ataxia, but we have had no experience with it. More convincing is the claim of experienced neurologists that the incoordination of gait and limb movements disappear with thyroid medication. There is no doubt that hypothyroidism is the basis of a slowness of movement, delayed relaxation of tendon reflexes, and rarely of a sensorimotor polyneuropathy.

Extreme *hyperthermia* from heat stroke may leave the patient with cerebellar ataxia due to loss of Purkinje cells.

METABOLIC DISEASES PRESENTING AS PSYCHOSIS AND DEMENTIA

Examples are chronic portal-systemic encephalopathy, Cushing disease and other corticosteroid psychoses, and the thyroid encephalopathies (thyrotoxic and myxedematous).

For a more detailed discussion of this topic, see Adams and Victor: *Principles of Neurology*, 4th ed, pp 846–869.

ADDITIONAL READING

Cooper AJL, Plum F: Biochemistry and physiology of brain ammonia. *Physiol Rev* 67:440, 1987.

Laureno R: Central pontine myelinolysis following rapid correction of hyponatremia. *Ann Neurol* 13:232, 1983.

McKee AC, Winkelman MD, Banker BQ: Central pontine myelinolysis in severely burned patients: Relationship to serum hyperosmolality. *Neurology* 38:1211, 1988.

Plum F, Posner JB: *Diagnosis of Stupor and Coma*, 3rd ed. Philadelphia, Davis, 1980.

Rosenblum JL, Keating JP, Prensky Al, Nelson JS: A progressive neurologic syndrome in children with chronic liver disease. *N Engl J Med* 304:503, 1981.

Shaywitz BA, Rothstein P, Venes JL: Monitoring and management of increased intracranial pressure in Reye syndrome: Results in 29 children. *Pediatrics* 66:198, 1980.

Victor M, Adams RD, Cole M: The acquired (non-wilsonian) type of chronic hepatocerebral degeneration. *Medicine* 44:345, 1965.

Victor M, Rothstein J: Neurologic complications of hepatic and gastrointestinal disease, in Asbury AK, McKhann G, McDonald WI (eds): *Diseases of the Nervous System*, 2nd ed. Philadelphia, Saunders, in press.

Wilkinson DS, Prockop LD: Hypoglycemia: Effects on the nervous system, in Vinken PJ, Bruyn BW (eds): *Handbook of Clinical Neurology*, vol 27: *Metabolic and Deficiency Diseases of the Nervous System*, pt I. Amsterdam, North-Holland, 1976, chap 4, pp 53–78.

Wright DG, Laureno R, Victor M: Pontine and extrapontine myelinolysis. *Brain* 102:361, 1979.

Zieve L: Pathogenesis of hepatic encephalopathy. *Metab Brain Dis* 2:147, 1987.

39 | Alcohol and Alcoholism

Ethyl alcohol or ethanol, in the form of whiskey, gin, vodka, wine, and beer, is the most widely used and abused of all intoxicant drugs. Its acute effects are known to everyone. As with all addictive drugs, tolerance develops with chronic usage and special symptoms develop upon withdrawal of the drug after a period of chronic abuse (withdrawal or abstinence syndrome).

The essential medical facts about the absorption, distribution, excretion, and metabolism of alcohol and its effects on nonneurologic organ systems are discussed in the *Principles*. Reviewed there also are the pharmacologic effects upon the nervous system and the theories of causation of alcoholism. Here, only the common neurologic problems will be considered; they are tabulated below.

CLINICAL EFFECTS OF ALCOHOL ON THE NERVOUS SYSTEM

I. Alcohol intoxication—drunkenness, coma, excitement (''pathological intoxication''), ''blackouts''
II. The abstinence or withdrawal syndrome—tremulousness, hallucinosis, seizures, delirium tremens
III. Nutritional diseases of the nervous system secondary to alcoholism
   A. Wernicke-Korsakoff syndrome
   B. Polyneuropathy
   C. Optic neuropathy (''tobacco-alcohol amblyopia'')
   D. Pellagra
   E. Cerebellar degeneration
IV. Diseases of uncertain pathogenesis, associated with alcoholism
   A. Central pontine myelinolysis
   B. Marchiafava-Bignami disease
   C. Alcoholic cardiomyopathy and myopathy
   D. Alcoholic dementia
   E. Cerebral atrophy
V. Fetal alcohol syndrome
VI. Neurologic disorders consequent upon Laennec cirrhosis and portal-systemic shunts
   A. Hepatic stupor and coma
   B. Chronic hepatocerebral degeneration

ALCOHOL INTOXICATION

The usual manifestations of alcohol intoxication are so common that they require no elaboration. The varying degrees of exhilaration and excitement, loss of restraint, loquacity, irregularity of behavior, slurred speech, incoordination of movement and gait, inattentiveness, drowsiness, stupor, and coma need only be mentioned. The usual forms of alcohol intoxication present little difficulty in diagnosis and management. In certain unusual forms, however, diagnosis may be difficult and urgent treatment is required.

Alcoholic coma In former times, alcohol was used as an anesthetic, but this was always a risky practice, since the margin of safety between a dosage that produces coma and one that seriously depresses respiration is much narrower than that of the common anesthetics. This fact adds an element of urgency to the diagnosis and treatment of alcoholic narcosis.

The diagnosis of alcoholic coma can be made with confidence only after exclusion of all other causes of coma; a flushed face and odor of alcohol are in themselves insufficient diagnostic criteria. The blood alcohol level is a useful but imperfect diagnostic measure. A concentration of 400 mg/dL may prove lethal in a nontolerant individual but cause only mild symptoms of intoxication in a chronic drinker. Relatively low blood levels in a comatose alcoholic (200 mg/dL or less) should always suggest the presence of associated drug intoxication (barbiturate, methyl alcohol), infection, or liver disease.

The main object in the *treatment* of alcoholic coma is to prevent respiratory depression and its complications and follows along the lines indicated in Chap. 16. Hemodialysis should be undertaken in patients with extremely high blood alcohol levels (>500 mg/dL), particularly those who are acidotic or have concurrently ingested methanol or ethylene glycol or some other dialyzable drug.

"Blackouts" At a certain stage of alcohol intoxication, an individual may cease to form memories, despite being able to carry out an array of complex activities. Later, when sober, the individual has no memory for these activities, which may have occupied a period of several hours. These are so-called blackouts, which may be taken as a measure of the severity of intoxication. Their occurrence is not an indicator of the development of alcohol addiction, as had commonly been assumed in the past.

Pathological intoxication (complicated intoxication, alcohol paranoid state, atypical intoxication) The boundaries of this syndrome have never been clearly drawn, as one might gather from its diverse designations. Well known are certain idiosyncratic reactions to alcohol, in which a few drinks predictably evoke behavioral abnormalities seemingly alien to the personality of the subject—argumentativeness, assaultiveness, acute paranoia, indiscriminate sexual advances, or criminality. All that can be said is that the disinhibitory effects of alcohol have exposed a latent sociopathic trait.

More often the term *pathological intoxication* is reserved for an outburst of blind fury with assaultive and destructive behavior, the patient being subdued only with difficulty and massive sedation; later the patient has no memory of the episode. This latter state needs to be distinguished from temporal lobe seizures and sociopathy, which occasionally take the form of explosive outbursts of rage and violence. A similar paradoxic reaction sometimes follows the administration of barbiturates.

ABSTINENCE OR WITHDRAWAL SYNDROME

This is a symptom complex consisting of tremulousness, hallucinations, seizures, confusion, and psychomotor and autonomic overactivity, which develops within several hours or days after an addictive drinker abstains from alcohol. The parts of the brain upon which alcohol acts and which come to tolerate increasing amounts of the drug appear to be released and become overactive when alcohol is withdrawn.

Clinical Features

These are depicted diagrammatically in Fig. 39-1. In effect, there are two syndromes: a minor and a major one.

The *minor or early syndrome* is characterized by tremulousness, nausea and vomiting, insomnia, flushed facies, mild diaphoresis, hallucinations (visual and auditory, rarely tactile and olfactory), and convulsions; disorientation and confusion are minimal in degree or absent altogether. These symptoms have their onset within 7 to 8 h after the cessation of drinking, reach their peak intensity within 24 h, and then subside over several days, usually without sequelae. Exceptionally, an alcohol withdrawal state that begins as an auditory hallucinosis fails to recover and settles into a chronic delusional-hallucinatory psychosis, which may be mistaken for paranoid schizophrenia. In a relatively small number of patients, the early symptoms of alcohol withdrawal (particularly withdrawal seizures) are a prelude to delirium tremens.

The *major withdrawal syndrome*, traditionally designated as *delirium tremens (DTs)*, is characterized by profound confusion, gross tremor and jactitations, delusions and hallucinations,

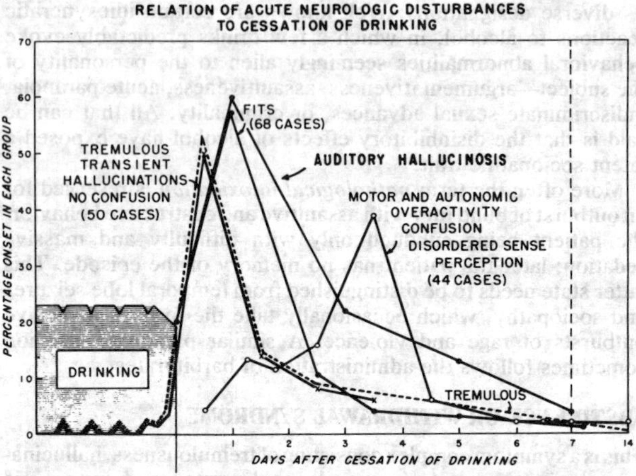

FIG. 39-1 Relation of acute neurologic disturbances to cessation of drinking. The shaded drinking period is greatly foreshortened and not intended to be quantitative. The periodic notching in the baseline represents the tremulousness, nausea, etc., that occur following a night's sleep. The time relations of the various groups of symptoms to withdrawal are explained in the text. (*From Victor and Adams, 1953.*)

and autonomic overactivity (fever, tachycardia, dilated pupils, marked diaphoresis). These symptoms have their onset between 48 and 96 h (peak onset, 72 h) after cessation of drinking. The major syndrome is much less frequent than the minor one, but far more serious, ending fatally in 5 to 10 percent of cases. Hyperthermia, circulatory collapse, infection, and injury are the conditions usually associated with a fatal outcome. Pathologic study of the brain in these cases has not disclosed any significant histologic abnormalities.

Withdrawal Seizures ("Rum Fits")

Early in the withdrawal period (7 to 48 h after cessation) there is a marked tendency to convulse, even in persons with no history or EEG evidence of epilepsy. Stated somewhat differently, alcohol withdrawal is an important cause of convulsive seizures occurring for the first time in adult life.

During the period of seizure activity, the EEG may be abnormal and the patient may be unusually sensitive to stroboscopic stimulation, but these abnormalities subside in a few days, even in patients who go on to develop DTs (this sequence occurs in almost 30 percent of patients with withdrawal seizures). As a rule, such seizures are grand mal in type; they may occur singly or there may be several seizures over a period of several hours, or rarely, status epilepticus. A focal seizure occurring in this setting indicates the presence of a focal cerebral lesion (most often traumatic), in addition to the effects of alcohol withdrawal.

In patients with idiopathic or post traumatic epilepsy, seizures may be precipitated by a short period of drinking, but here also the seizures occur not when the patient is intoxicated but in the "sobering-up" period.

Treatment of Alcohol Withdrawal Symptoms

Minor withdrawal symptoms The main considerations are replacement of fluids and electrolytes and the judicious administration of sedative drugs. In depleted alcoholics, the use of parenteral glucose solutions carries a special danger, namely, the precipitation of Wernicke disease, and should always be supplemented by B vitamins (Berroca-C is a useful IV preparation). A variety of sedative drugs are equally useful in allaying tremor, nervousness, and insomnia. In general, phenothiazine drugs should be avoided because they reduce the threshold to seizures. Chlordiazepoxide (Librium) and diazepam (Valium) are currently the most popular drugs, but their *oral* administration has no advantages over paraldehyde. The latter drug is extremely safe (8 to 12 mL in orange juice every 3 to 4 h), provided it is dispensed in ampoules, which prevent its deterioration.

Delirium tremens Treatment of this condition is a more compelling matter than treatment of the minor withdrawal syndrome. It begins with a careful search for an associated injury or infection, particularly cerebral laceration, subdural hematoma, pneumonia, and meningitis. A chest film, lumbar puncture, CT scan, and liver function tests should be obtained routinely.

The cornerstones of treatment are the administration of fluids and correction of electrolyte abnormalities. Severe diaphoresis requires the administration of as much as 10 L of fluid daily, of which about one-quarter should be normal saline. The importance of adding B vitamins has been mentioned above. The amounts of glucose and electrolyte to be added are governed by the laboratory findings. Very low Na concentrations should be corrected with caution, for the reasons given in Chap. 38.

In severe forms of DTs, vital signs need to be recorded frequently, in anticipation of shock and hyperthermia. Shock requires the urgent use of whole-blood transfusions, fluids, and vasopressor drugs, and hyperthermia requires the use of a cooling mattress in addition to the specific treatment of any infection that may be present.

Drugs must be used circumspectly. One's object is not the absolute suppression of agitation and tremor, which could seriously depress respiration, but simply the blunting of symptoms to the point of facilitating nursing care. Medication usually needs to be given parenterally—diazepam, 10 mg IV and repeated once or twice at 20- to 30-min intervals until the patient is calm but awake; or phenobarbital or amobarbital (120 mg) or haloperidal (10 mg) may be given at 3- to 4-h intervals, provided there is no serious liver disease. Corticosteroids have no place in the treatment of withdrawal symptoms.

Withdrawal seizures In most cases, anticonvulsant drugs are not required, since the seizures occupy only a brief circumscribed period in the early stages of withdrawal and often have ceased by the time the patient is seen by the physician. The parenteral administration of phenobarbital or chlordiazepoxide early in the withdrawal period might prevent seizures, but phenytoin is ineffective in this respect.

Also, the long-term administration of anticonvulsants is impractical. If patients remain abstinent, there will be no seizures; if they resume drinking, they usually abandon their medications.

Status epilepticus due to alcohol withdrawal should be managed like status of any other cause. Focal seizures need to be investigated and managed along the lines indicated in Chap. 15. In patients with idiopathic or posttraumatic epilepsy, drinking is interdicted, and such patients need to be maintained on their anticonvulsant regimen.

Nutritional Diseases of the Nervous System Secondary to Alcoholism

These do not differ in any particular from nutritional diseases in which alcohol plays no part. They have been described in Chap. 37.

Alcoholic Dementia (Alcoholic Deteriorated State)

These terms are used to designate a supposedly distinctive form of dementia that is attributable to the direct effects of alcohol on the brain. However, the clinical picture has been anything but clear, and the descriptions in current textbooks of psychiatry lack consistency. More importantly, no distinctive neuropathologic changes have ever been described. Such changes as have been attributed to the toxic effects of alcohol are artefactual or otherwise insignificant.

In our experience and that of others, most of the cases that come to autopsy with the label of alcoholic dementia or deteriorated state prove to have the lesions of the Wernicke-Korsakoff syndrome. Traumatic lesions are commonly added, as are the lesions of hepatic or anoxic encephalopathy, communicating hydrocephalus, or a variety of diseases unrelated to alcoholism. Practically always the clinical state can be accounted for by one or a combination of these diseases, and there has been no need to invoke a hypothetical toxic effect of alcohol on the brain.

"Alcoholic Cerebral Atrophy"

This disorder also does not constitute a clinical-pathologic entity. The diagnosis is essentially a radiologic one—the lateral ventricles are enlarged and the sulci are widened. The clinical correlates of these findings are quite unpredictable. About 25 percent of patients with the Wernicke-Korsakoff syndrome show dilated lateral ventricles and widened sulci, but we have not been able to find a histopathologic basis for these abnormalities. In other alcoholics, the radiologic findings are unassociated with any signs of neuropsychiatric disease. Moreover, in alcoholics who remain sober for a protracted period, the radiologic abnormalities are to a large extent reversible, suggesting that a shift of fluids had occurred in the brain rather than a loss of tissue (atrophy). Thus it would be more appropriate to refer to the asymptomatic ventricular enlargement and sulcal widening as such rather than as cerebral atrophy, at least until a consistent pathologic basis for this condition has been established.

Fetal Alcohol Syndrome

Infants born of a severely alcoholic mother who drinks throughout pregnancy are often smaller than expected for the duration of pregnancy, are slightly microcephalic, and have short palpebral fissures, epicanthal folds, heart abnormalities, micrognathia, and at times cleft palate. At birth, the infant sucks and sleeps poorly, is irritable, and hyperactive. Later in life, at school age, there are signs of psychomotor backwardness and learning difficulty. Developmental anomalies have been found in the brain.

Since alcohol readily crosses the placental barrier, it is generally assumed to be the factor that damages the brain. Whether alcohol is the sole cause is not completely settled, however. The condition is several times more frequent in blacks and American Indians than in whites. It is doubtful if alcoholic fathers produce infants with this syndrome. A genetic predisposition has been suspected, but no clear hereditary pattern or offending gene has been identified.

For a more detailed discussion of this topic, see Adams and Victor: *Principles of Neurology*, 4th ed, pp 871–888.

ADDITIONAL READING

Goldstein DB: *Pharmacology of Alcohol*. New York, Oxford University Press, 1983.

Grove WM, Cadoret RJ: Genetic factors in alcoholism, in Kissin B, Begleiter H (eds): *The Biology of Alcoholism*, vol 7: *The Pathogenesis of Alcoholism*. New York, Plenum, 1983, pp 31–56.

Isbell H, Fraser HF, Wikler A, et al: An experimental study of etiology of "rum fits" and delirium tremens. *Q J Stud Alcohol* 16:1, 1955.

Schenker S, Becker HC, Randall CL, et al: Fetal alcohol syndrome: Current status of pathogenesis. *Alcoholism: Clinical and Experimental Research* 14:635, 1990.

Victor M: Neurologic disorders due to alcoholism and malnutrition, in Baker AB, Joynt RJ (eds): *Clinical Neurology*. Philadelphia, Lippincott, 1986, chap 61.

Victor M: Alcohol withdrawal seizures. An overview, in Porter RJ, Mattson RH, Cramer JA, Diamond I (eds): *Alcohol and Seizures. Basic Mechanisms and Clinical Concepts*. Philadelphia, Davis, 1990, chap 15, pp 148–161.

Victor M, Adams RD: The effect of alcohol on the nervous system. *Res Publ Assoc Res Nerv Ment Dis* 32:526, 1953.

Victor M, Adams RD: The alcoholic dementias, in Vinken PJ et al (eds): *Handbook of Clinical Neurology*, vol 2: *Neurobehavioral Disorders*, 2nd ed. Amsterdam, North-Holland, 1985, pp 335–352.

Victor M, Adams RD, Collins GH: *The Wernicke-Korsakoff Syndrome and Other Disorders Due to Alcoholism and Malnutrition*. Philadelphia, Davis, 1989.

40 Disorders of the Nervous System Due to Drugs and Other Chemical Agents

Injurious or poisonous substances, customarily designated as toxins, exist in great number. Many of them affect the nervous system either directly or secondarily through damage to other organs. The scope of neurotoxicology is vast, and obviously one cannot do justice to it in a few pages. The most that can be done here is to draw attention to the major categories of neurotoxic agents and the manner in which they affect the nervous system.

OPIATES AND RELATED SYNTHETIC ANALGESICS

Opiates refer to the naturally occurring alkaloids of opium; morphine and codeine are the most common. *Opioids* designate all drugs with actions similar to those of opium: (1) chemical modifications of morphine or (2) purely synthetic analgesics. Compounds of the first group include diacetylmorphine or heroin (now the most regularly abused opioid), hydromorphone (Dilaudid), hydrocodone (Hycodan), oxymorphone (Numorphan), and oxycodone (Percodan). The best known synthetic analgesics are meperidine (Demerol), methadone (Dolophine or Amidone), *d*-propoxyphene (Darvon), and pentazocine (Talwin). All these drugs have been assigned a "controlled" status because of their addictive properties.

Apart from analgesia, the opioids produce a sense of well-being, a state conventionally referred to as *morphine euphoria* or a "high." For this reason they are sought by individuals to allay boredom and misery. Once introduced to the drug, the victim discovers that euphoria is soon followed by dysphoric symptoms—faintness, nausea, and vomiting—which can only be alleviated by repeated self-administration of the drug. This is the genesis of addiction, and the need becomes so compelling that crimes will be committed to obtain the drug.

Opioid poisoning, the result of a miscalculation of dosage or a suicidal attempt, results in varying degrees of unresponsiveness, slow and shallow or periodic breathing, pinpoint pupils, bradycardia, and hypothermia. In the most advanced stage of coma, the pupils dilate, the skin and mucous membranes are cyanotic, and circulation fails. Death results from respiratory depression and asphyxia. Survivors may show the effects of hypoxic encephalopathy.

Treatment of opioid poisoning consists of gastric lavage, maintenance of an adequate airway with a cuffed endotracheal tube, oxygenation, and the administration of naloxone (Narcan), the specific antidote to both opiates and synthetic analgesics. *Naloxone* is given IV in a dose of 0.7 mg/70 kg, repeated once or twice at 5-min intervals if necessary. If an adequate respiratory response is obtained, 1.0 mg of naloxone IM may then be given and repeated as needed.

Addiction to opiates or opioids afflicts more than 600,000 persons in the United States, half of them adolescents and young adults in New York City alone. It is characterized by a striking degree of tolerance to increasing doses and the development of typical symptoms and signs when the drug is withdrawn (abstinence syndrome). The latter appear within 8 to 16 h after the last dose of morphine (later with other opioids) and consist of yawning, rhinorrhea, sweating, lacrimation, diffuse pain, dilatation of pupils, waves of gooseflesh, muscle twitching, nausea and vomiting, diarrhea, insomnia, and an increase in temperature, respiratory rate, and blood pressure. These physical changes subside gradually over a period of 7 to 10 days but persist in mild form for several more weeks.

The *diagnosis* of opiate addiction, if history is not available, can be suspected from needle marks and the finding of opiate derivatives in the urine and is confirmed by the administration of naloxone (0.4 mg IV, repeated once if necessary), which induces some of the abstinence symptoms. Clonidine (5 mg/kg bid for a week) counteracts most of the noradrenergic withdrawal symptoms. An alternative method is to stabilize the patient on methadone for 3 to 5 days (10 to 20 mg bid orally) and then to withdraw the drug over a similiar period of time.

SEDATIVE-HYPNOTIC DRUGS

There are two main groups: (1) barbiturates, bromides, chloral hydrate, and paraldehyde and (2) meprobamate (and other glycerol derivatives) and the benzodiazepines, the most important of which are chlordiazepoxide (Librium) and diazepam (Valium).

Barbiturates

Medically, these drugs are now used very little. However, their nonmedical and illicit uses are still important causes of suicide, accidental death, and addiction. The following are the only barbiturates encountered with any regularity, and the first three are the ones most commonly abused: pentobarbital (Nembutal), secobarbital (Seconal), amobarbital (Amytal), thiopental (Pentothal), barbital (Veronal), and phenobarbital (Luminal).

Acute barbiturate coma Ingestion of 15 to 20 times the oral hypnotic dose of barbiturate induces coma, slow and shallow respiration, and flaccidity of the limbs with diminished or absent reflexes; however, pupillary light and corneal reflexes are retained (unless asphyxia has occurred). In the early hours of coma, a phase of decerebrate rigidity with hyperactive tendon reflexes and Babinski signs may be present. The *diagnosis*, if history is not available, is established by measurement of barbiturate levels in the blood. *Treatment* is directed along the lines indicated in Chap. 16—maintenance of respiration, prevention of atelectasis and infection, and in some instances, hemodialysis.

Chronic barbiturate intoxication This resembles alcohol intoxication, and the symptoms fluctuate with the time of self-administration of the drug. *Withdrawal* is followed by insomnia, generalized convulsions, and a confusional state, also resembling the alcohol withdrawal syndrome. Anxiety states and depression, for which many patients take barbiturates, may be uncovered and require psychiatric treatment. Often patients will have abused both alcohol and barbiturates or opioids and barbiturates.

Benzodiazepines

These are among the most commonly prescribed drugs in the world today. Chlordiazepoxide, diazepam, and related members of this group are particularly effective in the treatment of anxiety, insomnia, and (given parenterally) delirium, status epilepticus, and the muscle spasms of tetanus and the "stiff-man" syndrome. Flurazepam and triazolam are widely used in the management of insomnia (Chap. 18), and clonazepam, in the treatment of tremor and certain types of seizures.

The advantages of the benzodiazepines are their *relatively* low hypnotic effects and addictive potential and their minimal interactions with other drugs. Despite these attributes, the benzodiazepines are far from ideal. In large doses, they frequently cause drowsiness, unsteadiness of gait, and at times, hypotension and syncope, confusion, and impairment of memory, especially in the elderly. Also, these drugs can be addictive, and when discontinued, they sometimes give rise to a withdrawal syndrome much like that due to barbiturates.

ANTIPSYCHOTIC DRUGS

This heterogeneous group of drugs includes the phenothiazines, thioxanthines, butyrophenones, rauwolfia alkaloids, molindine, and a dibenzoxazepine, loxapine. The phenothiazines are the most popular and are recognized by their trade names—Thorazine, Sparine, Compazine, Vesprin, Trilafon, Mellaril, Stelazine, and Permitil, or Prolixin. The most familiar of the butyrophenones is haloperidol (Haldol). All these drugs are in common use for the control of psychotic behavior in schizophrenia, manic-depressive disease, and confusional-agitated states that complicate other brain diseases.

The *side effects* of these drugs are common and serious: Parkinson syndrome, buccolingual and oromasticatory dystonia, akathisia, choreoathetosis, and other dyskinesias. Some of the latter persist after the drug is discontinued (*tardive dyskinesia*). A severe and often fatal *neuroleptic malignant syndrome* (catatonic rigidity, stupor, unstable blood pressure, high fever, diaphoresis and other signs of autonomic dysfunction, and high creatine kinase levels) may also occur. The antipsychotic drugs must be given with great caution because some of the side effects are worse than the disease for which they are given. One uses the lowest possible dose for the shortest time, interspersing chronic administration with vacation periods. Neuroleptic drugs must be discontinued as soon as the adverse effects are recognized. The Parkinson syndrome usually improves under the influence of anticholinergic drugs, but tardive dyskinesia may persist for months or years. Dantrolene and the dopamine agonist bromocriptine have been used with some success in the neuroleptic malignant syndrome.

ANTIDEPRESSION DRUGS

These are monoamine oxidase (MAO) inhibitors such as isocarboxizide (Marplan), tranylcypromine (Parnate), phenelzine (Nardil); dibenzazepine derivatives such as imipramine (Tofranil), desipramine (Norpramin), amitriptyline (Elavil); and lithium. The MAO inhibitors need to be dispensed cautiously and with constant awareness of their potentially serious side effects—restlessness and agitation, insomnia, anxiety, and occasionally muscle twitching, mania, and convulsions. Also, sympathomimetic amines and tyramine, when taken in cheeses, beer, and wine, may induce hypertension, cardiac arrhythmias, pulmonary edema, and even death. Either desipramine or amitriptyline are preferable for endogenous depression, since they have considerably less side effects than the MAO inhibitors.

Lithium salts are of proven value in controlling and preventing mania. Less certain is their value in treating depression. Overdosage may result in delirious or confusional states with tremor, myoclonic twitching, dizziness, nystagmus, ataxia, and stuttering speech—symptoms that may persist for a week or two after cessation of lithium intake.

STIMULANTS

Drugs of this category have relatively limited medical uses. The most important ones are caffeine, amphetamine (Benzedrine), methylphenidate (Ritalin), and cocaine.

Methylphenidate and amphetamine are of value in the treatment of narcolepsy and cataplexy, and the former drug, for unexplained reasons, is helpful in controlling the hyperactivity syndrome of boys. Small doses of dextroamphetamine, in combination with sodium amytal, are useful in counteracting the fatigue of depression. The amphetamines also have an appetite-suppressant effect and have been widely and indiscriminately used for the control of obesity, as well as for the abolition of fatigue. Cocaine, originally utilized as a topical anesthetic, is now the most common illicitly used drug in the Western world.

Amphetamine and dextroamphetamine These drugs have been much abused. The toxic signs consist of restlessness, excessive speech and motor activity, tremor, hallucinations, paranoia, and alterations of thought and affect—a state that at times mimics paranoid schizophrenia. Chronic usage can lead to a high degree of tolerance and dependence. Withdrawal, after a period of sustained use, is followed by prolonged, predominantly REM sleep, from which the patient awakens with a ravenous appetite, muscle pains, and profound fatigue and depression.

Cocaine In chemical structure, cocaine resembles the amphetamines, and its toxic manifestations are also much the same. Formerly, cocaine was taken nasally ("snorting"), but in 1985, a relatively pure and heat-stable form of the drug ("free-base" or "crack"), suitable for smoking, became available. The relative cheapness and ready availability of crack have led to a veritable epidemic of cocaine use; there are, in the United States, an estimated 7 to 8 million persons who use the drug regularly.

Cocaine induces a state of well being, euphoria, restlessness, and loquacity. Psychologic dependence or habituation, i.e., an inability to abstain from frequent compulsive use ("craving") develops readily. Withdrawal, after a period of chronic abuse, is followed by restlessness, anorexia, depression, hyperprolactinemia, and signs of dopaminergic hypersensitivity. Severe intoxication causes seizures, coma, and death. Seizures in this setting are best treated with benzodiazepines. Coma requires emergency treatment in an ICU, along the lines indicated for barbiturate coma (Chap. 16).

With the widespread use of cocaine, serious new medical complications continue to appear—subarachnoid hemorrhage, myocardial infarction, cerebral and spinal cord infarction, acute rhabdomyolysis, acute renal failure, and disseminated intravascular coagulation.

PSYCHOACTIVE DRUGS

This group includes lysergic acid diethylamide (LSD), phenylethylamine derivatives (mescaline and peyote), psylocybin, certain indolic derivatives, cannabis (marijuana), and phencyclidine (PCP). All are loosely referred to as psychotomimetic or psychotogenic drugs, in that they can induce a psychosis that in some ways resembles schizophrenia. The psychosis of PCP may last several days or weeks.

Marijuana This is taken by inhaling the smoke from cigarettes. In low doses, its effects are like those of alcohol. With increasing amounts, the effects resemble those of LSD, mescaline, and psylocybin—vivid visual hallucinations, perceptual distortions, feelings of depersonalization, inattentiveness, paresthesias—an experience that many persons find pleasing. No definite withdrawal effects and no permanent abnormalities of the brain from excessive or prolonged usage have been documented. Often the smoking of marijuana has led to the abuse of other habit-forming drugs.

DISORDERS DUE TO BACTERIAL TOXINS

Diphtheria, botulism, and tetanus are the important diseases in this category. They are considered in Chaps. 44, 51, and 52, respectively.

POISONING DUE TO PLANTS, VENOMS, BITES, AND STINGS

Ergotism (fasciculations, myoclonus, muscle spasms, seizures) may be a problem in migraine patients who overuse ergotamine tartrate. *Lathyrism* has been described in Chap. 34, with the spinal cord diseases. *Mushroom poisoning*, the other important member of this category, is described in the *Principles*.

Neurologically, the most notable disorder consequent upon insect bites is *Lyme disease*, which is considered in Chap. 30, with the infectious diseases. The neurotoxic effects of other bites, stings, and venoms are discussed fully in *Harrison's Principles of Internal Medicine*.

HEAVY METALS

Lead, arsenic, mercury, manganese, bismuth, and thallium each affect the nervous system in a special way. Only plumbism, clinically the most important of the heavy metals, will be described here; the pathogenic properties of the others are summarized in Table 40-1. Restrictions of space preclude consideration of the toxic effects of other heavy metals (iron, antimony, zinc, silver, gold, platinum, etc.), certain nonmetalic elements

TABLE 40-1 Heavy-Metal Poisoning

Metal	Source	Clinical effects	Diagnostic tests	Treatment
Lead				
Children	Lead paint	Anorexia, apathy, vomiting, drowsiness, seizures, stupor, coma	↑ CSF pressure, protein, and cells; basophilic stippling of marrow normoblasts; ↑ blood Pb and urinary coproporphyrin	Chelation with BAL and EDTA; mannitol; IV diazepam for seizures
Adults	H_2O from lead pipes; burning or melting lead; leaded gasoline	Colic, anemia, wrist drop, polyneuropathy; delirium from organic lead	As above	As above
Arsenic (inorganic)	Ingestion of herbicides, insecticides, rodenticides	Encephalopathy, dermatitis, jaundice, Mees lines, sensorimotor polyneuropathy	↑ As levels in blood, urine, hair, nails	Vasopressor agents; BAL
Mercury	Exposure in manufacture of thermometers, mirrors, incandescent lights, x-ray machines, indoor (latex) paints	Tremor, ataxia of gait, confusion, blindness, sensory neuropathy	↑ Hg in blood and urine	*dl*-Penicillamine
Manganese	Mining Mn ore	Fatigue, drowsiness, progressive weakness, parkinsonism	Mn in blood and urine	L-Dopa
Thallium	Rodenticides, insecticides, depilatory agents	Acute polyneuropathy, optic atrophy, ophthalmoplegia, alopecia	Thallium in urine	KCl orally
Bismuth	Bi subgallate for gastrointestinal disorders	Subacute drowsiness, confusion, tremulousness, myoclonus, twitching, seizures, ataxia	Bi in urine; hyperdense concentration of Bi in cerebral and cerebellar cortices in CT scans	Nonspecific

(phosphorus), and certain industrial toxins (see suggested reading at end of chapter).

Lead Poisoning

In *young children*, lead poisoning continues to be observed in the slums of large urban centers. The indoor paint in many old houses contains lead and its sweetish taste appeals to young children, who nibble on it. The ingested lead induces anemia, with stippling of red blood cells, abdominal pain (colic), and deposits in the ends of the metaphyses of long bones, visible in radiographs. Headache, apathy, psychomotor regression, seizures, stupor, and coma are the main CNS effects. The CSF is under increased pressure, with an elevated protein content and often a low-grade pleocytosis. Lead levels are increased in the blood and urine.

Once the stage of coma is reached, the child may either die or survive blind and comatose. At autopsy the brain is swollen and edematous. Deposits of Pb salt are seen in the walls of arterioles in association with lymphocytes and perivascular ischemic lesions.

The main elements of *therapy* are (1) establishment of urinary flow, then maintenance of IV fluids at basal water and electrolyte requirements; (2) chelation therapy with BAL and $CaNa_2EDTA$ for 5 to 7 days followed by a course of oral penicillamine; (3) repeated administration of mannitol for relief of cerebral edema; and (4) use of IV diazepam to suppress seizures.

Lead poisoning in adults is less common than in children. Colic, anemia, and neuropathy (presenting as bilateral wrist drop or as a polyneuropathy) are the common manifestations. Ingestion of water or home brew that is conveyed in lead pipes or inhalation of fumes from the burning or melting of lead are the usual causes of intoxication. In adults, the treatment of inorganic lead poisoning with chelating agents follows along the same lines as in children.

The inhalation of fumes of tetraethyl and tetramethyl lead, used as additives in gasoline, has given rise to an acute delirious-confusional-hallucinatory state.

ANTINEOPLASTIC AGENTS

Several antineoplastic drugs affect the nervous system adversely, often requiring discontinuation of the drug or modification in its usage. Table 40-2 summarizes the most predictable of these complications.

TABLE 40-2 Neurotoxic Effects of Antineoplastic Agents

Drug	Clinical use	Adverse Neurologic Effects	Management
Vincristine	Lymphoblastic leukemia, lymphomas, some solid tumors	Paresthesias and sensory loss in feet, legs, and hands. Autonomic effects may be added. Cranial nerves may be affected.	Reduce dose to minimum effective levels or change to another drug.
Procarbazine	Hodgkin disease, other lymphomas, bronchogenic Ca, gliomas	Somnolence, confusion, agitation, mild polyneuropathy, orthostatic hypotension	Reduce dosage. Avoid alcohol, barbiturates, and narcotics.
L-Asparaginase	Lymphoblastic leukemia, multiple myeloma	Drowsiness, confusion, delirium, stupor, coma; cerebral venous thrombosis; other cerebrovascular complications	Discontinue drug
5-Fluorouracil	Ca of breast, ovary, gastrointestinal tract	Dizziness, nystagmus, dysarthria, cerebellar ataxia	Discontinue drug
Methotrexate	Meningeal leukemia or carcinomatosis; chorioepithelioma	Intrathecal use with x-radiation may cause focal necrotic lesions of brain or cord; ataxia, dementia, pseudobulbar palsy	Discontinue drug
Cisplatin	Ca ovary; head and neck tumors	Tinnitus, high-frequency hearing loss, retrobulbar neuritis, seizures, peripheral neuropathy	Discontinue drug
Carmustine (BCNU)	Malignant gliomas	Intracarotid injection—orbital and neck pain, focal seizures, transient confusion	Discontinue drug
Cytosine arabinoside (ARA-C)	Acute nonlymphocytic leukemia	Ataxia, dysarthria, nystagmus, usually transient	Discontinue drug

For a more detailed discussion of this topic, see Adams and Victor: *Principles of Neurology*, 4th ed, pp 889–920.

ADDITIONAL READING

Arena JM: *Poisoning: Toxicology-Symptoms-Treatments*, 5th ed. Springfield, IL, Charles C. Thomas, 1986.

Brust JCM: Drug dependence, in Baker AB, Joynt RJ (eds): *Clinical Neurology*, vol. 2. Hagerstown, MD, Harper & Row, 1986, chap 21.

Dreisbach RH: *Handbook of Poisoning: Prevention, Diagnosis and Treatment*, 12th ed. Los Altos, CA, Lang, 1987.

Gilman AG, Goodman LS, Gilman A, Murad F (eds): *The Pharmacological Basis of Therapeutics*, 8th ed. New York, Pergamon, 1990.

Goldfrank LR (ed): *Toxicologic Emergencies*, 4th ed. E Norwalk, CT, Appleton and Lange, 1990.

Le Quesne PM: Metal toxicity, in Asbury AK, McKhann GM, McDonald WI (eds): *Diseases of the Nervous System*, 2nd ed. Philadelphia, Saunders, in press.

Levy BS, Wegman DH: *Occupational Health: Recognizing and Preventing Work-Related Disease*, 2nd ed. Boston, Little Brown, 1988.

Proctor N, Hughes JP: *Chemical Hazards of the Workplace*, 2nd ed. Philadelphia, Lippincott, 1988.

41 Degenerative Diseases of the Nervous System

The diseases subsumed under this heading answer to the following criteria: (1) They begin insidiously after a long period of normal nervous system function and pursue a gradually progressive course for many years, often a decade or longer. (2) Some depend on genetic factors, or at least appear in more than one member of the same family (i.e., they are *heredodegenerative*). A larger number occur sporadically. (3) From a pathologic standpoint, the degenerative diseases consist of a gradual loss of neurons and replacement gliosis; often the neuronal loss is selective, i.e., it involves a functional system such as the anterior horn cells in ALS or the pigmented brainstem neurons in Parkinson disease. (4) This system atrophy is more or less symmetric once the disease has become fully established.

Why nerve cells that have functioned normally throughout most of an individual's lifetime should waste away (atrophy) remains a biologic mystery. Referring to the process as an *abiotrophy* (Gowers), or premature senescence, simply rephrases the same concept. Recently, with newer methods of cytologic study, changes that are not at all compatible with simple aging have been discovered.

DEGENERATIVE DISEASES CHARACTERIZED MAINLY BY PROGRESSIVE DEMENTIA

Alzheimer Disease

This is the most frequent of all degenerative diseases. It occurs in late adult life and the senium, and its prevalence in the population over 60 years of age is between 4 and 5 percent. Terry and Katzman estimate that there are more than 4 million such cases in the United States. The disease is familial in some 15% of cases and takes a progressive course that spans 5 to 10 years. The neuronal loss is mainly in the association areas of the frontal, temporal, and parietal cortices of both hemispheres; the primary motor, somatosensory, visual, and auditory cortices are spared. Apart from neuronal loss, the most distinctive pathologic features are senile (neural) plaques of amorphous material and a thickening and condensation of the neurofibrillary component of surviving and degenerating nerve cells (Alzheimer neurofibrillary change).

A slight degree of these two types of change is found with increasing age, but they are immeasurably greater in Alzheimer disease. Nevertheless, their ubiquity has led to the notion (incorrect in our view) that Alzheimer disease is merely an unusually advanced or premature senile change. The blood flow to the atrophied cortex is reduced, but there is no indication that this is due to arteriosclerosis. The disease is more frequent and occurs earlier in patients with the Down syndrome, a finding that has been explained by a genetic abnormality on chromosome 21.

Clinical features The syndrome of dementia, described in Chap. 20, is most faithfully portrayed by Alzheimer disease. It begins insidiously, with an impairment of memory, and as it worsens, other failures of cerebral function appear. Speech becomes halting with groping for words, comprehension is less quick, errors in calculation become frequent, and visuospatial orientation becomes defective. With progression of the disease, testing of mental status confirms the presence of manifest disorientation, amnesia, aphasia, apraxia, and agnosia. In variants of the disease, any one of these deficits may precede amnesia. By contrast, gait is preserved until late in the course of the illness; reflexes are normal, as are sensation, hearing, visual fields, ocular movements, and other brainstem functions. Later still, involuntary grasping and sucking responses become prominent, the step is shortened, and mild rigidity (sometimes myoclonus) and slowness of movement are evident. Finally, the patient sits all day, idle and mute, or lies immobile in bed until an infection or other illness terminates life.

The clinical picture enables one to make the diagnosis with an accuracy of 80 to 85 percent. CT scans and MRI reveal a greater degree of cerebral atrophy than expected for age. The EEG shows a diffuse slowing. The CSF is normal.

One or more cerebrovascular lesions, which are to be expected in 25 percent of individuals in the Alzheimer age group, may complicate the clinical picture. Differentiation of Alzheimer disease from treatable forms of dementia is the prime diagnostic consideration as indicated in Chap. 20.

There is no specific treatment for Alzheimer disease, but medical counseling and the use of drugs to counteract certain troublesome symptoms (e.g., insomnia, agitation, paranoia) are helpful to the patient's family.

Lobar Sclerosis (Pick Disease)

This rare disease consists of an extreme degree of atrophy (far greater than in Alzheimer disease) of the frontal or temporal lobes or both. Neurons are lost, and many of the surviving ones may show a peculiar swelling and argentophilic intracytoplasmic inclusions. The extreme loss of neurons and gliosis of the involved cortex is also associated with loss of myelinated nerve fibers in the central white matter.

A strong family history and the early and prominent affection of the frontal lobes (marked apathy and psychomotor slowing; grasping and sucking reflexes) or the temporal lobes (severe, early impairment of language function) suggest the diagnosis of Pick disease. Otherwise, the clinical picture resembles that of Alzheimer disease. CT scanning and MRI reveal the extreme sulcal widening. Pick disease is probably inherited as an autosomal dominant trait, but the matter is not settled. There is no treatment.

DISEASES IN WHICH DEMENTIA IS ASSOCIATED WITH OTHER NEUROLOGIC ABNORMALITIES

Huntington Chorea

This dominantly inherited neurologic disease usually begins in midadult life and progresses to death in 12 to 15 years. Either chorea or intellectual decline may be the initial manifestation; later on both are present. Often, emotional disturbances and disorders of behavior and personality precede the intellectual decline by many years. Variants consist of rigidity instead of chorea (Westphal form), and in children there may also be seizures, ataxia, dystonia, and bradykinesia.

A loss of certain classes of neurons in the caudate nuclei with replacement gliosis is the main pathologic abnormality. This is grossly evident in CT scans and MRI, which disclose a flattening of the normally rounded contour of the medial surfaces of the caudate nuclei. Less conspicuous neuronal loss is observed in the cerebral cortex. The gene abnormality is localized to the short arm of chromosome 4.

Treatment is unsatisfactory. L-Dopa makes the chorea worse. Reserpine and tetrabenazine, which block dopamine receptors, suppress the chorea to some extent but have unpleasant side effects. Haloperidol in doses of 2 to 10 mg daily is probably the most effective drug in suppressing the chorea, but it does not alter the course of the disease.

Special diagnostic problems are raised by nonfamilial cases of senile chorea, and by paroxysmal choreoathetosis, acanthocytosis with chorea, acquired hepatocerebral degeneration, and tardive dyskinesia.

Other diseases in this category are corticostriatospinal degeneration (Parkinson-dementia-ALS syndrome), cortical-basal ganglionic degeneration of non-Huntington type, and familial dementia with spastic paraparesis. These are all well-recognized entities but are too rare to be described here (see the *Principles*).

DISEASES CHARACTERIZED BY ABNORMALITIES OF POSTURE AND MOVEMENT

Paralysis Agitans (Parkinson Disease)

Akinesia, tremor at rest, rigidity, slowness of movement (best seen in alternating movements of hands), "masked" facies and unblinking stare, stooped posture, and festinating gait constitute the typical syndrome. Responsivity of the symptoms to L-dopa is another criterion. The disease usually appears in late adult life, sometimes as early as the fourth decade. About two-thirds of patients are disabled within 5 years, but the disease may drag on for as long as 20 years or longer. Familial coincidence is low. There is no ataxia or paralysis or other signs of corticospinal tract involvement. The proportions of tremor, rigidity, and akinesia vary from case to case. The Parkinson patient is often depressed. Also, dementia is not uncommon; in some instances, it proves to be due to an associated Alzheimer disease.

The distinguishing *pathologic features* are a loss of pigmented cells in the substantia nigra (pars compacta) and other pigmented nuclei in the brainstem and the presence of cytoplasmic inclusions—so-called Lewy bodies—in the remaining cells. The population of nigral cells falls from about 425,000 to less than 100,000. As a result, there is a deficiency of dopamine, both in the nigral cells, in which dopamine is synthesized, and at the synaptic endings of nigral fibers, in the striatum.

Treatment In past years this consisted of the administration of anticholinergic agents such as atropine and belladonna and later trihexyphenidyl (Artane) and related drugs such as benztropine mesylate (Cogentin). Early in the disease, when the tremor is strictly unilaterial, stereotaxic ventrolateral thalamotomy will relieve it, but this will not prevent other manifestations of the disease from appearing.

These methods of treatment have been superceded almost entirely by the use of L-dopa, which replaces the depleted striatal dopamine. L-Dopa is usually given in combination with a decarboxylase inhibitor (Sinemet), to prevent its rapid destruction, in doses of 10 to 25 mg inhibitor with 100 to 250 mg L-dopa, three to four times daily. Nausea, hypotension, and depression are common side effects that can usually be managed medically. The most troublesome effect is the induction of involuntary movements, which force a reduction in dosage. Useful adjunctive agents in patients who tolerate L-dopa poorly are the dopaminergic agents *bromocriptine* (10 mg daily in divided doses, increased slowly to 40 to 60 mg daily) and amantadine (50 to 100 mg tid). Selegiline (L-Deprenyl), 5 mg bid, if given early in the disease, may retard the evolution of Parkinson symptoms. Marked fluctuations in rigidity ("on-off" phenomenon), which characterize the late stages of the illness, demand careful titration of the drug dosages, literally hour by hour. The elimination of dietary protein from breakfast and lunch has been helpful in some patients. Transplantation of adrenal gland and embryonic nigral cells into the brain, to instill dopamine, are under investigation.

Striatonigral Degeneration

Extensive loss of both putaminal and nigral neurons evokes the picture of Parkinson disease. It is often combined with one type of olivopontocerebellar degeneration and dysautonomia due to degeneration of the lateral horn cells of the spinal cord (Shy-Drager syndrome). There are no Lewy bodies in the substantia nigra. Because of the striatal degeneration (loss of dopaminergic receptors), there is little or no response to L-dopa and related drugs. All the cases have been sporadic.

Progressive Supranuclear Palsy

Here, supranuclear gaze palsy (especially of vertical gaze) is combined with dystonia of the neck and trunk musculature, instability of balance with easy falling, pseudobulbar palsy, and a number of other components of Parkinson disease, which vary from case to case. Mental changes, usually mild, appear late in the disease, after several years. The affected neurons of subthalamus, thalamus, and basal ganglia contain masses of single-strand neurofilaments. L-dopa is only slightly beneficial.

Dystonia Musculorum Deformans (DMD; Torsion Spasm)

There are two main forms of this disease:

1. An autosomal recessive form, which affects young children, usually of Jewish extraction, and progresses slowly over a decade or longer. Limb, trunk, or cranial musculature is at first involved intermittently in tonic spasms, which later become widespread and persistent and cause grotesque deformities. Intellect is normal and there are no other neurologic abnormalities. There is uncertainty as to the pathologic basis of this disease. Stereotaxic ventrolateral thalamic surgery has been beneficial in some cases. Huge doses of Artane are said to alleviate the dystonia.
2. A dominant form of DMD begins in later childhood, is generally milder and more slowly progressive than the recessive type, and is not confined to a particular ethnic group.

In addition to DMD, there have been delineated a number of partial or restricted dystonic syndromes, described in Chap 5.

TABLE 41-1 The Hereditary Ataxias

- I. Predominantly spinal forms of hereditary ataxia
  - A. Friedreich ataxia
  - B. Non-Friedreich, predominantly spinal ataxias
- II. Predominantly cerebellar forms of hereditary ataxia
  - A. Cortical cerebellar atrophies
    1. Holmes type of cerebello-olivary atrophy
    2. Late cortical cerebellar atrophy of Marie-Foix-Alajouanine
  - B. Cerebellar-brainstem atrophies
    1. Olivopontocerebellar atrophy of Menzel and of Déjérine and André-Thomas (cerebellopetal)
    2. Other types of olivopontocerebellar atrophy (Konigsmark and Weiner) including cases with striatonigral degeneration, retinal degeneration, and dementia
    3. Dentatorubral atrophy (Ramsay-Hunt; Woods and Schaumburg; and others) (cerebellofugal)
- III. Idiopathic late-onset cerebellar ataxias

SYNDROME OF PROGRESSIVE ATAXIA

A large number of heredodegenerative diseases fall into this category. No single classification of these diseases is entirely satisfactory, but the one presented in Table 41-1, modified from Greenfield, has proved clinically useful. An account of these diseases, even the most clearly defined ones, is beyond the scope of this handbook; the reader is referred to the *Principles* and to the monographs of Greenfield and of Harding, listed in the references.

SYNDROME OF MUSCULAR WEAKNESS AND ATROPHY WITHOUT SENSORY CHANGES (MOTOR SYSTEM DISEASE)

The term *motor system disease* designates a progressive degenerative disorder of motor neurons of the spinal cord, brainstem, and motor cortex, manifested clinically by muscular weakness and atrophy (amyotrophy) and corticospinal tract signs, in varying combinations. Mainly it is a disease of middle life and progresses to death in 2 to 5 years, sometimes longer. Several readily recognizable subtypes of motor system disease have been identified.

Amyotrophic Lateral Sclerosis (ALS)

This is the most common form of motor system disease, with an annual incidence rate of 0.4 to 1.76 per 100,000 population, worldwide. In about 5 percent of cases the disease is inherited as an autosomal dominant trait, but this type differs in no other way from the sporadic type. It usually begins with weakness and wasting of hand muscles, associated with cramping and fasciculations of arm and then shoulder girdle muscles. Less often, the symptoms begin in one leg. Before long, the triad of atrophic weakness of the hands and forearms, slight spasticity of the legs, and generalized hyperreflexia—all in the absence of sensory changes—leaves little doubt as to the diagnosis. Early or late in the illness, dysarthria, dysphagia, and dysphonia set in, and the tongue may wither and fasciculate; or a spastic bulbar paralysis (pseudobulbar palsy) may become prominent. ALS is the only common condition in which a progressive atrophic and spastic bulbar paralysis coexist. The disease is inexorably progressive, leading to death in 2 to 5 years, usually from respiratory paralysis. There is no treatment.

At any stage of the disease, the EMG reveals the signs of widespread denervation atrophy while motor nerve conduction velocities are slowed only slightly or not at all. The CSF is normal as a rule; exceptionally, the total protein is slightly elevated. Serum CK is normal or slightly increased.

Neuropathologic examination discloses only atrophy and loss of cells in the anterior horns of the spinal cord and the motor nuclei of the lower brain stem, and of Betz cells, with secondary degeneration of corticospinal tracts.

Less Frequent Types of Motor System Disease

Weakness and atrophy may occur alone, without evidence of corticospinal tract affection. These cases are referred to as *progressive spinal muscular atrophy*. When weakness and wasting are more or less limited to the muscles innervated by the motor nuclei of the lower brainstem, the term *progressive bulbar paralysis* is used. Rarely, the degenerative process remains confined to the corticospinal pathways, in which case the disorder is designated *primary lateral sclerosis* (Beal and Richardson).

Special hereditary types of progressive muscular atrophy occur in infancy and childhood (*Werdnig-Hoffman disease* or *infantile muscular atrophy*) or as a separate spinal motor neuron degeneration in other age periods (see Chap. 50).

Familial spastic paraplegia, without amyotrophy, represents a special class of disease, to be distinguished from the forms of motor system disease described above. In the most common form of familial spastic paraplegia, only Betz cells and other cortical motor neurons and corticospinal tracts degenerate. In other types of this syndrome there may be optic atrophy or pigmentary retinal degeneration, or polyneuropathy, or signs of extrapyramidal, cerebral (dementia), or cerebellar disorder.

SYNDROME OF PROGRESSIVE BLINDNESS

Three important degenerative diseases present in this way. These are the male sex-linked hereditary optic atrophy of Leber; retinitis pigmentosa; and the tapetoretinal (macular) degeneration of Stargardt. Optic atrophy and retinitis pigmentosa overlap widely with other diseases, such as epilepsy, Refsum disease, Bassen-Kornzweig disease, Sjögren-Larsson syndrome, Kearns-Sayre syndrome, familial spastic paraplegia, and cerebellar degeneration, among others. The reader is referred to the *Principles* for details.

HEREDITARY HEARING LOSS WITH DISEASES OF THE NERVOUS SYSTEM

There is also a very large number of degenerative neurologic disorders that are linked to hereditary progressive cochleovestibular atrophies. They have been described in detail by Konigsmark, whose review is listed in the references.

For a more detailed discussion of this topic, see Adams and Victor: *Principles of Neurology*, 4th ed, pp 921–967.

ADDITIONAL READING

Beal MF, Richardson EP Jr: Primary lateral sclerosis: A case report. *Arch Neurol* 38:630, 1981.

Byers RK, Banker BQ: Infantile muscular atrophy. *Arch Neurol* 5:140, 1961.

Greenfield JG: *The Spino-Cerebellar Degenerations*. Springfield, IL, Charles C. Thomas, 1954.

Harding AE: *The Hereditary Ataxias and Related Disorders*. New York, Churchill Livingstone, 1984.

Konigsmark BW: Hereditary diseases of the nervous system with hearing loss, in Vinken PJ, Bruyn GW (eds): *Handbook of Clinical Neurology*, vol 22. Amsterdam, North-Holland, 1975, pp 499–526.

Leenders KL, Frackowiak SJ, Lees AJ: Steele-Richardson-Olszewski syndrome. *Brain* 111:615, 1988.

Martin JB: Huntington's disease: New approaches to an old problem. *Neurology* 34:1059, 1984.

Morris JC, Cole M, Banker BQ, Wright D: Hereditary dysphasic dementia and the Pick-Alzheimer spectrum. *Ann Neurol* 16:458, 1984.

Mulder DW, Kurland LT, Offord KP, Eard CM: Familial adult motor neuron disease: Amyotrophic lateral sclerosis. *Neurology* 36:511, 1986.

Schoenberg BS, Kokmen E, Okazaki H: Alzheimer's disease and other dementing illnesses in a defined United States population: Incidence rates and clinical features. *Ann Neurol* 22:724, 1987.

Snyder SH, D'Amato RJ: MPTP: A neurotoxin relevant to the pathophysiology of Parkinson's disease. *Neurology* 36:250, 1986.

Terry RD, Katzman R: Senile dementia of the Alzheimer type. *Ann Neurol* 14:497, 1983.

Whitaker PJ: The concept of subcortical and cortical dementia. *Ann Neurol* 19:1, 1986.

Woods BT, Schaumburg HH: Nigrospinodentatal degeneration with nuclear ophthalmoplegia, in Vinken PJ, Bruyn GW (eds): *Handbook of Clinical Neurology*, vol 22. Amsterdam, North-Holland, 1975, chap 7, pp 157–176.

42 Developmental Diseases of the Nervous System

Diseases of this type lie in the domain of pediatric neurology and are of particular interest to those concerned with mental retardation and cerebral palsy. The pathologic entities that constitute this category of disease have their basis in aberrations of brain development. Some derailment of the process of neuronal formation, migration, or organization has occurred. The primary cause may be genetic or some exogenous agent may have blighted the normal embryo or fetus during its intrauterine existence. Or something may have gone awry during parturition when the head and brain are exposed to forces never again duplicated. Whatever the cause, the final product is a deficient or malformed and malfunctioning brain with which the child must live for a lifetime and for which only inadequate substitutive or corrective measures are available. Identification and prevention of the pathogenic mechanisms are the primary goals of the medical profession.

The developmental anomalies of the brain assume many forms. Insofar as the size and shape of the cranium correspond closely to brain development in early life, it is not surprising that one group presents with craniospinal deformities. In another group, which includes neurofibromatosis, tuberous sclerosis, and cutaneous angiomatosis, an inherited disease affects both dermal structures and the brain, in multiple foci; by examining the skin, one can predict the pathologic changes in the brain. Chromosomal abnormalities, identifiable by karyotyping any cell in mitosis, is responsible for another group of developmental anomalies. Nevertheless, after careful analysis of any large group of mentally retarded and cerebral palsied children, the pathogenesis in approximately half of them cannot be ascertained. They present a major challenge to neuroscientists.

NEUROLOGIC DISORDERS ASSOCIATED WITH CRANIOSPINAL DEFORMITIES

The majority of such cases can be traced to a mutant gene or chromosomal abnormality, but many are of unknown etiology. In one group, the head is strikingly small (<45 cm in circumference) and the brain weight is only a few hundred grams in adult life (*microcephaly vera*). Both autosomal recessive and sex-linked inheritance patterns have been verified. Lesser degrees of smallness of the head and early closure of the fontanels also reflect the presence of cerebral disease of diverse type. Enlargement and rapid growth of the head is usually due to hydrocephalus (Chiari malformation, aqueductal stenosis) and less frequently to enlargement of the brain itself (Tay-Sachs disease, Alexander disease, spongy degeneration of infancy) or to subdural hematomas. Widespread destruction of the cerebrum, leaving only pial membranes in place of the hemispheres, also enlarges the head because of lack of resistance of the residual cerebral tissue to intraventricular pressure (*hydranencephaly*).

One of the most arresting types of cranial malformation, observed more frequently in males, is *craniostenosis*, in which the membranous junctions between the bones of the skull fuse prematurely, before the brain attains maximum growth. Early closure of the coronal suture causes the skull to be wide and short (*brachiocephalic*); closure of the sagittal suture results in a long, narrow skull (*scaphocephaly*); closure of the lambdoid and coronal sutures enlarges the skull in the vertical direction (tower skull, *oxycephaly* or *turricephaly*). In the latter instance, the orbits are shallow, the eyes bulge, and skull films show islands of bone thinning (Lückenschädel). If recognized early, the neurosurgeon can create artificial sutures and permit the skull to assume a more normal shape.

Many diseases that disrupt the development of the brain also deform the cranial and facial bones, the eyes, ears, nose, and fingers. The somatic stigmata serve as indicators of the cerebral abnormality. A catalogue of these is to be found in the monograph of Holmes and his colleagues (see references).

Rachischisis (dysraphism) is another important developmental fault. If for any reason the lower part of the neural tube fails to close, the baby is born with a spinal lumbar meningomyelocele or meningocele; or if the cephalic end remains deficient, a cranial encephalocele forms, or there is no brain at all (anencephaly). There is a small familial coincidence of these conditions, but exogenous factors are also under suspicion (excess vitamin A or folate, exposure to potato blight). In the *Chiari malformation* parts of the cerebellum and medulla are displaced into the cervical spinal canal. There are two types: type II with a meningomyelocele; type I without. The resulting syndrome is a combination of hydrocephalus, palsy of lower cranial nerves, and high cervical cord compression. Hydro- or syringomyelia is a frequent accompaniment.

CHROMOSOMAL ABNORMALITIES

With the discovery of methods for displaying chromosomes in cells that are undergoing mitosis, several abnormalities of the autosomal chromosomes (triplication, deletions, or translocations) and a lack or excess of sex chromosomes were identified: Down syndrome (mongolism, trisomy 21); one type of arrhinencaphaly (Patau syndrome, trisomy 13); trisomy 18 (Edwards syndrome); cri du chat syndrome (deletion of short arm of chromosome 5); Klinefelter syndrome (XXY); Turner syndrome (XO); and several others.

The *Down syndrome* is the most common, occurring once in every 700 births (more frequently in older women). The round head, open mouth, stubby hands, upward slanting of the palpebral fissure with medial epicanthal folds, poorly developed nasal bridge, low-set oval ears, enlarged tongue, gray-white specks of depigmentation of the irides (Brushfield spots), short incurved little fingers (clinodactyly), broad hands with single transverse palmar creases, and mental retardation (IQ 40 to 50) constitute the characteristic syndrome. The chromosomal abnormality can be demonstrated in cells of the amniotic fluid. The brain of such an individual is rounded and approximately 10 percent lighter than normal. The frontal lobes are relatively small, with a simplified convolutional pattern, and the superior temporal gyri are thin. Lenticular opacities and cardiac septal defects are frequent. Alzheimer neurofibrillary changes and senile plaques appear in most Down patients who die after their 40th year. Triplication and mosaic patterns of chromosome 21 account for variants of the Down syndrome.

See the *Principles* for details of the other chromosomal abnormalities.

THE PHAKOMATOSES (CONGENITAL ECTODERMOSES)

Encompassed by this term is a group of hereditary diseases affecting the skin and other organs as well as the brain. *Neurofibromatosis* and *tuberous sclerosis* are characterized by benign tumor-like formations in the CNS (hamartomas), which have the potential of undergoing neoplastic change. *Cutaneous angiomatosis* with abnormalities of the CNS is the other member of this group.

Tuberous sclerosis is an inherited disease (autosomal dominant) with a high mutation rate (1 in 20,000 to 1 in 50,000) and a prevalence of 5 to 7 per 100,000. It accounts for 0.1 to 0.7 percent of feebleminded patients in institutions. The abnormal gene has been localized on chromosome 9. Skin lesions, seizures, and retarded mental development represent a diagnostic triad. The brain lesions have been seen at birth by CT scan. The seizures begin in infancy and change pattern as the brain matures. The earliest skin lesions are white depigmented spots on trunk and limbs. Later the facial adenomas (of Pringle) appear and also thickened zones of subepidermal fibrosis (shagreen patches). The cerebral lesions produce relatively few focal signs. Postmortem examination discloses a variety of visceral lesions—rhabdomyoma of the heart and angiomyolipomas in many organs. In the brain some of the convolutions appear white in color and are enlarged and firm. Whitish masses protrude into the ventricles. Under the microscope these tuber-like structures are composed of plump astrocytes. Those in the cortex contain nerve cells, some of giant proportions, mixed with calcium deposits. Neoplastic transformation of these abnormal cells into gliomas may occur later in life in a small proportion of the patients.

Of clinical importance is the fact that not all components of the clinical triad need to be present in any given patient. Some patients with seizures and skin lesions remain mentally normal. In others a few trivial skin lesions or a rare retinal phakoma and a seizure or two may be the only manifestations to suggest the diagnosis, and some patients escape seizures altogether. Only the epilepsy can be treated, using anticonvulsant drugs selected in accordance with the seizure type.

Neurofibromatosis of Von Recklinghausen

In this hereditary disease, the skin, nervous system, bones, endocrine glands, and sometimes other organs are the sites of tumor-like masses of limited growth potential, i.e., hamartomas. Those of the skin and nerves are usually schwannomas. The prevalence of the disease is 40 per 100,000 population or about one case in every 2500 to 3000 births. The inheritance pattern is that of an autosomal dominant trait. The classic peripheral form, with widespread skin lesions, is due to an abnormal gene located on chromosome 17. A milder central form with few skin lesions and often bilateral acoustic neuromas has been linked to a DNA marker on chromosome 22.

Spots of hyperpigmentation of the skin (café au lait) and multiple cutaneous and subcutaneous tumors that increase in number during late childhood and adolescence are characteristic. Schwannomas and neurofibromas may form on spinal roots and cranial nerves, some in position to compress nerve roots and the spinal cord. Often such lesions are asymptomatic for a long time. Meningiomas are sometimes added to the syndrome. A hamartoma or glioma of one or both optic nerves is another serious complication. Some of the skin tumors, instead of extruding above the surface as papillomas, thicken the skin diffusely (plexiform neuroma) and disfigure the face or other parts of the body. About 2 to 5 percent of neurofibromas or central glial nodules undergo malignant degeneration. The treatment of the peripheral tumors, meningiomas, and gliomas is surgical excision, if possible, or radiation.

Cutaneous Angiomatosis with Abnormalities of the CNS

There are at least seven distinct conditions in which a cutaneous vascular anomaly is associated with an abnormality of the nervous system. Here only the most common one—meningofacial (encephalofacial) angiomatosis with cerebral calcification (Sturge-Weber syndrome)—will be described. In this condition a one-sided cutaneous hemangioma is seen at birth, extending from the forehead to the upper eyelid. It may or may not be elevated. Other parts of the face or body are involved in some patients. Later in childhood there may occur a progressive hemisensorimotor or visual field deficit and seizures, which are contralateral to the lesion. The vascular lesion in the brain lies in the meninges and is mainly venous. The underlying cortex undergoes a progressive laminar necrosis and calcification, the latter giving rise to characteristic double-contoured (''tram line'') radiographic images. Surgical excision of the lesion arrests the progressive ischemic neurologic deficit in some cases. Antiepileptic treatment is needed.

CONGENITAL PARAPLEGIA AND OTHER MOTOR DEFICITS (LITTLE'S DISEASE)

While hereditary forms of spastic paraplegia are well documented, most of the patients with this syndrome prove to have suffered parturitional or postparturitional damage to the brain. These conditions are much more frequent in premature infants. Hemiplegias at birth are usually of this type as well. Quadriplegia may also be an expression of hydranencephaly or of spinal cord trauma during delivery (especially breech delivery). Birth injury with paraparesis or paraplegia (diplegia) or double athetosis is usually referred to as Little's disease. The baby may have been born at term, but the greatest risk factors in every large series are birth weight below 2000 g, other fetal malformations in siblings, and maternal mental retardation, attesting probably to a multiplicity of types.

Clinically, two main groups of cases have been recognized. In one, the spastic diplegia, which gradually becomes apparent after 4 to 6 months of postnatal life, is associated with a slight diminution in head size and in intelligence. Its frequency increases with the degree of prematurity. Matrix hemorrhages and periventricular leukomalacia are the prominent types of neuropathologic change. In a second group, birth is difficult and severe intrapartum asphyxia and attendant fetal distress are evident. The difficulty may arise in either full-term or premature infants. Such infants will usually require resuscitation and have low Apgar scores, which in this instance are of predictive value. The clinical picture, later to emerge, is tetraparesis and pseudobulbar palsy, with signs of bilateral corticospinal involvement or double athetosis, or both. The pathologic lesions are those of hypoxia-ischemia in the distal arterial fields in gray and white matter (lobar sclerosis, i.e., ulegyria) or *état marbré* of the lenticular nuclei and thalamus.

Hemiplegia and, less often, double hemiplegia may also develop at a later time in infancy or childhood, usually from embolic or thrombotic arterial occlusion or venous thrombosis. The resulting lesions are often epileptic.

Kernicterus

Erythroblastosis fetalis is secondary to Rh and ABO incompatibilities between mother and fetus. This results in a high postpartum concentration of bilirubin, which damages the brain, particularly the basal ganglia and thalamus. At autopsy, dead neurons are stained a canary yellow color, hence the name of the brain lesion—Kern (nucleus) icterus. The clinical picture in survivors consists of double athetosis, gaze palsies, and deafness. Control of hyperbilirubinemia by phototherapy has virtually eliminated this category of disease.

INTRAUTERINE AND NEONATAL INFECTIONS

The best known are rubella, cytomegalic inclusion disease, toxoplasmosis, herpes simplex encephalitis, and neurosyphilis. The clinical characteristics are summarized in Table 42-1.

MENTAL RETARDATION

This is a condition of impaired psychomotor development of diverse etiology. The most glaring defects are in learning and in scholastic achievement in general. Two groups are recognized. In the first group, which is relatively small (comprising about 10 percent of all retarded individuals), the retardation is severe and usually nonfamilial. The diagnosis in these patients is usually not difficult because of the obvious somatic and neurologic abnormalities and is made soon after birth. (The congenital anomalies of development described in the preceding pages fall into this category.) In almost all cases of this type, pathologic changes can be found in the brain—hence this group is spoken of as the "*pathologically retarded*."

TABLE 42-1 Intrauterine and Neonatal Infections of the CNS

Disease	Time of infection	Clinical manifestations	Diagnostic tests	Prevention and treatment
Rubella	First 10 weeks of intrauterine life	*Mother:* ± symptomatic *Infant:* mental retardation, cataracts, neurocochlear deafness, congenital heart disease, pigmentary degeneration of retina; cloudy cornea; hepatosplenomegaly	IgM antibodies or viral isolation in neonate	Vaccination of all women against rubella
Cytomegalic inclusion disease	First trimester	*Mother:* asymptomatic *Infant:* Jaundice, mental retardation, convulsions, sensorineural deafness, chorioretinitis, optic atrophy, microcephaly	↑ Cells and protein in CSF; cytomegalic changes in cells in urine	No treatment
Toxoplasmosis	Intrauterine—probably third trimester	*Mother:* usually asymptomatic *Infant:* Foci of retinal destruction, spastic paralysis, severe retardation, hydrocephalus. Affects only one pregnancy	↑ Cells and protein in CSF; ↑ antibody titers in mother	Spiramycin to mother; pyrimethamine plus sulfadiazine to neonate

Neurosyphilis	Last half of pregnancy	*Mother:* recent 1^{ry} or 2^{ry} syphilis *Infant:* stillbirth or syphilitic infection	Positive serology in mother; ↑ cells and protein and positive serology in CSF of neonate	Penicillin G to mother and infant
Herpes simplex	At or near birth	*Mother:* genital herpes infection *Infant:* Skin lesions, salivary gland infection; encephalitis; diminished responsiveness and neonatal automatisms	↑ Antibodies in mother and fetus	Acyclovir (?)
Neonatal bacterial meningitis	First days after birth	*Mother:* usually infected *Infant:* fever, bulging fontanels, reduced responsivity; ↓ brainstem automatisms	↑ Cells and protein, ↓ glucose, and bacteria in CSF	Antibiotics
Viral infection: Coxsackie B, poliomyelitis, arboviruses	Late in pregnancy or at term	Signs of encephalitis or encephalomyelitis	↑ Cells and protein in CSF	

TABLE 42-2 Categories of Disease Causing Mental Retardation (in 1372 Patients at the W. E. Fernald State School)

Disease category	Number of patients		Percentage of all patients
	IQ < 50	IQ > 50	
Acquired destructive lesions	278	79	26.0
Chromosomal abnormalities	247	10	18.7
Multiple congenital anomalies	64	16	5.8
Developmental abnormality of brain	49	16	4.7
Metabolic and endocrine diseases	38	5	3.1
Progressive degenerative disease	5	7	0.9
Neurocutaneous diseases	4	0	0.3
Psychosis	7	6	1.0
Mentally retarded (cause unknown)	385	156	39.5

The second group, comprising the large majority of mentally retarded, does not have a recognizable cerebral pathology. In general, the mental retardation is less severe than in the first group and may not be fully appreciated until school age, when scholastic incompetence becomes apparent. Since early motor, sensory, visual, and auditory functions have developed at more or less the usual times, an unfavorable environment (e.g., poverty and poor nutrition, lack of parental affection and social stimulation) is blamed for the scholastic failure—a condition referred to as "*subcultural retardation*." To what extent genetic factors are operative in this group is not yet fully known. The noteworthy fact is that in this group, much more often than in the severely retarded, one or both parents are mentally backward. At least one segment of this "subcultural" group lies at the lowest end of the Gaussian curve of intelligence, the opposite of genius.

The main categories of disease that cause mental retardation are indicated in Table 42-2. The diverse diseases constituting these categories are listed in Table 42-3.

TABLE 42-3 Diseases Associated with Mental Retardation

I. Mental defect with associated developmental abnormalities in nonnervous structures
  A. Those affecting cranioskeletal structures
    1. Microcephaly
    2. Macrocephaly
    3. Hydrocephalus (including myelomeningocele with Chiari malformation and associated cerebral anomalies)
    4. Down syndrome (mongolism)
    5. Cretinism (congenital hypothyroidism)
    6. Mucopolysaccharidoses (Hurler, Hunter, and Sanfilippo types)
    7. Acrocephalosyndactyly (craniostenosis)
    8. Arthrogryposis multiplex congenita (in certain cases)

TABLE 42-3 Diseases Associated with Mental Retardation (*continued*)

9. Rare specific syndromes: De Lange
10. Dwarfism: Russell-Silver dwarf, Seckel bird-headed dwarf, Rubinstein-Taybi dwarf, Cockayne-Neel dwarf, etc.
11. Hypertelorism, median cleft face syndromes, agenesis of corpus callosum

B. Those affecting nonskeletal structures
1. Neurocutaneous syndromes: tuberous sclerosis, Sturge-Weber, neurofibromatosis (uncommon)
2. Congenital rubella syndrome (deafness, blindness, congenital heart disease, small stature)
3. Chromosomal disorders: Down syndrome, some cases of Klinefelter syndrome (XXY), XYY, Turner (XO) syndrome (occasionally), and others.
4. Laurence-Moon-Biedl syndrome (retinitis pigmentosa, obesity, polydactyly)
5. Eye disorders: toxoplasmosis (chorioretinitis), galactosemia (cataract), congenital rubella
6. Prader-Willi syndrome (obesity, hypogenitalism)

II. Mental defect without developmental anomalies in nonnervous structures, but with focal cerebral and other neurologic abnormalities
A. Cerebral spastic diplegia
B. Cerebral hemiplegia, unilateral or bilateral
C. Congenital choreoathetosis or ataxia
1. Kernicterus
2. Status marmoratus
D. Congenital ataxia
E. Congenital atonic diplegia
F. Syndromes resulting from hypoglycemia, trauma, meningitis, and encephalitis
G. Associated with other neuromuscular abnormalities (muscular dystrophy, Friedreich ataxia, etc.)
H. Cerebral degenerative diseases (lipidoses)
I. Lesch-Nyhan syndrome
J. Rett syndrome

III. Mental defect without signs of other developmental abnormality or neurologic disorder (epilepsy may or may not be present)
A. Simple mental retardation, familial mental retardation, subcultural mental retardation
B. Some cases of encephaloclastic disease (hypoxia, hypoglycemia)
C. Infantile autism
D. Associated with inborn errors of metabolism (phenylketonuria, other aminoacidurias, organic acidurias)
E. Congenital infections (some cases of congenital syphilis, cytomegalic inclusion disease)

For a more detailed discussion of this topic, see Adams and Victor: *Principles of Neurology*, 4th ed, pp 968–1005.

ADDITIONAL READING

Adams RD: Neurocutaneous diseases, in Fitzpatrick TB et al (eds): *Dermatology in General Medicine*, 3rd ed. New York, McGraw-Hill, 1987, chap 172, pp 2022–2062.

Baker RS, Ross PA, Bauman RJ: Neurologic complications of the epidermal nevus syndrome. *Arch Neurol* 44:227, 1987.

Banker BQ, Larroche J-C: Periventricular leukomalacia of infancy. *Arch Neurol* 7:386, 1962.

Barlow CF: *Mental Retardation and Related Disorders*. Philadelphia, Davis, 1978.

Dyken P, Krawiedki N: Neurodegenerative diseases of infancy and childhood. *Ann Neurol* 13:351, 1983.

Fenichel GM: *Neonatal Neurology*, 2nd ed. New York, Churchill Livingstone, 1985.

Gomez MR: *Neurocutaneous Disease (a Practical Approach)*. Boston, Butterworth, 1987.

Gorlin RS, Pindborg JJ, Cohen MM Jr: *Syndromes of the Head and Neck*. New York, McGraw-Hill, 1976.

Hagberg V, Aicardi J, Dias K, et al: A progressives syndrome of autism, dementia, ataxia and loss of purposeful hand movements in girls. Rett's syndrome. *Ann Neurol* 14:471, 1983.

Holmes LB, Moser HW, Halldorsson S, et al: *Mental Retardation: An Atlas of Disease with Associated Physical Abnormalities*. New York, Macmillan, 1972.

Kalter H, Warkany J: Congenital malformations: Etiologic factors and their role in prevention. *New Engl J Med* 308:424, 1983.

Martuza RL, Eldridge R: Neurofibromatosis 2 (bilateral acoustic neurofibromatosis). *N Engl J Med* 318:684, 1988.

Volpe JJ: *Neurology of the Newborn*, 2nd ed. Philadelphia, Saunders, 1986.

Winick M: *Malnutrition and Brain Development*. New York, Oxford University Press, 1976.

V DISEASES OF PERIPHERAL NERVE AND MUSCLE

43 Laboratory Aids in the Diagnosis of Neuromuscular Disease

This chapter and succeeding ones (Chaps. 44 to 52) are concerned with diseases of the peripheral and cranial nerves and of muscle. Certain laboratory tests are particularly helpful in the diagnosis of these diseases and can suitably be discussed by way of introduction to this subject. The intelligent use of these laboratory procedures requires some knowledge of the biochemistry and physiology of nerve action potentials and muscle contraction; this information is reviewed in the *Principles*. Essential to good neurologic practice, and to medical practice in general, is the resourceful and wise selection of the laboratory test(s) most applicable to the disease at hand. This, of course, should be dictated by the clinical phenomena under investigation.

ALTERED BLOOD CHEMISTRY AND NEUROMUSCULAR DISEASE

Diffuse muscular weakness or muscle twitching, spasms, and cramps may be due to underactivity or overactivity of motor neurons as well as to impaired neuromuscular transmission and muscle activation (contraction and relaxation). The occurrence of any such abnormality should always raise the question of an alteration of serum electrolytes, which in turn reflects a change in their concentration in intra- and extracellular fluids. Endocrinopathies are less common causes of such abnormalities.

Abnormalities of Serum Electrolytes

A fall in serum *potassium* below 2.5 meq/L or a rise above 7 meq/L results in weakness of limb and trunk muscles. Below a serum concentration of 2.0 meq/L and above 9.0 meq/L, there is almost always complete paralysis of these muscles and later of the respiratory muscles as well. In addition, tendon reflexes are diminished or absent and the reaction of muscle to percussion is abolished.

Hypocalcemia of 7.0 mg/dL or less (as occurs in rickets or hypoparathyroidism) or a reduction in the proportion of ionized calcium (as in hyperventilation) causes increased irritability and spontaneous discharge of sensory and motor nerve fibers, i.e., tetany (instability of polarization of neurilemma). Sometimes convulsions result from similar changes in cerebral neurons. The effects upon muscle, which are secondary, appear in the EMG as frequent repetitive discharges and later as prolonged spontaneous discharges. Convulsive effects are recorded in the EEG.

Hypercalcemia, above 12.0 mg/dL (as occurs in vitamin D intoxication, hyperparathyroidism, and metastatic bone disease), causes weakness and lethargy, probably on a central basis.

Hypomagnesemia results in muscle weakness, tremor, tetanic spasms, and convulsions. An increase in plasma Mg also leads to muscle weakness, the result of the depressant action of Mg on lower motor neurons.

Marked *hyponatremia* (Na $<$ 115 meq/L) may be attended by confusion and stupor. The rapid correction of hyponatremia may lead to the development of central pontine myelinolysis (Chap. 38).

Endocrinopathies

Muscle weakness may be a prominent feature of excessive secretion of ACTH or prolonged corticosteroid therapy. High and low thyroxin (T_4) levels in the blood are reflected in diffuse muscle weakness, the result of chemical alterations in the contractile process of muscle fibers. In hyperthyroidism the contraction and relaxation of muscle are abbreviated and in hypothyroidism they are prolonged.

Changes in Serum Levels of Muscle Enzymes

Release of muscle enzymes into the blood [elevated creatine-kinase (CK), aldolase, etc.] is indicative of destruction of muscle fibers, especially if the destruction is acute. For unclear reasons, however, CK may be elevated in hypothyroidism, in which there is no myonecrosis. For serum CK to be interpretable, one must be certain that it is derived from skeletal muscle and not from heart or brain. The source of the isoenzymes can be determined by quantitation. The MM form of CK is found in highest concentration in striated muscle, and in patients with acute destructive lesions (e.g., alcoholic rhabdomyolysis; neuroleptic malignant syndrome) it often exceeds 1000 units and may reach 40,000 units.

Myoglobinuria

Red urine is an uncommon but important finding in muscle disease. With destruction of muscle fibers, the red pigment, myoglobin, is released into the serum, and in sufficient amounts it will color the urine. Unlike hemoglobin, myoglobin is a small molecule which is cleared rapidly from the serum by the kidneys. Hence in myoglobinuria the *serum* retains its normal color. Approximately 200 g of muscle must be destroyed to color the urine. Smaller quantities, insufficient to color the *urine*, can be detected spectroscopically or preferably by radioimmunoassay techniques. The commonly used urine dipstick test for hemoglobin will also detect myoglobin, because both contain iron. Thus a positive Hgb dipstick in the absence of hematuria should suggest myoglobinuria in the appropriate clinical situation.

ELECTRODIAGNOSTIC TESTS

Muscle weakness and atrophy may be due to a primary disease of muscle (dystrophy or a myopathy of metabolic, traumatic, or inflammatory type) or to denervation (from disease of anterior horn cells or peripheral nerves), and the two can be readily differentiated by electrodiagnostic methods. The two standard procedures are (1) the demonstration of fibrillation potentials and changes in the size and shape of motor unit potentials (MUPs) by the insertion of needle electrodes into muscles (*electromyogram*, or EMG) and (2) the percutaneous stimulation of peripheral nerve fibers and recording of muscle and sensory action potentials (motor and sensory *nerve conduction studies*), expressed as amplitudes, conduction velocities, and distal latencies.

The EMG findings in primary muscle disease are characteristic. During voluntary contraction of muscle, one can detect many motor units of small size (short duration and diminished voltage) because the motor units are depleted of their quota of muscle fibers.

In acutely denervated muscle there is a reduced number of MUPs. The individual muscle fibers of motor units, released from nerve control, *fibrillate* independently, and increased irritability of affected motor nerve fibers or cells, not yet degenerated, may cause *fasciculation* (independent random contraction of all or most of the fibers of a motor unit). After several months, the remaining MUPs tend to increase in amplitude and duration and become polyphasic because collateral sprouts from surviving axons re-innervate the denervated muscle fibers.

EMG is also useful in demonstrating myotonia and defects in neuromuscular transmission, as occur in myasthenia gravis and in the myasthenic syndrome of Lambert-Eaton (see *Principles* for details).

Nerve conduction studies are standard procedures in the study of peripheral nerve disease. Slowing of velocity of nerve conduction indicates that the denervative weakness is of demyelinative type. In axonal disease the velocity of nerve conduction is slowed only slightly because the preservation of only a few large fibers is sufficient to transmit an induced impulse at normal speed.

Special nerve conduction studies (H reflex and F wave) provide information about disease of proximal sensory and motor nerves and roots. Localized slowing or multifocal blocks in conduction are particularly useful in the diagnosis of entrapment syndromes, e.g., of the median nerve at the wrist (carpal tunnel) or the ulnar nerve at the elbow, and of vascular and inflammatory diseases of nerves.

BIOPSY PATHOLOGY

Biopsy of muscle and nerve can be of considerable help in differentiating muscle, nerve, and spinal cord disease and sometimes in specifying the disease process.

Both surgical and microscopic techniques must be exacting. The muscle to be studied should be easily accessible; there should be evidence that it has been affected but not too severely damaged and that it has not been the site of recent injections or needle EMG study.

Myopathies and dystrophies are expressed by random loss of muscle fibers and their replacement by fat and connective tissue. If the sample is well chosen, one may actually see muscle fibers in the process of degeneration and regeneration. The process does not respect motor units. In the *polymyositides*, inflammatory changes are usually evident. In *denervation atrophy* there is a great reduction in the size of muscle fibers within affected motor units and enlargement of intact motor units. This is best demonstrated by ATPase and other histochemical stains for fiber types, since all the fibers of a motor unit are derived from one anterior horn cell and are therefore of one histochemical type. Histochemical stains showing an excess of lipid or glycogen within surviving muscle fibers are diagnostic of the lipid and glycogen storage diseases.

Electron microscopy can be done on specially fixed bits of muscles and will expose some of the characteristic morphologies of the mitochondrial and other myopathies (central core, nemaline, myotubular, etc.) and also lipid and glycogen storage products (lipidoses and glycogenoses). Also, by the study of specimens from the innervation point of a muscle fiber, one can find abnormalities that are diagnostic of disorders of the neuromuscular junction (myasthenia gravis; Lambert-Eaton syndrome).

Nerve biopsy is of less value. Usually the sural nerve is selected, since it is purely sensory, and its interruption results in no disability. By teasing apart single nerve fibers, the status of myelin and axon and the length of internodal segments can be determined. Light and electron-microscopic sections may show demyelination, onion bulb formations of Schwann cells and fibroblasts (recurrent demyelination), axon degeneration of several types, wallerian degeneration, inflammatory reactions, arteritis, and amyloid deposition.

Finally, it must be pointed out that none of these laboratory tests is infallible. In biopsy studies there is a prodigious sampling problem so that a bit of nerve or muscle may be normal even though the clinical data indicating disease are indubitable. Also, each procedure is subject to technical error and the findings may be misinterpreted.

For a more detailed discussion of this topic, see Adams and Victor: *Principles of Neurology*, 4th ed, pp 1009–1027.

ADDITIONAL READING

Aminoff MJ: *Electromyography in Clinical Practice*, 2nd ed. New York, Churchill Livingstone, 1987.

Engel AG, Banker BQ: *Myology: Basic and Clinical*. New York, McGraw-Hill, 1986.

Fischbeck K: Structure and function of striated muscle, in Asbury AK, McKhann GM, McDonald W (eds): *Diseases of the Nervous System*. Philadelphia, Saunders, 1986, chap 15, pp 185–196.

Kimura J: *Electrodiagnosis in Diseases of Nerve of Muscle: Principles and Practice*, 2nd ed. Philadelphia, Davis, 1989.

Kuffler, SW, Nicholis JG, Martin AR: *From Neuron to Brain*, 2nd ed. Sunderland, MA, Sinauer Associates, 1984.

Rowland LP: Myoglobinuria. *Can J Neurol Sci* 11:1, 1984.

44 | Diseases of the Peripheral Nerves

The peripheral nervous system (PNS) includes all neural structures lying outside the pial membranes of the spinal cord and brainstem. The optic and olfactory nerves are not included, for they are special extensions of the brain. Unlike all other nerves, in which the myelin sheaths are enclosed by Schwann cells and supported by fibroblasts, the optic and olfactory fibers lie within oligodendroglia and are supported by astrocytes. The parts of the PNS that are within the spinal canal and are attached to the ventral and dorsal surfaces of the spinal cord are called the *spinal nerve roots* and those attached to the ventrolateral surface of the brainstem, the *cranial nerve roots*. The dorsal (afferent or sensory) roots consist of the central axonal processes of dorsal root ganglion cells; they synapse in the dorsal gray matter of the spinal cord or ascend directly in the posterior columns (funiculi). Similarly, the central processes of cranial ganglion cells extend into the spinal trigeminal and other tracts in the pons and medulla. The peripheral axons of dorsal root ganglion cells are the sensory nerve fibers. They terminate as fine, freely branching fibers or in specialized corpuscular endings in the skin, joints, and other tissues. The ventral (efferent or motor) roots are composed of the emerging fibers of anterior horn cells, which terminate on muscle fibers, and of lateral horn cells or brainstem motor nuclei, which terminate on sympathetic and parasympathetic ganglion cells, respectively. Traversing the subarachnoid space and lacking epineurial sheaths, the cranial and spinal roots are bathed in and are susceptible to toxic agents in the CSF, the lumbosacral roots having the longest exposure.

Other notable features of the PNS are that (1) it is composed of the axons of five systems of nerve cells—spinal anterior and intermediolateral horn cells, cranial motor nuclei cells, dorsal root ganglia cells, and sympathetic and parasympathetic ganglion cells; (2) the axons are of different sizes; (3) some axons are myelinated and some unmyelinated; (4) all fibers are enclosed in epineurial and perineurial sheaths of fibrous connective tissue; (5) the blood supply is sparse in nerves, in which there is an anastomosing chain of longitudinally oriented nutrient arteries and veins; and (6) most nerves and plexuses are mixtures of motor, sensory, and autonomic fibers.

With these anatomic facts in mind, one can conceptualize the targets of diseases affecting the PNS. Each type of nerve cell has its special susceptibilities as do the myelin sheaths, axoplasm, Schwann cells, blood vessels, connective tissue, and spinal-cranial leptomeninges and CSF. The following are examples of disease in which each of these elements is affected predominantly:

Poliomyelitis	Anterior horn cells
Herpes zoster	Dorsal root ganglion cells
Shy-Drager syndrome	Intermediolateral horn cells
Autonomic polyneuropathy	Sympathetic and parasympathetic ganglion cells
Botulinus toxin	Presynaptic endings, interfering with acetylcholine transmission at neuromuscular junctions and in autonomic ganglia
Diphtheria; Guillain-Barré syndrome	Myelin sheaths in the most vascular parts of the PNS
Heavy metals, e.g., arsenic	Axons of sensory and motor nerves
Alcoholic-nutritional diseases	Myelin sheaths and axons beginning in distal segments ("dying back" neuropathy)
Diabetes; polyarteritis	Blood vessels
"Connective tissue" diseases; amyloidosis	Blood vessels, connective tissue
Tabes dorsalis	Spinal meninges, CSF, and sensory roots

Pathologic reactions Despite the fact that more than 100 distinct diseases are known to affect the PNS, there are essentially only three pathologic processes by which nerves react to disease. The basic pathologic processes, illustrated in Fig 44-1, are referred to as wallerian degeneration, segmental demyelination, and axonal degeneration. These processes are not disease specific and may be present in different combinations in any given patient.

In *wallerian degeneration*, there is degeneration of both the axis cylinder and the myelin sheath, distal to the site of axonal interruption. The cell body becomes rounded and its chromatin disperses (chromatolysis).

In *segmental demyelination*, axons are preserved so that there is no wallerian degeneration and no chromatolysis in nerve cell

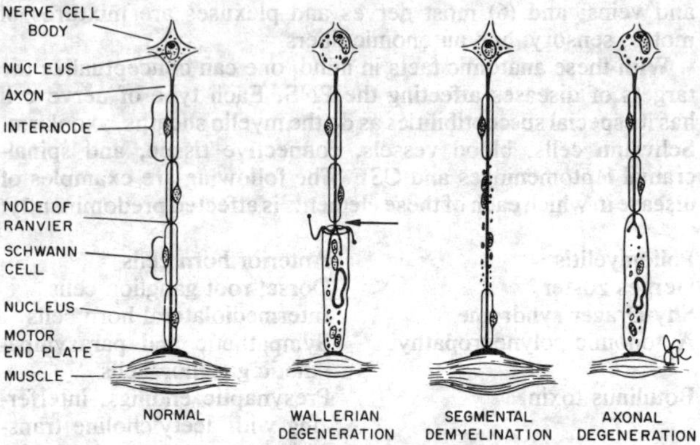

FIG. 44-1 Diagram of the basic pathologic processes affecting peripheral nerves. In wallerian degeneration, there is degeneration of the axis cylinder and myelin distal to the site of axonal interruption (arrow), and central chromatolysis. In segmental demyelination the axon is spared. In axonal degeneration there is a distal degeneration of myelin and axis cylinder as a result of neuronal disease. Both wallerian and axonal degeneration cause muscle atrophy. Further details in text. *(Courtesy of A Asbury.)*

bodies. Remyelination restores function. This process is most prominent in diphtheritic and Guillain-Barré polyneuropathies.

Axonal degeneration is characteristic of metabolically determined polyneuropathies. There is degeneration of myelin as well as axis cylinders, progressing from distal to proximal segments ("dying-back" neuropathy).

Both wallerian and axonal degeneration cause muscle atrophy.

In addition to these three reaction types, ultrastructural studies have revealed a number of more or less specific changes in Schwann cell cytoplasm and axoplasm, e.g., storage products such as sulfatide, galactocerebroside, ceramide, etc.

Terminology

In discussing PNS disease, the following terms are employed. *Polyneuropathy* refers to a bilaterally symmetric affection of the peripheral nerves, usually involving the legs more than the arms, and the distal segments earlier and more severely than the proximal ones. Involvement of the roots is referred to as *radiculopathy*. *Mononeuropathy* designates involvement of a single nerve, and *mononeuropathy multiplex*, the random involvement of multiple nerves. The term *axonal* or *demyelinative* specifies the nature of the principal lesion.

SYMPTOMATOLOGY

Affection of the peripheral nerves is characterized by a number of motor, sensory, reflex, autonomic, and trophic symptoms and signs, various combinations of which stand as the clinical criteria for diagnosis.

Most polyneuropathies are marked by weakness and reflex loss and, if chronic, by denervation atrophy (severe) or by disuse atrophy (relatively slight). The pattern of motor loss varies. The common one is a symmetric involvement of the muscles of the feet and legs, followed by those of the hands and arms, because the largest and longest fibers are the most susceptible. This principle does not apply to mononeuropathy or mononeuropathy multiplex, in which any nerve or combination of nerves may be affected. Another pattern, observed in the Guillain-Barré syndrome (GBS), is one in which all nerves and roots of the limbs, trunk, and cranial musculature may be involved, leading to respiratory paralysis.

Sensory loss duplicates the pattern of motor weakness, but in any given neuropathy it may be more or less severe than the motor affection, hence sensorimotor or motor-sensory. The loss of proprioceptive fibers gives rise to sensory ataxia and tremor; loss of pain and thermal fibers, to impaired pain and temperature sensation; and a loss of autonomic fiber, to a number of trophic changes (ulcers, osteomyelitis, loss of digits, Charcot joints). The large sensory fibers subserving touch-pressure, vibration, and postural senses are more frequently affected than the small ones subserving pain, temperature, and autonomic functions.

Autonomic deficits are manifest mainly by dryness and warmth of the skin (sometimes by hyperhidrosis), orthostatic hypotension, impotence, and impairment of bladder and bowel function.

PNS diseases not only destroy fibers leading to sensory, motor, and autonomic deficits but may increase the irritability of residual fibers. This is the basis of sensations of numbness, tingling, burning and pressure, and fascicular twitching and spasms.

The multitude of diseases that cause neuropathy and the principal syndromes by which they present are listed in Table 44-1. Space permits only the briefest consideration of representative examples from each of the major categories.

Guillain-Barré Syndrome (GBS)

This is a nonseasonal, nonepidemic, inflammatory polyradiculoneuropathy occurring worldwide at an annual rate of about 1.5

TABLE 44-1 Principal Neuropathic Syndromes

I. Syndrome of acute ascending motor paralysis with variable disturbance of sensory function
   A. Acute idiopathic polyneuritis (inflammatory demyelinative polyradiculoneuropathy), Landry-Guillain-Barré syndrome (GBS)
   B. Infectious mononucleosis and polyneuritis
   C. Hepatitis and polyneuritis
   D. Diphtheritic polyneuropathy
   E. Porphyric polyneuropathy
   F. Certain toxic polyneuropathies (triorthocresyl phosphate, thallium)
   G. Acute axonal polyneuropathy (rare)
   H. Rarely, paraneoplastic, vaccinogenic (smallpox, rabies), serogenic, polyarteritic, or lupus polyneuropathy
   I. Acute panautonomic neuropathy
II. Syndrome of subacute sensorimotor paralysis
   A. Symmetric polyneuropathies
      1. Deficiency states: alcoholism (beriberi), pellagra, vitamin B_{12} deficiency, chronic gastrointestinal disease
      2. Poisoning with heavy metals and industrial solvents: arsenic, lead, mercury, thallium, methyl *n*-butyl ketone, *n*-hexane, methyl bromide, organophosphates (TOCP, etc.), acrylamide.
      3. Drug intoxications: isoniazid, ethionamide, hydralazine, nitrofurantoin and related nitrofurazones, disulfiram, carbon disulfide, vincristine, chloramphenicol, phenytoin, amitriptyline, dapsone, stilbamidine, trichlorethylene, thalidomide, Clioquinol, etc.
      4. Uremic polyneuropathy
   B. Asymmetric neuropathies (mononeuropathy multiplex)
      1. Diabetes
      2. Polyarteritis nodosa and other inflammatory angiopathic neuropathies
      3. Subacute idiopathic polyneuropathies
      4. Sarcoidosis
      5. Ischemic neuropathy with peripheral vascular disease.
III. Syndrome of chronic sensorimotor polyneuropathy, acquired forms
   A. Carcinoma, myeloma, and other malignancies
   B. Paraproteinemias
   C. Uremia (occasionally subacute)
   D. Beriberi (usually subacute)
   E. Diabetes
   F. Hypothyroidism
   G. Connective tissue diseases
   H. Amyloidosis
   I. Leprosy
   J. Benign form in the elderly
   K. Sepsis and chronic illness

TABLE 44-1 Principal Neuropathic Syndromes *(continued)*

IV. Syndrome of chronic polyneuropathy, genetically determined forms
- A. Inherited polyneuropathies of predominantly sensory type
  1. Dominant mutilating sensory neuropathy in adults
  2. Recessive mutilating sensory neuropathy of childhood
  3. Congenital insensitivity to pain
  4. Other inherited sensory neuropathies, including those associated with spinocerebellar degenerations and Riley-Day syndrome and the universal anesthesia syndrome
- B. Inherited polyneuropathies of mixed sensorimotorautonomic types
  1. Idiopathic group
     - a. Dominant peroneal muscular atrophy (Charcot-Marie-Tooth)
     - b. Dominant hypertrophic polyneuropathy of Déjerine-Sottas, adult and childhood forms
     - c. Roussy-Lévy polyneuropathy
     - d. Polyneuropathy with optic atrophy, with spastic paraglegia, with spinocerebellar degeneration, with mental retardation, and with dementia
  2. Inherited polyneuropathies with a recognized metabolic disorder (see also Chap. 36)
     - a. Refsum disease
     - b. Metachromatic leukodystrophy
     - c. Globoid-body leukodystrophy (Krabbe disease)
     - d. Adrenoleukodystrophy
     - e. Amyloid polyneuropathy of Andrade
     - f. Porphyric polyneuropathy
     - g. Anderson-Fabry disease
     - h. Abetalipoproteinemia and Tangier disease

V. Syndrome of recurrent or relapsing polyneuropathy
- A. Idiopathic polyneuritis (GBS)
- B. Porphyria
- C. Chronic inflammatory polyradiculoneuropathy
- D. Certain forms of mononeuritis multiplex
- E. Beriberi or intoxications
- F. Refsum disease, G. Tangier disease

VI. Syndrome of mononeuropathy or multiple neuropathies
- A. Pressure palsies
- B. Traumatic neuropathies (including irradiation and electrical injuries)
- C. Idiopathic brachial and sciatic neuropathy
- D. Serum and vaccinogenic (smallpox, rabies) neuropathy
- E. Herpes zoster
- F. Neoplastic infiltration of roots and nerves
- G. Leprosy
- H. Diphtheritic wound infections with local neuropathy
- I. Migrant sensory neuropathy

cases per 100,000 population. In about two-thirds of cases, some type of respiratory or gastrointestinal infection or surgical operation precedes the onset of weakness by 1 to 3 weeks. The major manifestation is muscle weakness, which evolves more or less symmetrically over a period of several days or a week or two. Usually, the legs are affected first and then the trunk, intercostal, neck, and cranial muscles; occasionally progression is in the reverse direction. Invariably tendon reflexes are reduced and then lost. Pain and aching in muscles, sensory symptoms and signs, and autonomic disturbances occur frequently but tend to be slight and evanescent. CSF protein rises after a few days, and nerve conduction velocities are characteristically slowed.

GBS is the most rapidly evolving form of polyneuropathy and is potentially fatal (progression to complete paralysis and death from respiratory failure in a few days). For these reasons it needs to be distinguished from poliomyelitis and other acute polyneuropathies (diphtheritic, porphyric, toxic).

As to *treatment*, the patient needs to be in a hospital where intensive respiratory care is available. Respiratory assistance should be instituted at the first sign of dyspnea or atelectasis (arterial Po_2 < 70 mmHg). In patients with rapidly evolving paralysis and respiratory failure, a course of plasmapheresis hastens recovery. We have observed that large doses of steroids may improve the chances of recovery, but not all neurologists agree on this point.

Most patients recover spontaneously and completely, although this may take several months or a year or longer. About 3 percent of patients do not survive, even in the best equipped hospitals and 10 percent are left with some degree of disability. Approximately 3 percent suffer one or more recurrences of the disease.

Chronic Inflammatory Polyradiculoneuropathy (CIP)

This disorder is in some respects similar to GBS—both are symmetric polyneuropathies and both are characterized by an increased CSF protein (usually without cells), a demyelinative type of nerve conduction abnormality, and an inflammatory pathology. However, there are important differences. A preceding illness is relatively uncommon in patients wih CIP. Whereas GBS is an acute monophasic illness, CIP evolves much more slowly, either in a steadily progressive or stepwise manner, and only attains its maximum severity after several months or a year or longer, following which it tends to run a relapsing or fluctuating course. Also, in distinction to GBS, most cases of CIP respond favorably to the prolonged administration of corticosteroids and to intravenous immune globulin.

Nutritional Polyneuropathy (Neuropathic Beriberi)

In the Western world, this form of neuropathy is usually associated with chronic alcoholism and is the most common example of subacute sensorimotor polyneuropathy. This and rarer forms of deficiency neuropathy (Strachan syndrome, pellagra, vitamin B_{12} deficiency, and malabsorption syndromes) are described in Chap. 37.

Carcinomatous and Myelomatous Polyneuropathy

A predominantly distal, symmetric sensorimotor polyneuropathy, affecting first the legs and then the hands and arms and evolving over a period of months, may occur as a remote effect of carcinoma or multiple myeloma and, rarely, of lymphoma. A pure sensory polyneuropathy, with severe ataxia and retention of strength, is much less common. These forms of polyneuropathy are manifest clinically in 2 to 5 percent of all patients with malignant disease, and more than half of these cases are associated with carcinoma of the lung. More importantly, the paraneoplastic syndrome may be present for months or even a year or longer before the malignant tumor is discovered. Sometimes the polyneuropathy improves if the primary tumor is effectively treated.

Peroneal Muscular Atrophy (Charcot-Marie-Tooth Disease)

This, the most common form of inherited neuropathy, is transmitted as an autosomal dominant trait. Onset is in late childhood or adolescence, with atrophy of the feet and legs and later the hands and arms. The early involvement of the peronei and extensors of the toes produces an equinovarus deformity and claw foot. Deep and superficial sensation are impaired, usually to a slight degree, and tendon reflexes are absent in the involved limbs. The illness progresses very slowly, with long periods of stability. Wasting seldom extends above the elbows and the middle third of the thighs.

The walking difficulty, which is the main disability, is due to a combination of sensory ataxia and weakness. Foot drop and instability of the ankles are additional handicaps and can be treated by arthrodeses and light leg braces.

There are several variants of this disorder, and in some families the signs of spastic weakness or spinocerebellar disease are conjoined (see the *Principles* for details).

The Diabetic Neuropathies

Neuropathic complications of diabetes mellitus are exceedingly common, particularly in patients over 50 years of age.

Several clinical syndromes are recognized, occurring singly or in various combinations:

1. Diabetic ophthalmoplegia: This is due to infarction of the sixth or third cranial nerve, more often the latter. The oculomotor palsy is acute in onset and is accompanied by severe pain around the eye and forehead. The pupilloconstrictor fibers, located peripherally in the third nerve, are spared by the infarction, which characteristically involves the central portion of the nerve; hence pupillary function is intact. (Contrariwise, compressive lesions of the third nerve, e.g., aneurysm or temporal-tentorial herniation, tend to cause pupillary dilatation.)
2. Acute mononeuropathy: Affection of practically all the major peripheral nerves has been described in diabetes, but the ones most commonly involved are the femoral and sciatic. The acute peripheral mononeuropathies, like the cranial ones, are presumably due to infarction of nerve and in both the outlook for recovery is good.
3. Mononeuropathy multiplex: This takes the form of a rapidly evolving, painful, asymmetric, predominantly motor neuropathy, affecting multiple nerves in a random distribution. It tends to occur in older patients with mild (or unrecognized) diabetes, but it may complicate long-standing diabetes as well. Muscle weakness and atrophy are most evident in the pelvic girdle and thigh muscles, for which reason the condition is sometimes referred to as "diabetic amyotrophy." Recovery is to be expected but may take many months.
4. A second type of proximal diabetic neuropathy is characterized by a *symmetric* weakness and wasting of the pelvic and proximal thigh muscles, of insidious onset and gradual evolution. Scapular and upper arm muscles are affected less frequently. Pain is not a consistent feature and sensory changes, if present, are mild in degree and of the distal symmetric type.
5. The most common type of diabetic neuropathy takes the form of a persistent and often distressing numbness and tingling, affecting the feet and lower legs symmetrically. In severe cases, the hands may be involved. Occasionally deep sensation is impaired, with ataxia and bladder atony (*diabetic pseudotabes*).
6. Symptoms of *autonomic involvement* include pupillary and lacrimal dysfunction, impairment of sweating and vascular reflexes, nocturnal diarrhea, atonicity of the gastrointestinal tract and bladder, impotence, and postural hypotension. These symptoms are frequently combined with other forms of diabetic neuropathy, particularly with the distal sensory type.

7. A relatively uncommon complication of diabetes takes the form of severe pain and dysesthesia in a segmental distribution over the chest or abdomen. Superficial sensory loss can be detected over the involved area. This complication is observed in long-standing diabetics and is usually accompanied by marked weight loss. It is presumably due to a *widespread radiculopathy*, on the basis of the EMG changes (fibrillations of paraspinal muscles in multiple myotomes).

In all forms of diabetic neuopathy the *CSF* protein may be elevated, 50 to 200 mg/dL, and sometimes even higher.

As to treatment there is controversy. Careful control of the blood glucose is indicated. One seldom observes quick improvement, but symptomatic treatment over a period of months usually allows some of the most unpleasant manifestations to recede. Aldose reductase inhibitors are being tried.

DIFFERENTIAL DIAGNOSIS

Once it has been ascertained from existent symptoms and signs that there is disease involving many peripheral nerves, three questions must be answered: (1) Is the disease in question a polyneuropathy or a random affection of multiple nerves (mononeuropathy multiplex)? (2) What is the time course? (3) Is the deficit due to demyelination or axonal degeneration?

The features that distinguish polyneuropathy from mononeuropathy multiplex have already been described, and from Table 44-1 it is apparent that the two categories are of different causation. The multiple neuropathies usually prove to have a systemic vascular or arteritic cause whereas the polyneuropathies are of inflammatory, toxic, nutritional, or heredodegenerative nature. The time course provides helpful clues as to etiology. Most acute polyneuropathies, developing over 2 to 3 days, are inflammatory (GBS) or toxic (rare). Those evolving over a period of weeks may be inflammatory, but a toxic factor or nutritional deficiency is more likely. Neuropathic diseases evolving over months tend to be paraneoplastic or metabolic. Any polyneuropathy progressing over 5 to 10 years will probably prove to be a familial metabolic or degenerative disease. The only exceptions to this statement are the paraproteinemic and a few of the diabetic polyneuropathies.

The most helpful ancillary procedures in differential diagnosis are the electrodiagnostic tests. They provide data as to the presence of sensory nerve deficits, assuming that this is not clear from the clinical examination. They separate a group of slow-conducting motor nerve (demyelinative) diseases from ones that are primarily axonal and yield data concerning multifocality of lesions causing conduction block. The relative degree of

TABLE 44-2 Principal Mononeuropathies and Plexopathies

Nerve or plexus (derivation)	Symptoms and signs	Usual causes
Entire brachial plexus (C4–C8, T1)	All arm muscles paralyzed and tendon reflexes lost; sensation lost to upper third of arm	Vehicular accidents; rare familial forms
Upper brachial plexus (C5, C6)	Paralysis of deltoid, biceps, brachialis, supinator longus, supraspinatus, rhomboids; hand unaffected	Difficult birth (Erb-Duchenne), injection of serum and vaccines, "neuralgic amyotrophy"
Lower brachial plexus (C7, C8, T1)	Amyotrophy of hand muscles; ulnar sensory loss; sometimes Horner syndrome	Traction on abducted arm; apical lung tumor; cervical rib or band; breech delivery (Déjerine-Klumpke); radiation injury
Cords of brachial plexus:		
Lateral	Weakness of flexion and pronation of forearm	Dislocation of head of humerus, axillary trauma, cervical rib or band; supraclavicular compression
Medial	Combined median and ulnar palsy	
Posterior	Weakness of deltoid, extensors of elbow, wrist and fingers; sensory loss on outer surface of upper arm	
Long thoracic nerve (C5, C6, C7)	Winging of medial border of scapula; inability to raise arm over head	Heavy weights on shoulder; serum neuritis; neuralgic amyotrophy
Suprascapular (C5, C6)	Atrophy of supra- and infraspinatus, weakness of first 15° abduction and external rotation of arm	Part of brachial neuritis; entrapment in spinoglenoid notch
Axillary nerve (*C5*,* C6)	Deltoid atrophy; weakness of arm abduction, between 15° and 90°	Dislocations and fractures of shoulder joint; serum and vaccine injections; brachial neuritis
Musculocutaneous nerve (C5, C6)	Wasting of biceps, brachialis, and coracobrachialis; weakness of flexion of supinated arm; ↓ sensation along radial and volar forearm	Fracture of humerus
Radial nerve (C6, *C7*, C8)	Paralysis of extension and flexion of the elbow, supination of forearm, extension of wrist, fingers, abduction of thumb; ↓ sensation over radial aspect of dorsum of hand	Compression in axilla and around humerus; part of brachial neuritis
Median nerve (C5, *C6*, C7, C8, T1)	Weakness of pronation of forearm and flexion of fingers, abduction and opposition of thumb; ↓ sensation over radial aspect of palm and dorsum of distal index and third fingers	Injuries between axilla and wrist; compression at wrist (*carpal tunnel*)

TABLE 44-2 Principal Mononeuropathies and Plexopathies (*continued*)

Nerve or plexus (derivation)	Symptoms and signs	Usual causes
Ulnar nerve (C8, T1)	Wasting of hand muscles with weakness of ulnar flexor of wrist and abductors and adductors of fingers; hyperextension of fingers at metacarpophalangeal joints and flexion at interphalangeal joints ("claw hand"); ↓ sensation over fifth and ulnar parts of fourth fingers and ulnar border of palm	Fracture-dislocation of elbow with cubitus valgus deformity; compression in cubital tunnel or ulnar tunnel at wrist
Entire lumbosacral plexus (T12, L1–L5, S1–S3)	Amyotrophy of all leg muscles; areflexia; anesthesia from toes to perianal region; warm dry skin	Neuralgic amyotrophy, rarely carcinomatous infiltration
Upper plexus	Weakness of flexion and abduction of thigh and extension of leg; ↓ sensation anterior thigh and leg	Abdominal and pelvic operations; aortic aneurysm; Ca and lymphoma; lumbosacral plexitis; diabetic and other arteritic lesions
Lower plexus	Weakness posterior thigh, leg, and foot muscles; ↓ sensation first and second sacral segments	
Lateral cutaneous nerve of thigh (L2, L3)	Paresthesias and sensory loss over anterolateral aspect of thigh	Compression by lateral part of inguinal ligament
Obturator nerve (L2–L4)	Weakness of abduction, flexion, internal and external rotation of thigh	Injury by fetal head or forceps; obturator hernia; infarction; Ca
Femoral nerve (L2–L4)	Weakness of extension of leg; atrophy of quadriceps; weakness of flexion of leg with proximal lesions; loss of knee jerk	Diabetes; pelvic tumors and operations; bleeding into iliacus muscle
Sciatic nerve (L4, L5, S1, S2)	Weakness of leg flexors and all muscles below knee. Weakness of gluteal muscles with pelvic lesions; ↓ sensation posterior thigh, posterior and lateral leg, and sole	Fractures of pelvis and femur; lower gluteal injections; compression; diabetes; ruptured discs
Common peroneal nerve	Weakness of dorsiflexion of foot and toes; ↓ sensation dorsum of foot and lateral aspect of lower aspect of leg	Compression or fracture at head of fibula; diabetes
Tibial nerve	Weakness of plantar flexion and inversion of foot and flexion of toes; ↓ sensation over plantar aspect of foot	Diabetes; compression in tarsal tunnel

* Italics indicate major nerve involved.

involvement of proximal nerves and roots can be determined by H and F responses. And finally, electrical tests help to identify primary muscle diseases and diseases of the neuromuscular junctions.

The predominantly demyelinative polyneuropathies are few—mainly the acute (GBS) and chronic recurrent inflammatory polyneuritides and the familial hypertrophic polyneuropathies.

Nerve biopsy is undertaken only when etiologic diagnosis remains in doubt, after clinical and electrodiagnostic studies have been completed.

MONONEUROPATHIES AND PLEXOPATHIES

Here the diagnosis rests on the finding of motor, reflex, or sensory changes confined to the territory of a single nerve (or a plexus of nerves) and the presence of other data pointing to the causation. Table 44-2 provides a perspective on the most frequent entities comprising this category of peripheral nerve disease.

For a more detailed discussion of this topic, see Adams and Victor: *Principles of Neurology*, 4th ed, pp 1028–1076.

ADDITIONAL READING

Asbury AK, Arnason BGW, Adams RD: The inflammatory lesion in acute idiopathic polyneuritis. *Medicine* 48:173, 1969.

Dawson DM, Hallett M, Millender LH: *Entrapment Neuropathies*, 2nd ed. Boston, Little Brown, 1990.

Dyck PJ, Thomas PK, Lambert EH, Bunge R (eds): *Peripheral Neuropathy*, 2nd ed. Philadelphia, Saunders, 1984.

Gruener G, Bosch P, Strauss R, et al: Prediction of early beneficial response to plasma exchange in Guillain-Barré syndrome. *Arch Neurol* 44:295, 1987.

Guarantors of Brain: *Aids to the Examination of the Peripheral Nervous System*. London, Bailliere-Tindall, 1986.

Haymaker W, Woodhall B: *Peripheral Nerve Injuries*, 2nd ed. Philadelphia, Saunders, 1953.

Henson RA, Urich H. *Cancer and the Nervous System*. Oxford, Blackwell, 1982, pp 368–405.

Layzer RB: *Neuromuscular Manifestations of Systemic Disease. Contemporary Neurology Series*, vol 25. Philadelphia, Davis, 1984.

McKhann GM, Griffin JW, Cornblath DR, et al: Plasmapheresis and Guillain-Barré syndrome: Analysis of prognostic factors and effect of plasmapheresis. *Ann Neurol* 23:347, 1988.

Ropper AH, Wijdicks EFM, Truax BT: *Guillain-Barré Syndrome*. Philadelphia, Davis, 1991.

Schott GD: Mechanisms of causalgia and related clinical conditions. *Brain* 109:717, 1986.

45 | Diseases of the Cranial Nerves

The effects of lesions of the olfactory, optic, ocular-motor, cochlear, and vestibular nerves have already been described in Chaps. 11, 12, 13, and 14 and certain facial pain syndromes referable to the trigeminal and oculomotor nerves were commented upon in Chap. 9. There remain the disorders of the fifth, seventh, and lower (IX to XII) cranial nerves.

Fifth, or Trigeminal, Nerve

Owing to the wide anatomic distribution of this nerve, complete ablation of both its sensory and motor functions is rarely observed. However, branch lesions, with pain and sensory loss, are common.

Trigeminal neuralgia (tic douloureux) This is the most frequent disturbance of fifth-nerve function. The idiopathic form occurs mainly in the elderly but also in the middle-aged. It consists of brief paroxysms of stabbing pain in the distribution of the mandibular and maxillary divisions of the nerve, intense enough to cause the patient to wince (hence the term *tic*). The paroxysms recur frequently for weeks on end. A characteristic feature of the pain is its initiation by tactile stimuli to the face, lips, or gums or by movement of these parts in chewing, talking, shaving, etc. ("trigger zones"). As a rule, the pain is unaccompanied by sensory loss. The cause of this condition is still unsettled, though the trigeminal nerve root is sometimes found to be compressed by a tortuous artery.

The majority of patients respond favorably to the administration of carbamazepine (Tegretol), which either suppresses the attack or shortens its duration and permits a spontaneous remission to occur; phenytoin, clonazepam, or baclofen may be useful in patients who cannot tolerate carbamazepine. These drugs are administered in the same dosages and with the same precautions as in epilepsy. Persistent, severe pain requires surgery; stereotactically controlled thermocoagulation of the trigeminal roots using an RF generator is one of the most popular procedures. Some neurosurgeons favor a posterior craniotomy and removal of a vessel apposed to the trigeminal root.

Idiopathic trigeminal neuralgia needs to be distinguished from *symptomatic trigeminal neuralgia*, in which paroxysmal facial pain is a manifestation of some other neurologic disease. In the latter type the neuralgia is often accompanied by variable degrees of sensory loss and weakness of the muscles of mastication (if the mandibular division is involved). Branches of the fifth nerve may be compressed by a cerebellopontine angle tumor or by a tortuous basilar artery or posterior cerebellar artery aneurysm. A discrete area of infarction or demyelination (multiple sclerosis) at the sensory root entry zone in the pons may give rise to typical tic douloureux. Of the inflammatory lesions, *herpes zoster* is the most frequent. Middle ear infections and petrositis may involve the gasserian ganglion and root and also implicate the sixth cranial nerve (Gradenigo syndrome). This and other combinations of cranial nerve disorders are summarized in Table 45-1.

Cases of acute or chronic trigeminal sensory neuropathy of idiopathic type, affecting one or both sides of the face, are infrequent but well documented. Even less common is a pure trigeminal motor neuropathy. The prognosis for recovery in all these instances is good.

The Seventh, or Facial, Nerve

Bell's palsy (idiopathic facial paralysis) This is the most common disorder of the facial nerve (annual incidence rate of 23 per 100,000). It affects men and women equally and occurs at all ages and at all times of the year. It has an acute onset, attaining maximum severity in a few hours or a few days, and it is commonly preceded for a day or two by pain behind the ear.

All the muscles of facial expression on one side are weakened or paralyzed. The eyelids cannot be closed, the corner of the mouth droops, and the forehead will not wrinkle. There is no demonstrable sensory loss, though the affected side of the face may feel "heavy" or otherwise unnatural. Taste will be lost on the anterior two-thirds of the tongue if the lesion extends proximal to the point where the chorda tympani joins the facial nerve. Hyperacusis or distortion of sound indicates involvement of the nerve to the stapedius muscle.

The nerve is believed to be implicated in an acute inflammatory process of unknown etiology. The pathologic changes have not been studied carefully but the nerve is manifestly swollen in MRI of the petrous bone.

About 80 percent of patients recover within several weeks or months. Incomplete paralysis in the first 5 to 7 days is a favorable sign. Complete and persistent paralysis, meaning complete interruption of the nerve, indicates a long delay in the onset

TABLE 45-1 Cranial Nerve Syndromes

Site	Cranial nerves involved	Eponymic syndrome	Usual cause
Sphenoidal fissure	III, IV, ophthalmic, V, VI	Foix	Invasive tumors of sphenoid bone, aneurysms
Lateral wall of cavernous sinus	III, IV, ophthalmic (occasionally maxillary) V, VI	Tolosa-Hunt, Foix	Aneurysms or thrombosis of cavernous sinus, invasive tumors from sinuses and sella turcica; sometimes recurrent, benign granulomatous reactions, responsive to steroids
Retrosphenoidal space	II, III, IV, V, VI	Jacod	Large tumors of middle cranial fossa
Apex of petrous bone	V, VI	Gradenigo	Petrositis, tumors of petrous bone
Internal auditory meatus	VII, VIII	—	Tumors of petrous bone (dermoids, etc.), acoustic neuroma
Pontocerebellar angle	V, VII, VIII, and sometimes IX		Acoustic neuromas, meningiomas
Jugular foramen	IX, X, XI	Vernet	Tumors and aneurysms
Posterior laterocondylar space	IX, X, XI, XII	Collet-Sicard	Tumors of parotid gland, carotid body, secondary and lymph node tumors, tuberculous adenitis
Posterior retroparotid space	IX, X, XI, XII, and Bernard-Horner syndrome	Villaret, MacKenzie	Same as above, and granulomatous lesions (sarcoid, fungi), chordoma
Posterior retroparotid space	X and XII, with or without XI	Tapia	Parotid and other tumors of, or injuries to, the high neck

of recovery (up to 3 months). Recovery in such cases is by regeneration, which may take as long as 2 years and is often incomplete and associated with spasms and contractures of facial muscles and signs of aberrant regeneration of nerve fibers (crocodile tears, dyskinesias).

The cornea should be protected with artificial tears or ointment and a patch until recovery allows closure of the lids. There is some evidence that 40 mg of prednisone daily during the first 10 days of the illness is beneficial.

Other causes of facial palsy. These are considerably less common than Bell's palsy and are tabulated below. Descriptions of their characteristic features should be sought in the *Principles* or other neurology texts.

Compression of facial nerve by tumor: Schwannoma, meningioma, cholesteatoma, dermoid, carotid body tumor, mixed tumor of the parotid.

Herpes zoster: Inflammation of facial nerve and geniculate ganglion and contiguous ganglia (Ramsay-Hunt syndrome).

Facial diplegia: Due to GBS or rarely to sarcoid (uveoparotid fever or Heerfordt syndrome) or Lyme disease.

Melkersson-Rosenthal syndrome: Recurrent facial palsy, labial edema, and plication of tongue—a rare disorder of unknown cause.

Facial palsy with pontine lesions (must be distinguished from supranuclear facial weakness): Infarcts, tumors, demyelinative lesions.

Hemiatrophy of Romberg (pseudofacial palsy): A lipodystrophy without muscle weakness.

Hemifacial spasm: Idiopathic or may follow Bell's palsy. Responds to periodic injections of affected muscles with botulinus toxin and in some instances to intracranial decompression of the nerve root.

Ninth, or Glossopharyngeal, Nerve

This nerve is seldom affected separately, except possibly in glossopharyngeal neuralgia. The latter consists of severe paroxysmal pain originating in the tonsillar fossa and provoked mainly by swallowing but also by talking, chewing, etc. The pain may be localized to the ear or radiate from throat to ear, implicating the auricular branch of the vagus (hence vagoglossopharyngeal neuralgia). Occasionally the pain activates afferent fibers in the ninth nerve, which in turn activate brainstem vasomotor mechanisms and induce bradycardia and syncope. This condition should be treated like trigeminal neuralgia, i.e., with carbamazepine or other antiepileptic drugs. If unsuccessful, the glossopharyngeal nerve and upper rootlets of the vagus need to be interrupted surgically.

More often, cranial nerve IX is compressed together with nerves X and XI by a tumor (neurofibroma, meningioma, plasmacytoma, metastatic Ca) at the jugular foramen. Then there is hoarseness, difficulty in swallowing, deviation of the soft palate to the sound side, anesthesia of the posterior wall of the pharynx, and weakness of the upper trapezius and sternomastoid muscles (see Table 45-1). The lesion is often visible by MRI.

The Tenth, or Vagus, Nerve

Complete interruption of one vagus nerve intracranially results in ipsilateral weakness of the soft palate, deviation of the uvula to the normal side, unilateral loss of the gag reflex, hoarse voice and immobile vocal cord on one side, and loss of sensation in the pharynx, external auditory meatus, and back of the pinna. The vagus nerve may be implicated at the meningeal level by tumors and infective processes and within the medulla by vascular lesions (Wallenberg syndrome), motor system disease, and occasionally herpes zoster.

The left recurrent laryngeal nerve, which has a longer course in the mediastinum than the right, may be compressed by an aneurysm of the aorta or a mediastinal or lung tumor. There is no dysphagia with such lesions because the branches to the pharynx leave the vagus nerve more proximally; only the vocal cord is paralyzed. Bilateral vagal lesions occur in some cases of familial hypertrophic polyneuropathy and the Chiari malformation (defects in phonation and laryngeal stridor). Bilateral destruction of the nucleus ambiguus (motor system disease, poliomyelitis) is probably incompatible with life.

The Eleventh, or Accessory, Nerve

This nerve has two parts: a spinal one, derived from the anterior horn cells of the upper cervical cord, and a medullary one, which issues with the lower bundles of the vagus (vagal-accessory nerve). A complete lesion paralyzes the sternocleidomastoid and upper part of the trapezius muscles. Motor system disease, poliomyelitis, syringobulbia, and Chiari malformation are well-documented causes. Intracranially it may be affected with cranial nerves IX and X and sometimes with XII (see Table 45-1). An idiopathic accessory nerve palsy akin to Bell's palsy is also a known entity. Polymyositis may affect the trapezius and sternomastoid muscles bilaterally as well as those of the pharynx and larynx and needs to be distinguished from bilateral eleventh-nerve lesions.

TABLE 45-2 Brainstem Syndromes Involving Cranial Nerves

Eponym	Site	Cranial nerves involved	Tracts and nuclei involved	Signs	Usual cause
Weber syndrome	Base of midbrain	III	Corticospinal tract	Oculomotor palsy with crossed hemiplegia	Vascular occlusion, tumor, aneurysm
Claude syndrome	Tegmentum of midbrain	III	Red nucleus and brachium conjunctivum	Oculomotor palsy with contralateral cerebellar ataxia and tremor	Vascular occlusion, tumor, aneurysm
Benedikt syndrome	Tegmentum of midbrain	III	Red nucleus, cortico-spinal tract, and brachium conjunctivum	Oculomotor palsy with contralateral cerebellar ataxia, tremor and corticospinal signs	Infarction, hemorrhage, tuberculoma, tumor
Nothnagel syndrome	Tectum of midbrain	Unilateral or bilateral III	Superior cerebellar peduncles	Ocular palsies, paralysis of gaze, and celebellar ataxia	Tumor
Parinaud syndrome	Dorsal midbrain		Supranuclear mechanism for upward gaze and other structures in periaqueductal gray matter	Paralysis of upward gaze and accommodation; fixed pupils	Pinealoma, hydrocephalus and other lesions of dorsal midbrain

Millard-Gubler syndrome and Raymond-Foville syndrome	Base of pons	VII and often VI	Corticospinal tract	Facial and abducens palsy and contralateral hemiplegia; sometimes gaze palsy to side of lesion	Infarction or tumor
Avellis syndrome	Tegmentum of medulla	X	Spinothalamic tract; sometimes descending pupillary fibers, with Bernard-Horner syndrome	Paralysis of soft palate and vocal cord and contralateral hemianesthesia	Infarction or tumor
Jackson syndrome	Tegmentum of medulla	X, XII	Corticospinal tract	Avellis syndrome plus ipsilateral tongue paralysis	Infarction or tumor
Wallenberg syndrome	Lateral tegmentum of medulla	Spinal V, IX, X, XI	Lateral spinothalamic tract Descending pupillodilator fibers Spinocerebellar and olivocerebellar tracts	Ipsilateral V, IX, X, XI palsy, Horner syndrome and cerebellar ataxia; contralateral loss of pain and temperature sense	Occlusion of vertebral or posterior-inferior cerebellar artery

Hypoglossal Nerve

Lesions of this nerve alone are rare. It may be compressed by metastatic or meningeal tumor at or near the hypoglossal foramen, by the bony overgrowth of Paget disease of the clivus, or by dissecting aneurysm of the carotid artery. Complete interruption causes unilateral weakness and atrophy of the tongue, with fasciculations. On protrusion, the tongue deviates to the affected side. Intracranial and intramedullary lesions, e.g., vertebral and anterior spinal artery thrombosis, simultaneously affect the pyramid, medial lemniscus, and hypoglossal nerve; the result is paralysis and atrophy of one side of the tongue together with spastic weakness and loss of deep sensation in the opposite arm and leg.

Involvement of multiple cranial nerves may be due to intracranial extramedullary leptomeningeal carcinomatosis or fibrosis, tumors and granulomas, or lesions of the brainstem (infarcts, tumors, hemorrhages), in which case they are conjoined with signs of long tract disease. The extramedullary cranial nerve syndromes are listed in Table 45-1, and the brainstem syndromes in Table 45-2.

For a more detailed discussion of this topic, see Adams and Victor: *Principles of Neurology*, 4th ed, pp 1077–1089.

ADDITIONAL READING

Devinsky O, Feldmann E: *Examination of the Cranial and Peripheral Nerves*. New York, Churchill Livingstone, 1988.

Karnes WE: Diseases of the seventh cranial nerve, in Dyck PJ et al (eds): *Peripheral Neuropathy*, 2nd ed. Philadelphia, Saunders, 1984, chap 55, pp 1266–1299.

Kennedy RH, Bartley GB, Flanagan JC, Waller RR: Treatment of blepharospasm with botulinum toxin. *Mayo Clinic Proc* 64:1085, 1989.

Lecky BRF, Hughes RAC, Murray NMF: Trigeminal sensory neuropathy. *Brain* 110:1463, 1987.

Mayo Clinic and Mayo Foundation: *Clinical Examinations in Neurology*, 6th ed. St. Louis, Mosby-Year Book, 1991.

Sweet WH: The treatment of trigeminal neuralgia (tic douloureux). *New Engl J Med* 315:174, 1986.

Wilson-Panels L, Akesson EJ, Stewart PA: *Cranial Nerves: Anatomy and Clinical Comments*. St. Louis, Mosby-Year Book, 1988.

46 Principles of Clinical Myology: Diagnosis and Classification of Muscle Diseases

The symptoms and signs of diseases of muscle, the diagnostic methods utilized in their detection, and the various means of treating them constitute a relatively new branch of medicine known as *clinical myology*.

As one would expect from a tissue of uniform structure and function, the symptoms and signs by which diseases of striated muscle express themselves are relatively few in number. Weakness, fatigue, limpness or stiffness, spasm, pain, a muscle mass, or change in muscle volume constitute the clinical manifestations. This explains the fact that many different muscle diseases share certain symptoms and syndromes. It is expedient, therefore, to discuss here the symptoms and signs common to all the diseases of striated muscle and in later chapters to specify those peculiar to certain diseases.

Myopathic Weakness and Fatigue

These two symptoms are often confused. While fatigue is a prominent feature of a few muscle diseases, the complaint of fatigue, without demonstrable weakness, is far more often indicative of anxiety, depression, or an endocrine or other systemic disease (see also Chap. 23). To distinguish between weakness and fatigue, it is necessary to assess the patient's capacity to walk or climb stairs and to arise from a sitting, kneeling, squatting, or reclining position. Difficulty in performing these tasks, either as a single test or repeatedly (in tests of endurance), signifies weakness rather than fatigue. The same applies to difficulty in working with the arms above shoulder level. More localized muscle weakness is manifested by drooping of the eyelids, diplopia and strabismus, changes in facial expression and voice, difficulty in chewing and swallowing, closing the mouth, and pursing the lips and by failure of contraction of single muscles or groups of muscles in the extremities. Of course, impairment of muscle function may be due to a neuropathic or CNS disorder rather than a myopathic one, but usually these conditions can be separated by the methods indicated further on in this chapter and in Chap. 3.

Ascertaining the pattern of muscle weakness, whether restricted or generalized, and its degree requires the systematic testing of all the major muscle groups. The actions of the various muscle groups and their innervation are shown in Table 46-1.

Grading of Muscle Weakness

Grading of muscle weakness by using a standard scale permits the accurate recording of the severity of weakness and comparison from one examination to another. The most widely used rating scale recognizes the following grades of muscle strength:

0 = complete paralysis
1 = minimal contraction
2 = active movement, with gravity eliminated
3 = weak contraction, against gravity
4 = active movement against gravity and resistance
5 = normal strength

Finer degrees of weakness can be denoted by a plus or minus sign, e.g., 4+ means barely detectable weakness.

Such tests of peak power require the full cooperation of the patient, and the examiner must watch for signs of lack of effort. Pain during contraction may also hamper tests of strength (antalgic contraction).

Topography or Patterns of Muscle Weakness

Each muscle disease exhibits a particular pattern of involvement. That is to say, a given pattern of muscle involvement tends to be similar in all patients with the same disease. Thus, topography or pattern of muscle affection becomes an important diagnostic attribute of myopathic disease, as indicated in Table 46-2.

Qualitative Changes in Muscle Contractility

Apart from simple weakness and proportionate reflex loss, affected muscles undergo a number of special (qualitative) changes in function, mostly in relation to sustained activity. *In myasthenia gravis* (MG), continuing contraction rapidly induces increasing weakness and resting restores power. Thus, looking upward for 2 to 3 min causes a progressive ptosis, which is quickly relieved by resting the eyes; diplopia and strabismus increase with persistent horizontal or upward gaze; talking for a few minutes causes progressive dysarthria and nasality of the voice. These phenomena, by themselves, establish the diagnosis of MG.

A state of weakness in which a series of successive contractions actually increases the power of a group of muscles (e.g., abduction of the arm) is diagnostic of the *myasthenic syndrome of Lambert-Eaton*. Slowness and stiffness of contraction of the handgrip, which lessens with each contraction, is typical of *myotonia*; the opposite—increasing slowness and stiffness with each contraction (*paradoxical myotonia*)—occurs in some cases of von Eulenberg paramyotonia.

The fixed shortening of muscle that follows a series of strong contractions, especially under ischemic conditions (BP cuff on arm), is characteristic of McArdle disease (phosphorylase deficiency). This state, referred to as *true contracture*, needs to be distinguished from cramp and *pseudocontracture* (myostatic contracture), which occurs whenever muscle is immobilized for a long period in a shortened position (in a cast, for fracture).

Myotonia, a persistence of contraction (for several seconds) during attempted relaxation, is characteristic of myotonic dystrophy and congenital myotonia. This phenomenon may also be elicited by a sharp tap on the muscle belly (*percussion myotonia*). (By contrast, the *myoedema* of cachexia and hypothyroidism is a localized bulge in muscle, appearing at the point struck, without contraction of the entire muscle.) Forceful voluntary contraction is necessary to evoke myotonia; thus, the eyelids open immediately after an ordinary blink but not after forceful closure, and the hand will not open after being firmly fisted. Myotonia needs to be distinguished from the spreading tautness and gradual failure of relaxation that occur in mild or localized tetanus. In the tetany of hypocalcemia, the muscle, once excited in any way, may remain in spasm.

Other Features of Muscle Disease

A loss of normally innervated motor units causes a decrease in muscle tone. Infants with *hypotonia* are said to be "floppy." This is an especially valuable sign in infants with neuromuscular disease, in whom graded tests of voluntary contraction cannot be performed.

Diminution or increase in muscle bulk are other useful indices of neuromuscular disease. Extreme atrophy is a mark of muscle dystrophy or of spinal or neural denervation. In the former, the atrophy is due to a reduction in the number of muscle fibers and in the latter, to a reduction in their size. Enlargement of muscle may be the result of persistent overactivity (work hypertrophy) or an early sign of some dystrophies. Usually the enlargement in dystrophy is due to infiltration of fat cells, leaving the muscle in a weakened condition; this is called *pseudohypertrophy*.

TABLE 46-1 Tests of Muscle Action

Action tested	Roots*	Nerves	Principal muscles
Cranial			
Closure of eyes, pursing of lips, exposure of teeth	Cranial 7	Facial	Orbicularis oculi Orbicularis oris
Elevation of eyelids, movement of eyes	Cranial 3, 4, 6	Oculomotor, trochlear, abducens	Extraocular
Closing and opening of jaw	Cranial 5	Motor trigeminal	Masseters Pterygoids
Protrusion of tongue	Cranial 12	Hypoglossal	Lingual
Phonation and swallowing	Cranial 9, 10	Glossopharyngeal, vagus	Palatal, laryngeal, and pharyngeal
Elevation of shoulders, anteroflexion and turning of head	Cranial 11	Spinal accessory	Trapezius, sternomastoid
Brachial			
Adduction of extended arm	*C5*, C6	Brachial plexus	Pectoralis major
Fixation of scapula	C5, 6, 7	Brachial plexus	Serratus anterior
Initiation of abduction of arm	*C5*, C6	Brachial plexus	Supraspinatus
External rotation of flexed arm	*C5*, C6	Brachial plexus	Infraspinatus
Abduction and elevation of arm up to 90°	*C5*, C6	Axillary nerve	Deltoid
Flexion of supinated forearm	C5, C6	Musculocutaneous	Biceps, brachialis
Extension of forearm	C6, *C7*, C8	Radial	Triceps
Extension (radial) of wrist	C6	Radial	Extensor carpi radialis longus
Flexion of semipronated arm	C5, *C6*	Radial	Brachioradialis
Adduction of flexed arm	C6, *C7*, C8	Brachial plexus	Latissimus dorsi
Supination of forearm	C6, C7	Posterior interosseous	Supinator

Extension of proximal phalanges	C7, C8	Posterior interosseous	Extensor digitorum
Extension of wrist (ulnar side)	C7, C8	Posterior interosseous	Extensor carpi ulnaris
Extension of proximal phalanx of index finger	C7, C8	Posterior interosseous	Extensor indicis
Abduction of thumb	C7, C8	Posterior interosseous	Abductor pollicis longus and brevis
Extension of thumb	C7, C8	Posterior interosseous	Extensor pollicis longus and brevis
Pronation of forearm	C6, C7	Median nerve	Pronator teres
Radial flexion of wrist	C6, C7	Median nerve	Flexor carpi radialis
Flexion of middle phalanges	C7, C8, T1	Median nerve	Flexor digitorum superficialis
Flexion of proximal phalanx of thumb	C8, T1	Median nerve	Flexor pollicis brevis
Opposition of thumb against fifth finger	C8, T1	Median nerve	Opponens pollicis
Extension of middle phalanges of index and middle fingers	C8, T1	Median nerve	First, second lumbricals
Flexion of terminal phalanx of thumb	C8, T1	Anterior interosseous nerve	Flexor pollicis longus
Flexion of terminal phalanx of second and third fingers	C8, T1	Anterior interosseous nerve	Flexor digitorum profundus
Flexion of distal phalanges of ring and little fingers	C7, C8	Ulnar	Flexor digitorum profundus
Adduction and opposition of fifth finger	C8, T1	Ulnar	Hypothenar
Extension of middle phalanges of ring and little fingers	C8, T1	Ulnar	Third, fourth lumbricals
Adduction of thumb against index finger	C8, T1	Ulnar	Adductor pollicis
Flexion of proximal phalanx of thumb	C8, T1	Ulnar	Flexor pollicis brevis
Abduction and adduction of fingers	C8, T1	Ulnar	Interossei

(*continued*)

TABLE 46-1 Tests of Muscle Action (*continued*)

Action tested	Roots*	Nerves	Principal muscles
		Crural	
Hip flexion from semiflexed position	*L*1, *L*2, L3	Femoral	Iliopsoas
Hip flexion from externally rotated position	L2, L3	Femoral	Sartorius
Extension of knee	L2, *L*3, *L*4	Femoral	Quadriceps femoris
Adduction of thigh	*L*2, *L*3, L4	Obturator	Adductor longus, magnus, brevis
Abduction and internal rotation of thigh	*L*4, *L*5, S1	Superior gluteal	Gluteus medius
Extension of thigh	*L*5, *S*1, *S*2	Inferior gluteal	Gluteus maximus
Flexion of knee	L5, *S*1, *S*2	Sciatic	Bicepts femoris, semitendinosus, semimembranosus
Dorsiflexion of foot (medial)	*L*4, L5	Peroneal (deep)	Anterior tibial
Dorsiflexion of toes (proximal and distal phalanges)	*L*5, S1		Extensor digitorum longus and brevis
Dorsiflexion of great toe	*L*5, S1		Extensor hallucis longus
Eversion of foot	L5, S1	Peroneal (superficial)	Peroneus longus and brevis
Plantar flexion of foot	*S*1, S2	Tibial	Gastrocnemius, soleus
Inversion of foot	L4, *L*5	Tibial	Tibialis posterior
Flexion of toes (distal phalanges)	L5, *S*1, *S*2	Tibial	Flexor digitorum longus
Flexion of toes (middle phalanges)	*S*1, *S*2	Tibial	Flexor digitorum brevis
Flexion of great toe (proximal phalanx)	S1, S2	Tibial	Flexor hallucis brevis
Flexion of great toe (distal phalanx)	L5, *S*1, *S*2	Tibial	Flexor hallucis longus
Contraction of anal sphincter	S2, S3, S4	Pudendal	Perineal muscles

* Italics indicate major nerve root involved.

TABLE 46-2 Pattern of Weakness Diseases of Muscle

Pattern of weakness	Causative disease
1. Bilateral ocular palsies, strabismus, ptosis, and impaired closure of eyelids—diplopia prominent, pupils spared	Myasthenia gravis; oculopharyngeal dystrophy; exophthalmic ophthalmoplegia of thyroid disease; myotonic dystrophy; Kearns-Sayre syndrome; botulism (autonomic symptoms are added)
2. Bifacial weakness—inability to smile, expose teeth, and close eyelids	Myasthenia gravis; myotonic dystrophy; facioscapulohumeral dystrophy; centronuclear, nemaline, and carnitine myopathies; Guillain-Barré syndrome (neuropathic); Lyme disease; Moebius syndrome
3. Bulbar palsy—dysphonia, dysarthria, dysphagia, amyotrophy of tongue; weak masseter and facial muscles in some	Myasthenia gravis; progressive bulbar palsy; myotonic dystrophy; botulism; rarely polymyositis, Chiari malformation and basilar invagination
4. Cervical muscle palsies—inability to lift head or extend neck	Polymyositis; muscular dystrophy; rarely progressive spinal muscular atrophy (motor system disease)
5. Weakness of respiratory and trunk muscles	Motor system disease; glycogen storage disease; muscular dystrophy; GBS; myasthenia gravis
6. Bibrachial palsy—dangling arms	Motor system disease (ALS); rarely GBS or porphyric polyneuritis; *not* usually a manifestation of muscle disease
7. Bicrural palsy	Usually a polyneuropathy or motor system disease
8. Limb-girdle palsies	Polymyositis; congenital myopathies Progressive muscular dystrophy: Shoulder girdle and proximal arms (Landouzy-Déjerine) Pelvic girdle (Leyden-Moebius)
9. Distal limb palsies—footdrop, steppage gait, wrist drop, weak hands	Distal muscular dystrophies Familial polyneuropathies (Charcot-Marie-Tooth, Déjerine-Sottas, Refsum disease); chronic polyneuropathies
10. Generalized or universal paralysis	*Episodic*: Hypo- or hyperkalemic paralysis *Persistent*: Werdnig-Hoffmann disease (infants); progressive spinal muscular atrophy (children); rarely advanced dystrophy; Guillain-Barré syndrome (acute)
11. Paralysis of single muscles or groups of muscles	Almost always neuropathic or spinal

Twitches, spasms, and cramps are other natural phenomena that may assume prominence in certain muscle diseases. Fibrillations and fasciculations have been described in Chap. 3. Fibrillations are an EMG change and are due to denervation. Fasciculations and cramps are due to hyperexcitability of motor units and, though ordinarily benign, become pronounced in motor system disease. In the latter condition they are always accompanied by weakness, atrophy, and reflex changes. Cramps also become more frequent and severe as a result of excessive sweating and salt loss and in hypocalcemic tetany. *Continuous muscle activity*, wherein parts of many muscles or whole muscles are continually twitching, may be due to excessive irritability of motor units and may also be part of the more generalized twitch-myoclonus-convulsive syndrome of renal failure and hypocalcemia.

Pain is a rare complaint in primary muscle disease. Even polymyositis is in most cases painless. The pain that follows intense overactivity of unconditioned muscles is probably due to single-fiber necrosis. However, when aching discomfort, especially after every attempt at exercise, is a major complaint, there may be some subtle disorder of muscle contraction, such as one caused by an enzyme deficiency, e.g., a Ca-ATPase deficiency, or by hypothyroidism. More often, when pain is associated with evidence of neuromuscular disease, the lesion involves the nerves or blood vessels within muscles or the connective tissue or periarticular structures (e.g., polymyalgia rheumatica, Lyme disease). Of course, cramps of whatever causation are painful and leave the muscle tender. The majority of patients who come to muscle clinics complaining only of fatigue and aching muscles will be found to suffer from neurasthenia and depression, though chronic viral infections are under suspicion.

Lumps in muscle are due to hemorrhage, infarction, or tumors. In so-called fibromyositis, tender lumpy areas can be palpated, but biopsy seldom reveals a recognizable change.

Diagnosis of Muscle Disease

The findings described in the preceding pages are of diagnostic importance, and when considered in connection with the age of the patient at the time of onset, their mode of evolution and time course, and the presence or absence of familial coincidence, they enable one to identify all of the more common diseases. The EMG is of assistance, particularly in differentiating the atrophies, myopathies, and dystrophies. One can resort to biopsy if there is still uncertainty as to diagnosis.

TABLE 46-3 Syndromic Classification of Muscle Diseases

I. Acute (evolving in days) or subacute (weeks) paretic or paralytic disorders of muscle*
  A. Rarely fulminant myasthenia gravis or myasthenic syndrome from a "mycin" antibiotic or hypokalemia
  B. Idiopathic polymyositis and dermatomyositis
  C. Viral polymyositis
  D. Acute paroxysmal myoglobinuria (several types)
  E. "Alcoholic" polymyopathy
  F. Familial (malignant) hyperpyrexia precipitated by anesthetic agents
  G. First attack of episodic weakness may enter into differential diagnosis (see below)
  H. Botulism
  I. Organophosphate poisoning
II. Chronic (i.e., months to years) weakness or paralysis of muscle usually with severe atrophy
  A. Progressive muscular dystrophy
    1. Duchenne type
    2. Facioscapulohumeral type (Landouzy-Déjerine)
    3. Limb-girdle types
    4. Distal type (Gowers, Welander)
    5. Myotonic dystrophy
    6. Progressive ophthalmoplegic, oculopharyngeal, and Kearns-Sayre types
  B. Chronic idiopathic polymyositis (may be subacute)
  C. Chronic thyrotoxic and other endocrine myopathies
  D. Chronic, slowly progressive, or relatively stationary polymyopathies†
    1. Central core and multicore diseases
    2. Rod-body and related polymyopathies
    3. Mitochondrial and centronuclear polymyopathies
    4. Other congenital myopathies (reducing-body, fingerprint, zebra body, fiber-type disproportion)
    5. Glycogen storage diseases
    6. Lipid myopathies (carnitine deficiency myopathy, undefined lipid myopathies)
III. Episodic weakness of muscle
  A. Familial (hypokalemic) periodic paralysis
  B. Normokalemic or hyperkalemic familial periodic paralysis
  C. Paramyotonia congenita (von Eulenberg)
  D. Nonfamilial hyper- and hypokalemic periodic paralysis (including primary hyperaldosteronism)
  E. Acute thyrotoxic myopathy (also thyrotoxic periodic paralysis)
  F. Conditions in which weakness fluctuates
    1. Myasthenia gravis, immunologic type
    2. Myasthenia associated with
      a. Lupus erythematosus
      b. Polymyositis
      c. Rheumatoid arthritis
      d. Nonthymic carcinoma
    3. Familial and sporadic nonimmunologic types of myasthenia
    4. Myasthenia due to antibiotics and other drugs
    5. Lambert-Eaton syndrome
IV. Disorders of muscle presenting with myotonia, stiffness, spasm, and cramp
  A. Congenital myotonia (Thomsen disease), paramyotonia congenita, myotonic dystrophy, and Schwartz-Jampel syndrome

TABLE 46-3 Syndromic Classification of Muscle Diseases (*continued*)

- B. Hypothyroidism with pseudomyotonia (Debré-Semelaigne and Hoffmann syndromes)
- C. Tetany
- D. Tetanus
- E. Black widow spider bite
- F. Myopathy resulting from myophosphorylase deficiency (McArdle syndrome), phosphofructokinase deficiency, and other forms of contracture
- G. Contracture with Addison disease
- H. Idiopathic cramp syndromes
- I. Myokymia and syndromes of continuous muscle activity

IV. Myalgic states‡

- A. Connective tissue diseases (rheumatoid arthritis, mixed connective tissue disease, Sjögren syndrome, lupus erythematosus, polyarteritis nodosa, scleroderma, polymyositis)
- B. Localized fibrositis or fibromyositis
- C. Trichinosis
- D. Myopathy of myoglobinuria and McArdle syndrome
- E. Myopathy with hypoglycemia
- F. Bornholm disease and other forms of viral polymyositis
- G. Anterior tibial syndrome
- H. Other
  - 1. Hypophosphatemia
  - 2. Hypothyroidism
  - 3. Psychiatric illness (hysteria, depression)

VI. Localized muscle mass(es)

- A. Rupture of a muscle
- B. Muscle hemorrhage
- C. Muscle tumor
  - 1. Rhabdomyosarcoma
  - 2. Desmoid
  - 3. Angioma
  - 4. Metastatic nodules
- D. Monomyositis multiplex
  - 1. Eosinophilic type
  - 2. Other
- E. Localized and generalized myositis ossificans
- F. Fibrositis (myogelosis)
- G. Granulomatous infections
  - 1. Sarcoidosis
  - 2. Tuberculosis
  - 3. Wegener granulomatosis
- H. Pyogenic abscess
- I. Infarction of muscle in the diabetic

* The acute and subacute primary disorders of muscle need to be differentiated from acute spinal cord or peripheral nerve diseases, in which paralysis is often severe and widespread and atrophy may or may not be present (poliomyelitis, acute idiopathic polyneuritis, or other forms of polyneuropathy; see Chap. 44).

† The chronic myopathies need to be distinguished from the progressive muscular atrophies and other forms of motor system disease (amyotrophic lateral sclerosis, progressive bulbar palsy) and infantile spinal muscular atrophy (Werdnig-Hoffmann disease), as well as chronic neural muscular atrophies such as peroneal muscular atrophy (Charcot-Marie-Tooth), hypertrophic polyneuritis (Déjerine-Sottas), amyloid polyneuropathy, chronic nutritional, arsenical, leprous, and other polyneuropathies (see Chap. 44).

‡ Pain and tenderness of muscle are characteristic also of many forms of polyneuropathy (see Chap. 44).

The clinical recognition of myopathic diseases is facilitated by a prior knowledge of a few syndromes. The ones listed in Table 46-3 occur with regularity. A description of these syndromes and the diseases of which they are a manifestation forms the content of the chapters that follow (Chaps. 47 to 52).

For a more detailed discussion of this topic, see Adams and Victor: *Principles of Neurology*, 4th ed, pp 1090–1103.

ADDITIONAL READING

Adams RD: Thayer lectures: I. Principles of myopathology. II. Principles of clinical myology. *John Hopkins Med J* 131:24, 1972.

Brooke MH: *A Clinician's View of Neuromuscular Diseases*, 2nd ed. Baltimore, Williams & Wilkins, 1986.

Engel AG, Banker BQ (eds): *Myology*. New York, McGraw-Hill, 1986.

Walton JN (ed): *Disorders of Voluntary Muscle*, 5th ed. Edinburgh, Churchill Livingstone, 1988.

47 Polymyositis and Other Acute and Subacute Myopathic Paralyses

Seldom is a primary disease of muscle the cause of an acute widespread paralysis; the usual causes of such a syndrome are acute polyneuropathy, poliomyelitis, or some other spinal cord disease. Exceptionally, certain disorders of neuromuscular transmission (botulinus poisoning and rare instances of myasthenia gravis), hypo- or hyperkalemia, or an episode of paroxysmal myoglobinuria may be associated with a rapidly evolving diffuse weakness or paralysis.

Paresis of widespread distribution and subacute evolution (over a period of weeks) are attributable to a much wider spectrum of diseases, including some that are clearly myopathic, such as the infective and idiopathic polymyositides, dermatomyositis, and several of the metabolic myopathies.

Infective Forms of Polymyositis

Of these, only trichinosis is likely to occur with sufficient frequency to be of concern. Toxoplasmosis, cysticercosis, trypanosomiasis, and certain viral infections—group B coxsackie (pleurodynia or Bornholm disease), influenza, Epstein-Barr (EB)—and *Mycoplasma pneumoniae* do affect muscles, but other aspects of these infections are far more prominent.

Trichinosis This infection results from the ingestion of undercooked pork containing the encysted larvae of *Trichinella spiralis*. Following an initial gastroenteritis, there may be widespread invasion of skeletal muscles, but weakness is limited mainly to the cranial ones—tongue, masseters, and extraocular and pharyngeal muscles. The involved muscles may be slightly swollen and tender and accompanied by conjunctival, orbital, and facial edema. Other muscles are tender as well. Rarely, in the acute phase of the disease there may be cerebral symptoms, probably due to embolism from a trichinal myocarditis.

Eosinophilia is the most helpful laboratory finding. Serum antibodies (bentonite flocculation assay) become evident within 3 to 4 weeks after infection. Muscle biopsy is confirmatory but seldom required.

Usually the symptoms subside spontaneously, but in severe

cases, thiobendazole, 25 mg/kg bid, and prednisone, 40 to 60 mg daily, for 10 to 14 days, are recommended.

Idiopathic Polymyositis and Dermatomyositis

These are rather frequent diseases in tertiary referral centers. They involve proximal limb and trunk muscles and, to a lesser degree, those of the neck, pharynx, and larynx. If only muscles are involved, the condition is called polymyositis (PM); if skin and muscle, dermatomyositis (DM). If other connective tissue diseases are associated, the designation is PM or DM with rheumatoid arthritis, lupus erythematosus, scleroderma, or mixed connective tisue disease ("overlap group"), as the case may be.

Clinically, PM presents as a symmetric weakness of the proximal limb and girdle muscles developing over a period of weeks to months. It affects individuals of both sexes and all ages, the middle-aged and elderly somewhat disproportionately. *Usually there is no pain, fever, or recognizable initiating event*. Weakness of the hip and thigh muscles is expressed by difficulty in climbing or descending stairs and arising from a deep chair or from a kneeling or squatting position. Less often, the shoulder and upper arm muscles are affected first, in which case working with the arms above the head (combing hair, putting objects on a high shelf) becomes increasingly difficult. Lolling of the head (weakness of posterior neck muscles), dysphagia, and dysphonia are frequent. The affected muscles are not tender, the reflexes are only slightly reduced, and atrophy is not marked. Restricted forms, affecting only the shoulder or pelvic girdle, are well known. Rarely, in the beginning, the symptoms predominate in one limb. Sometimes the myocardium is affected.

In DM, the skin lesions may precede, accompany, or follow the polymyositis. They vary from a few patches of erythematous or scaling eczematoid dermatitis to a diffuse exfoliative dermatitis or scleroderma. A lilac (heliotrope) discoloration over the bridge of the nose, cheeks, and forehead and around the fingernails and mild periorbital and perioral edema are characteristic.

One-third to one-half of our cases of PM and DM have occurred sometime in the course of connective tissue disease. And in 8 to 30 percent in different series, more in the older age group, PM and particularly DM have occurred in association with a malignant tumor (most often of lung and colon in males, breast and ovary in female).

A special form of DM is observed in children, in whom, in addition to involvement of skin and muscle, there is pain, intermittent fever, melena and hematemesis, and sometimes perforation of the gastrointestinal tract.

Inclusion body myositis is another special and common type of inflammatory muscle disease. It is characterized by an increased incidence in males, a disproportionate affection of the distal limb muscles, rarity of dysphagia, only slight elevation of CK, and a lack of response to corticosteroids. The muscle biopsy findings are distinctive: intranuclear and intracytoplasmic inclusions, comprised of masses of filaments and subsarcolemmal whorls of membranes, combined with fiber necrosis, cellular infiltrates, and regeneration. A viral origin has been suggested, but such a causation has never been established.

Laboratory tests Serum concentrations of transaminase, aldolase, and CK are greatly increased. The sedimentation rate may or may not be elevated. Tests of rheumatoid factor and antinuclear antibodies are positive in fewer than half the cases. Eosinophilia and neutrophilic leucocytosis are usually absent. The EMG is myopathic, but there are also fibrillation potentials. The ECG may be abnormal.

Muscle biopsy discloses widespread infiltrates of lymphocytes, mononuclear cells, and plasma cells and scattered muscle fibers undergoing necrosis and regeneration. Probably because of biopsy sampling error, the proportions of inflammation and necrosis vary widely. DM is characterized by a number of additional changes (degeneration and atrophy of perifascicular muscle fibers and tubular aggregates in endothelial cells). In childhood DM, vasculitis and occlusion of intramuscular vessels by fibrin thrombi are prominent changes.

The cause of these diseases is unknown. As to *pathogenesis*, there is considerable evidence that an autoimmune mechanism is operative—predominantly a humoral response directed against intramuscular vessels in DM and a T-cell-mediated attack on the muscle fiber in PM (see *Principles* for details).

Treatment The following program has been adopted in most centers: (1) *Prednisone*, 60 mg in three or four divided doses daily. Once recovery begins, as judged by an increase in muscle power and decrease in serum CK, the dose is reduced in steps of 5 mg every 2 to 3 weeks. When prednisone has been reduced to 20 mg daily, administration of 40 mg every other day is preferred. A dose of 7.5 to 20 mg/day should be continued for 6 to 12 months or longer. If relapse occurs, the dose is again increased. Potassium and antacids must be given with prednisone. (2) *Physiotherapy*, in the form of gentle massage, passive movement, and stretching of muscles is needed to prevent pseudocontractures.

In patients who do not respond to steroids alone, *methotrexate*, 25 to 30 mg IV each week, or oral *azathioprine*, up to 150 to 300 mg/day combined with a low dose of prednisone, may be successful.

With treatment, prognosis for survival is favorable, except in those with malignant tumors. Approximately 20 percent of our patients have recovered completely. Most of the others improve and are more or less functional but may need continuous therapy.

OTHER ACUTE AND SUBACUTE MYOPATHIES

Necrotizing Polymyopathy (Rhabdomyolysis) with Myoglobinuria

Any disease that results in rapid destruction of muscles may cause myoglobin to enter the bloodstream and to appear in the urine. The muscles become painful, tender, and weak, and serum CK is greatly elevated. In most cases recovery occurs spontaneously, within a few days or weeks, but severe degrees of myoglobinuria may damage the kidneys and lead to anuria that is sometimes fatal.

The following conditions may give rise to rhabdomyolysis and myoglobinuria:

1. Extensive crushing, compression, or infarction of muscle.
2. Excessive use of certain muscles, especially those in the tight pretibial compartment.
3. PM and DM, when necrosis is exceptionally severe.
4. Ingestion of toxins, such as resins, in poisoned fish (Haff disease), and particularly *alcohol*, in some individuals (see below).
5. Several *hereditary disorders of muscle glycolysis* have been incriminated, all of them rare: myophosphorylase deficiency (McArdle disease); phosphofructose kinase deficiency (Tarui disease); lipid storage myopathy; palmityl transferase deficiency; and phosphoglycerate kinase deficiency. The first two of these diseases have other myopathic features and will be described in Chap. 49; the others are so rare that the reader should turn to textbooks on myology for details.
6. Familial recurrent, or *paroxysmal*, *myoglobinuria* (Meyer-Betz and related diseases), occurring in families with or without chronic myopathy or dystrophy. Usually the episodes of myoglobinuria occur under conditions of intense physical activity, often associated with infection or fasting.
7. *Malignant hyperthermia* is essentially an anesthesia accident in patients with an inherited (autosomal dominant) metabolic muscle defect, which renders them sensitive to certain agents, particularly halothane and succinylcholine. A sudden stiffening of the masseters and other muscles and severe hyperthermia (up to 42 to 43° C) with circulatory collapse and failure of brainstem reflexes are the main clinical features. Unless the anesthesia is discontinued and the body cooled, many of the patients die. Dantrolene given intravenously may be

lifesaving. There is widespread muscle fiber necrosis and a dramatic rise in serum CK. A primary defect of the enzyme phosphodiesterase is suspected. The *neuroleptic malignant syndrome* (Chap. 40) has many similar features.

Alcoholic Myopathy

Alcoholism is complicated by several types of muscle disease. One type is a focal *compressive-ischemic myopathy* of a buttock, leg, or shoulder muscle, the result of lying immobile and insensate for a prolonged period. Severe degrees of *hypokalemia* (<2 meq/L), due to diarrhea and vomiting, may develop in the course of a prolonged drinking bout and give rise to a painless and predominantly proximal weakness of limb musculature. Still other patients, in the course of a sustained drinking bout, develop muscle cramps and mild diffuse weakness, for which there is no apparent explanation.

Yet another type of myopathic syndrome occurs acutely at the height of a prolonged drinking bout and is manifested by severe pain, tenderness, and edema of muscles of the limbs and trunk accompanied in severe cases by myoglobinuria and renal damage. The muscle affection may be focal, giving the appearance of a deep phlebothrombosis. This syndrome is probably the most common form of rhabdomyolysis seen in a general hospital. Haller and Drachman have presented evidence that a period of fasting, after a prolonged drinking spree, is the factor that precipitates the myonecrosis.

The subacute or chronic evolution of painless weakness and atrophy of the proximal muscles of the lower limbs, commonly referred to as "chronic alcoholic myopathy," is probably neuropathic in nature (see references).

For a more detailed discussion of this topic, see Adams and Victor: *Principles of Neurology*, 4th ed, pp 1104–1116.

ADDITIONAL READING

Banker BQ, Engel AG: The polymyositis and dermatomyositis syndromes, in Engel AG, Banker BQ (eds): *Myology*. New York, McGraw-Hill, 1986, chap 46, pp 1385–1422.

Currie S: Polymyositis and related disorders, in Walton JN (ed): *Disorders of Voluntary Muscle*, 5th ed. Edinburgh, Churchill Livingstone, 1988, chap 17, pp 588–610.

Haller RG, Drachman DB: Alcoholic rhabdomyolysis: An experimental model in the rat. *Science* 208:412, 1980.

Victor M: Toxic and nutritional myopathies, in Engel AG, Banker BQ (eds): *Myology*. New York, McGraw-Hill, 1986, pp 1807–1842.

48 | The Muscular Dystrophies

The *muscular dystrophies* are progressive, hereditary degenerative diseases of skeletal muscles. These diseases have their origin in the muscle fibers; spinal motor neurons, muscular nerves, and nerve endings are intact. Common to all members of this group of diseases are the symmetric distribution of muscular weakness and atrophy, intact sensibility, preservation of cutaneous reflexes, and heredofamilial occurrence.

By consensus, other primary degenerative diseases of muscle, sometimes traceable to vitamin E deficiency, a viral infection, a hereditary metabolic disorder (e.g., myophosphorylase deficiency), or a congenital and relatively nonprogressive disorder with distinctive morphologic features (e.g., central-core disease), are called *myopathies* or *polymyopathies*.

In Table 48-1 are listed all the known types of progressive muscular dystrophy. Only a few of the more common ones will be described here.

Duchenne Muscular Dystrophy (Severe Generalized Muscular Dystrophy of Childhood, Erb Childhood Type)

This type of dystrophy begins in early childhood, or even in infancy, and progresses to complete incapacity and death by early adult life. The incidence rate ranges from 13 to 33 per 100,000 annually. The disease is inherited as a sex-linked recessive trait and is transmitted to male children by the mother, who is usually asymptomatic but who displays, on careful examination, subtle signs of muscle involvement (see further on).

The clinical presentation varies somewhat. Most of the boys will have begun to walk or even run before it is noticed that they have trouble climbing stairs and arising from the floor. The pelvifemoral muscles are affected before those of the shoulder girdle. Almost invariably the calf muscles and sometimes the quadriceps and deltoids are enlarged and firm, but soon they become weaker than normal (pseudohypertrophy). Other muscles such as those of the thighs, pelvis, and shoulder girdles become atrophied. Characteristically, the gait is waddling because of weak gluteal support of the hips. The back becomes lordotic and

TABLE 48-1 The Progressive Muscular Dystrophies

Type of dystrophy	Age of onset	Pattern of muscular involvement	Special features	Increase in CK	Inheritance
Duchenne	Infancy or early childhood	Pelvifemoral, later pectoral girdle	Hypertrophy-pseudohypertrophy, cardiac involvement, mental retardation	Marked	X-linked recessive
Becker	Childhood, adolescence, or early adult	Pelvifemoral, later pectoral girdle	Cardiac involvement, slight; mentation normal	Moderate	X-linked recessive
Emery-Dreifuss	Childhood, adolescence	Humeroperoneal	Contractures posterior neck and biceps muscles	Moderate	X-linked recessive
Landouzy-Déjerine	Late childhood, adolescence	Facioscapulohumeral; pelvic girdle, late	Heart normal, mentation normal	Slight to moderate	Dominant
Scapulohumeral (Seitz)	Childhood or adult	Spinati and humeral, later pelvic girdle	Cardiomyopathy	Slight to moderate	Dominant
Limb-girdle (Erb)	Childhood, adolescence, sometimes adult	Pectoral or pelvic or both	Heart usually normal, mentation normal	Slight to moderate	Autosomal recessive, or dominant

von Graefe-Fuchs	Childhood, adolescence	Ocular (sparing pupils); later facial and other muscles (slight)	Kearns-Sayre patients have retinitis pigmentosa, heart block, stunting of growth, and ovarian dysgenesis	Slight to moderate	Dominant; Kearns-Sayre recessive
Oculopharyngeal	Middle or late adult	Levators of lids, then other ocular-pharyngeal muscles; pectoral and pelvic muscles later	—	Slight or normal	Dominant
Myotonic (Steinert)	Infancy, childhood, adult	Ocular, facial, sternomastoid, forearm, peroneal	Cataracts, testicular atrophy	Slight or normal	Dominant
Congenital	Birth, infancy	Pectoral and pelvic girdles, or diffuse	Arthrogryposis, congenital abnormalities of brain (Fukuyama type)	Slight or moderate	Dominant or recessive

the abdomen protuberant, and later, affection of all paravertebral muscles results in kyphoscoliosis. The tendon reflexes diminish in proportion to muscle weakness; Achilles reflexes are usually retained because of the relative escape of calf muscles. The weakness of respiratory muscles and the kyphoscoliotic deformity become a threat to life once the patient becomes bedfast. Some of the patients are mentally backward. Cardiac muscle is usually involved late in the course of the illness, leading to enlargement of the heart, conduction defects, and congestive failure.

Ancillary findings The serum CK concentrations are invariably elevated, and this may precede manifest muscle weakness. The EMG is myopathic. The female carrier can be identified in almost all cases by a slight enlargement of calf muscles, a mild degree of muscular weakness, elevation of serum CK values, and mild abnormalities in the EMG and muscle biopsy.

Muscle biopsy discloses a loss of muscle fibers in a random distribution, i.e., without respect to motor units, and their replacement by fat cells and fibrous tissue; some of the remaining fibers are hypertrophied. In less affected parts of the muscle one can observe single or small groups of fibers in various stages of degeneration and attempted regeneration.

Becker-type muscular dystrophy This is another form of male sex-linked dystrophy, considerably less common and less severe than the Duchenne type. The incidence rate is 3 to 6 per 100,000. It causes weakness and hypertrophy in the same muscles as Duchenne dystrophy but the age of onset is much later (mean age 11 years; range 5 to 45 years) and long survival is the rule. Cardiac and mental disturbances are hardly ever observed.

Another relatively benign sex-linked dystrophy, slightly different in topography and lacking hypertrophy, is that described by Emery and Dreifuss. Also included as a variant is an X-linked *scapuloperoneal dystrophy*. In these latter forms the cardiac involvement may be severe.

Etiology of Duchenne-Becker dystrophy An important advance in our understanding of these dystrophies has been the recent discovery by Louis Kunkel and his colleagues of the abnormal gene that is shared by these disorders and also the protein product of the affected gene. In Duchenne dystrophy, the gene product, called *dystrophin*, is absent; in the Becker type, it is greatly reduced and structurally abnormal. In intermediate ("outlier") phenotypes, the amounts of dystrophin fall between those of the classic types.

Unfortunately, these new findings have as yet given no direction to therapy. In Duchenne and other forms of dystrophy only supportive measures are possible. Maintaining activity for as long as possible is desirable.

Facioscapulohumeral (Landouzy-Déjerine) Dystrophy

Like many dominantly inherited diseases, the onset is during late childhood or adolescence and rarely in early adult life. Usually the first manifestations are difficulty in lifting the arms above the head and winging of the scapulae, although bifacial weakness may have been present since early childhood. The eyelids cannot be closed firmly and the lips are loosely pursed. The atrophy and weakness affect mainly the muscles of the shoulder girdle (trapezii, pectorals, sternomastoids, serrati, rhomboids) and the proximal arm muscles. As a general rule, pelvifemoral muscles are involved later and to a lesser degree. In one subvariety of this disease the facial muscles are spared, and in another the pelvic and proximal lower-limb muscles are disproportionately involved.

The disease is slowly progressive and may appear to be arrested for long periods, so that many of the patients attain an advanced age. Cardiac function and mentation are unaffected. Serum CK is slightly elevated. The EMG is myopathic.

Restricted Ocular and Oculopharyngeal Dystrophies

The best-known form is *progressive external ophthalmoplegia*, described in the nineteenth century by Von Graefe and Fuchs. There is a paralysis of all the external ocular muscles, beginning in childhood and progressing slowly. Paralysis of the levator muscles of the eyelids is an early and troublesome symptom. In middle and late adult life, other muscles become affected, usually to a slight degree. Inheritance can be autosomal recessive or dominant. If combined with retinitis pigmentosa, short stature, elevated CSF protein, and heart-block, the condition is classed as the *Kearns-Sayre syndrome*, which is essentially a widespread disorder of mitochondria.

Oculopharyngeal dystrophy is inherited as an autosomal dominant trait and is unique in respect to its late onset, usually after 45 years of age, and the restricted muscular weakness, which is initially manifest as ptosis and dysphagia. Blepharoplasty and cutting the cricopharyngeus muscles provides symptomatic relief for variable periods of time, but progression is inexorable, involving other extraocular muscles and then shoulder and pelvic muscles as well. Like other relatively mild and restricted myopathies, serum CK and aldolase levels are normal, and the EMG is abnormal only in the affected muscles.

Myotonic Dystrophy (Steinert Disease)

In this form, the most frequent of all types of muscular dystrophy, there are more widespread dystrophic changes in addition to myotonia. Slight mental retardation may be present. Often the heart is affected; there is a peculiar type of cataract and, in the male, hypogonadism. The distribution of the muscle weakness and atrophy are unlike the other dystrophies. The thin, narrow face, temporal atrophy, drooping eyelids, and thin sternomastoid muscles reflect the cranial muscle involvement and, together with frontal baldness, impart a diagnostic physiognomy. The weak pharyngeal and laryngeal muscles give the voice a soft, monotonous nasal quality. In the limbs, the distal muscles are mainly affected, placing the condition in a class of distal dystrophies, but different from the others with respect to myotonia. The gene abnormality is on chromosome 19. Mild incomplete forms run in certain families. In general, progression is slow.

The myopathology is distinctive by virtue of long rows of central sarcolemmal nuclei and sarcoplasmic masses and many circular arrangements of myofibrils in addition to the usual dystrophic changes. Serum CK is slightly elevated. The EMG is diagnostic because of the combination of myopathic changes and myotonic discharges.

There is no specific treatment. The myotonia can be relieved to some extent by quinine, 0.3 to 0.6 g, or by procaine amide, 0.5 to 1.0 g, four times daily. Androgens may offer symptomatic benefit when gonadal deficiency is apparent. Cataracts can be managed surgically. The common complications of all dystrophies—notably fractures, pulmonary infections, and cardiac decompensation—need to be treated symptomatically.

A distinctive and potentially lethal form of this disease may be present at birth (*congenital myotonic dystrophy*). The affected parent is almost always the mother, who need not be severely affected. Drooping eyelids, tented upper lip ("carp mouth"), and open jaw allow recognition of the disease in the newborn infant. Difficulty in sucking and swallowing, bronchial aspiration, and respiratory distress are present in varying degrees of severity. In surviving infants, delayed motor and speech development, mental retardation, and arthrogryposis are common. Interestingly, myotonia does not become evident until later in childhood.

Other Forms of Muscular Dystrophy

These comprise the limb-girdle dystrophies, late-onset distal dystrophy, and congenital dystrophy of nonmyotonic types. These forms are less common than the ones described above;

their main features are summarized in Table 48-1. Comprehensive accounts of these and other dystrophies can be found in the Engel and Banker monograph, *Myology* (see references).

For a more detailed discussion of this topic, see Adams and Victor: *Principles of Neurology*, 4th ed, pp 1117–1132.

ADDITIONAL READING

Engel AG, Banker BQ (eds): *Myology*. New York, McGraw-Hill, 1986.

Harper PS: *Myotonic Dystrophy*. Philadelphia, Saunders, 1979.

Hoffman EP, Fischbeck KH, Brown RH, et al: Characterization of dystrophin in muscle-biopsy specimens from patients with Duchenne's or Becker's muscular dystrophy. *N Engl J Med* 318:1363, 1988.

Rowland LP: Dystrophin. A triumph of reverse genetics and the end of the beginning. *N Engl J Med* 318:1392, 1988.

Walton JN (ed): *Disorders of Voluntary Muscle*, 5th ed. Edinburgh, Churchill Livingstone, 1988.

49 | The Metabolic Myopathies

Subsumed under this title are two classes of metabolic diseases. In one, striated muscle fibers are affected by a disorder of an endocrine gland—thyroid, parathyroid, pituitary, or adrenal. In the other, the polymyopathy is based on a primary biochemical abnormality of the muscle cell. Due to limitations of space, only a few of the more frequent and representative examples will be described here.

Thyroid Myopathies

These are (1) chronic thyrotoxic myopathy, (2) exophthalmic ophthalmoplegia (infiltrative ophthalmopathy), (3) hyper- or hypothyroidism with myasthenia gravis, (4) periodic paralysis associated with hyperthyroidism, and (5) muscle hypertrophy and slow muscle contraction and relaxation associated with hypothyroidism.

Thyroxin influences the contractile mechanism of the striated muscle fiber but has no influence on nerve fiber conduction, neuromuscular transmission, or propagation of impulse over the sarcolemma (muscle cell membrane). In *hyperthyroidism*, the duration of the contractile process is somewhat reduced, and the effect is a diminution of muscle power and an increased fatigability. In *hypothyroidism*, the duration of muscle contraction and relaxation is prolonged. The speed of the contractile process is thought to be related to the quantity of myosin ATPase, which is increased in hyperthyroidism and decreased in hypothyroidism. The speed of relaxation depends on the rate of release and reaccumulation of calcium in the sarcoplasmic reticulum.

In *chronic hyperthyroid or thyrotoxic myopathy* there is a progressive weakness and wasting of muscles, particularly those of the thighs (Basedow paraplegia) and shoulders. This may progress to a degree that suggests a diagnosis of motor system disease—especially when tremor and twitching during contraction are prominent. Yet there are no fasciculations at rest, and serum levels of muscle enzymes are not increased. Muscle biopsy discloses slight atrophy of Type I and II fiber groups. The EMG is usually normal. Full recovery follows treatment of the thyrotoxicosis.

In *exophthalmic ophthalmoplegia*, the eye muscles become thickened and infiltrated by lymphocytes, monocytes, and lipocytes and many of the muscle fibers degenerate. There is strabismus and diplopia, most prominent on upward gaze, because of disproportionately greater thickening and shortening of the medial and inferior recti. These muscle abnormalities, which can be seen in ultrasonograms or CT scans of the orbit, are thought to be due to the formation of serum antibodies that react with components of eye muscles. The exophthalmia, which may affect one or both eyes, is due to thickening of the orbital tissue and needs to be distinguished from pseudotumor of the orbit.

In hyperthyroidism, an autoimmune disease, there is an increased incidence of *myasthenia gravis*. The latter is the typical autoimmune prostigmine-responsive form of the disease. Either the hyperthyroidism or myasthenia gravis may appear first; each may pursue an independent course and each must be treated separately.

Hypokalemic periodic paralysis, appearing for the first time as the patient develops hyperthyroidism, is particularly frequent among Orientals. Correction of the thyroid dysfunction relieves the patient of periodic paralysis.

In *hypothyroidism*, *myxedema*, and *cretinism* the muscles enlarge and movements become slow, stiff, and clumsy. The tongue partakes of the muscle enlargement, resulting in dysarthria. Slowness in the relaxation phase of the tendon reflexes is readily demonstrable, but contraction is slowed as well. Myoedema and spreading myospasm may sometimes be elicited. Serum CK is elevated. Muscle action potentials in the EMG may be myopathic, but the biopsy shows no consistent abnormality.

Corticosteroid Myopathy

Weakness and atrophy of girdle and proximal limb muscles, particularly those of the lower limbs, complicate Cushing disease and the prolonged use of corticosteroids. Climbing stairs, arising from a chair, and using the arms above the shoulders are difficult, and thigh and leg muscles become soft and thin. Yet the serum CK and aldolase levels are normal, and the muscle biopsy discloses only slight atrophy and increased variation in size of muscle fibers. Type IIB fibers are the most affected. Discontinuation of steroids or a reduction in their dosage and treatment of Cushing disease lead to improvement and recovery.

TABLE 49-1 Glycogen Storage Diseases

Type	Clinical and laboratory findings	Enzyme defiency	Heredity	Proper name
I	Enlarged liver and kidneys, hyperlipidemia, hypoglycemia, ketoacidosis, hypotonia in infants	Glucose-6-phosphatase	Autosomal recessive	von Gierke
II	*Infantile form:* cardiomegaly, hypotonia and weakness; dysphagia, respiratory difficulty; death in infancy *Childhood:* proximal weakness, enlarged calves, atonic anal sphincter, respiratory difficulties *Adult:* slowly progressive proximal myopathy; respiratory failure	α-1,4-Glucosidase (acid maltase)	Autosomal recessive	Pompe
III	Hepatomegaly, hypoglycemia, growth retardation, proximal and distal myopathy in some patients	Amylo-1,6-glucosidase (debranching)	—	Illingworth-Cori-Forbes
IV	Failure to thrive and growth failure, hepatosplenomegaly, cirrhosis, hypotonia with muscle atrophy in lower limbs in some patients	α-1,4-Glucan 6-glucosyltransferase (branching)	Autosomal recessive	Anderson
V	Cramp, pain, and weakness of muscles with exercise, sometimes myoglobinuria, lack of rise in blood lactate after ischemic exercise	Myophosphorylase	Probably autosomal recessive; autosomal dominant (rare)	McArdle
VI	Growth retardation, hepatosplenomegaly, hypoglycemia and mild ketosis	Hepatic phosphorylase	—	Hers
VII	Same as type V	Muscle phosphofructokinase,	Same as type V	Tarui
Other	—	phosphohexoisomerase, phosphorylase-*b*-kinase, phosphoglucomutase		

Other Endocrine Myopathies

A proximal myopathy, with weakness and fatigability, is a frequent complication of hyperparathyroidism, hypophosphatemia, and the late stages of acromegaly.

POLYMYOPATHY OF PRIMARY TYPE

Glycogen Storage Myopathies

There are several entities in which glycogen accumulates in muscle fibers and weakens their contractile power. Each is a manifestation of an enzymatic defect that blocks one step in the conversion of intramuscular glycogen to glucose and its further metabolism. Because of the rarity of these diseases, their clinical attributes are summarized only briefly in Table 49-1.

Mitochondrial Myopathies

This interesting group of hereditary myopathies, first recognized in hypotonic infants, has been expanded in recent years to include syndromes that involve the retinae, peripheral nerves, and brain. In the *Kearns-Sayre* syndrome, which is characterized by weakness of eye muscles, retinitis pigmentosa, cardiomyopathy, and other organ affections, there is a great increase in mitochondria and storage of lipid in muscle fibers. Oxygen transport through the cytochrome oxidative system is blocked at any one of several points. Muscle biopsies using the Gomori trichrome stain shows masses of subsarcolemmal mitochondria ("ragged red fibers").

For a more detailed discussion of this topic, see Adams and Victor: *Principles of Neurology*, 4th ed, pp 1133–1139.

ADDITIONAL READING

DiMauro S, Miranda AF, Sakoda D, et al: Metabolic myopathies. *Am J Med Genet* 25:635, 1986.

Engel AG: Metabolic and endocrine myopathies, in Walton JN (ed): *Disorders of Voluntary Muscle*, 5th ed. Edinburgh, Churchill Livingstone, 1988, pp 811–868.

Engel AG, Banker BQ (eds): *Myology*. New York, McGraw-Hill, 1986.

50 The Congenital Neuromuscular Disorders

Like all cells and tissues, muscle is subject to complex sequences of growth and development as well as aging. Derangements of these sequences give rise to a number of characteristic neuromuscular disorders, usually, but not always, at an early age.

NORMAL DEVELOPMENT AND AGING OF MUSCLE

The commonly accepted view of the embryogenesis of muscle, in its briefest form, is that muscle fibers are derived from mesenchymal cells. These cells are transformed into primitive myoblasts, which in turn fuse to form myotubes, and the latter gradually acquire the properties of fully constituted muscle fibers. Each of these steps is under genetic control, as is also the varying number of fibers that comes to constitute each muscle. A localized embryologic failure at one point in development may result in the congenital absence of a muscle, often occurring in association with aplasia of other tissues as well [e.g., absence of a pectoral muscle and a mammary gland; agenesis of abdominal muscle(s) with a defect in the ureters, bladder, or genital organs]. Inherent faults in the fine structure of the muscle fiber, such as persistence of the myotubular state, central nucleation, or central-core or nemaline body formation, retard the natural growth processes. Defective maturation of motor innervation will also impair the growth of one or other muscle fiber type (congenital fiber-type disproportion).

Once the full complement of muscle fibers has been reached, presumably by the middle trimester of intrauterine life, the main process then is one of fiber growth (volumetric increase) in each muscle. This follows a predictable time scale up to adult years. At puberty, the growth of certain muscles in the male is greater than in the female.

During late life there occurs a gradual loss of anterior horn cells, amounting to 30 percent of the lumbar motor neurons between the sixth and ninth decades. This leads to group atrophy, which is observed in 90 percent of gastrocnemii in individuals more than 60 years of age. In addition, there are an increasing accumulation of lipofuscin and signs of degeneration of single muscle cells. Some of the remaining ones hypertrophy so that there is greater than normal variation in fiber sizes. Possibly these aging processes, occurring before their expected time (a kind of presenile polymyopathy), might explain diseases such as oculopharyngeal dystrophy.

This subject is elaborated in the *Principles*.

CONGENITAL FIBROUS CONTRACTURES OF MUSCLES AND JOINT DEFORMITIES

Infants may be born with fixed deformities of discrete parts of the body (e.g., club foot or congenital torticollis) or more widespread fixation and deformity of joints (arthrogryposis). Sometimes both joints and muscles are affected. The underlying developmental defect may be a purely spinal or muscular one. If certain groups of anterior horn cells fail to develop or are otherwise developmentally disorganized, the muscles which they normally innervate retain their fetal size and are powerless. The unopposed actions of normally innervated muscles may then lead to a fixed deformity. This is the most common basis of arthrogryposis multiplex, which is often associated with a variety of developmental anomalies of the cerebrum and mental retardation. However, a primary muscular defect, whereby certain muscles fail to form or muscle fibers are destroyed by a congenital dystrophy, may have more or less the same effect. Congenital polyneuropathy is another cause, though extremely rare.

THE CONGENITAL POLYMYOPATHIES

In these diseases, which are usually but not always recognized in infancy and early childhood, there is a structural abnormality of muscle from the time of embryogenesis. Their identification has been made possible by the histochemical study of frozen (cryostat) sections of muscle biopsies and by electron microscopy. In most instances, the affected infant shows less than the usual power of muscle contraction, hypotonia (floppiness and lack of resistance to passive movement of the limbs), and delay in the attainment of the milestones of motor development. With growth, there is some improvement, but always a degree of muscular subnormality remains. In many cases, a slight increase in the motor deficit occurs later in life for unknown reasons. Fiber degeneration is not found and the CK levels are usually normal, but the EMG is likely to be myopathic.

The members of this group of relatively nonprogressive congenital myopathies are central-core myopathy, nemaline myopathy, the mitochondrial myopathies, myotubular myopathy, and other even rarer types (reducing body, fingerprint, zebra body, sarcotubular). An account of the distinguishing features of the congenital myopathies, many of them still problematic, cannot be undertaken here. They are considered in detail by Banker in the Engel and Banker monograph, *Myology*.

THE SPINAL MUSCULAR ATROPHIES OF INFANCY AND CHILDHOOD

The effects of an inherited (usually autosomal recessive) degeneration of anterior horn cells may be apparent at birth, but more often they express themselves in the first and second years of life. Progressive enfeeblement of movement of the limb, trunk and cranial muscles (excepting ocular) interfere with motor development. Tendon reflexes are absent, but sensation, perception, and various cognitive acquisitions are unscathed.

In the common, early-life, autosomal recessive form of spinal muscular atrophy (*Werdnig-Hoffman disease*) the child seldom survives more than 2 or 3 years, owing to involvement of the bulbar muscles and resultant dysphagia, inanition, and respiratory insufficiency. Such children usually never attain the capacity to sit, stand, or walk. The EMG reveals fibrillation potentials and reduced numbers of motor units. Serum CK is normal, and the muscle biopsy discloses grouped atrophy of both fiber types. Some patients, with onset in late infancy or early childhood, may survive to adolescence or to early adult life (Byers and Banker).

An even milder form of inherited spinal muscular atrophy, in which the onset is between 2 and 17 years and walking is still possible in adult life, was described by Wolfahrt et al and by Kugelberg and Welander. These cases and some beginning even later in life (Emery) affect mainly the proximal muscles or cranial muscles (Fazio-Londe syndrome). Other sex-linked and dominant modes of inheritance are known.

Only supportive measures are possible.

For a more detailed discussion of this topic, see Adams and Victor: *Principles of Neurology*, 4th ed, pp 1140–1149.

ADDITIONAL READING

Adams RD, Kakulas BA: *Diseases of Muscle: The Pathological Foundations of Clinical Myology*, 4th ed. Philadelphia, Harper & Row, 1985.

Banker BQ: Congenital muscular dystrophy, in Engel AG, Banker BQ (eds): *Myology*. New York, McGraw-Hill, 1986a, chap 45, pp 1367–1382.

Banker BQ: Congenital deformities, in Engel AG, Banker BQ (eds): *Myology*. New York, McGraw-Hill, 1986b, chap 73, pp 2109–2159.

Byers RK, Banker BQ: Infantile muscular atrophy. *Arch Neurol* 5:140, 1961.

Emery AEH: The nosology of the spinal muscular atrophies. *J Med Genet* 8:481, 1971.

Kugelberg E, Welander L: Heredofamilial juvenile muscular atrophy simulating muscular dystrophy. *Arch Neurol Psychiatry* 5:500, 1956.

Wohlfart G, Fex J, Eliasson S: Hereditary proximal spinal muscular atrophy. A clinical entity simulating progressive muscular dystrophy. *Acta Psychiat Scand* 30:395, 1955.

51 Myasthenia Gravis and Episodic Forms of Muscular Weakness

Considered in this chapter are two categories of disease, related only loosely by virtue of the fluctuating or episodic nature of the muscle weakness. In *myasthenia gravis and other myasthenic states*, the fundamental abnormality is one of neuromuscular transmission; usually, some degree of weakness of certain muscles is present at all times, but it is worsened strikingly by activity. In *the periodic paralyses*, discrete attacks of weakness occur in association with disturbances of serum electrolytes. In view of the fluctuating or episodic nature of the weakness in these diseases, it is not surprising that structural changes are subtle and that physiologic mechanisms predominate.

MYASTHENIA GRAVIS (MG)

This disease occurs sporadically in individuals of all ages and both sexes. As the name implies, it may be of grave import. Characteristically, the contractile power of affected muscles is exhausted by repeated or persistent activity and is restored by rest, though not to a normal level. As indicated in Chap. 46, the pattern of muscle involvement is unique—the ocular, facial, and bulbar muscles bear the brunt of the disease (hence its old name—myasthenic bulbar paralysis). Only in advanced cases are limb and trunk muscles weakened. The onset is usually insidious and the progression is subacute, over a period of weeks. Drooping of the eyelids, diplopia and strabismus, dysphonia, dysarthria, and dysphagia occur in various combinations. The rate of progression varies. In most patients the symptoms improve with treatment, but in a few weakness progresses to the point where the patient is bedfast and in need of respiratory support.

MG is of several clinical types, which vary in respect to the pattern and severity of muscle involvement. The following classification, introduced by Osserman, is now in general use and has proved to be useful in judging the prognosis and in treating the disease.

I. Ocular myasthenia
II. A. Mild generalized myasthenia with slow progression; no crises; drug responsive
B. Moderate generalized myasthenia; severe bulbar and some skeletal involvement, but no crises; drug response less than satisfactory
III. Fulminant myasthenia; rapid progression of severe weakness with respiratory crises and poor drug response; high incidence of thymoma; high mortality
IV. Late severe MG; same as III, but with progression over two years from Class I to II

The close relationship of MG to the thymus gland is another important but incompletely understood feature of the disease. In children, adolescents, and young adults, thymic hyperplasia is usually found. In older individuals, thymic tumors become increasingly frequent. The latter may precede the appearance of MG by years.

A special form of transient MG, lasting several weeks, occurs in newborn infants of myasthenic mothers.

Not infrequently, the younger myasthenic suffers from some other type of autoimmune disease—thyrotoxicosis, rheumatoid arthritis, lupus erythematosus, or polymyositis. These diseases are also more frequent in first-degree relatives of patients with MG. However, familial occurrence of MG is rare and is usually of nonimmunologic type.

The course of the illness is extremely variable. In mild form it may remain stationary for years. In the early stage of the disease, spontaneous remission and relapse are not infrequent.

Pathology and pathogenesis Aside from the thymic pathology, the only definite abnormality is at the neuromuscular junction, where there is a simplification of the postsynaptic region and a widening of the primary synaptic cleft. The number and size of the presynaptic vesicles and their quanta of acetylcholine (ACh) neurotransmitter are normal. However, on the postsynaptic side of the neuromuscular junction, the number of ACh receptor (AChR) sites is greatly decreased and immune complexes (1gG and complement components) are deposited on the postsynaptic membrane.

Antibodies to ACh receptor protein are found in approximately 85 percent of patients with generalized MG, although the level of serum antibodies does not correlate precisely with the severity of weakness. These antibodies, transferred across the placenta from the myasthenic mother, also account for the transient weakness in infants with neonatal MG. Exactly where these antibodies are formed, what stimulates their formation, and how they damage the receptor surface of the end plate are incompletely known.

Diagnosis The EMG reveals a highly characteristic decrementing response in the amplitude of compound muscle action potentials in response to 3-per-second nerve stimulation. In single-fiber EMG, there is an increased variability in the firing of individual muscle fibers of a motor unit ("jitter") when the nerve is stimulated. Equally diagnostic is the edrophonium (Tensilon) test. Initially 2 mg of Tensilon are injected intravenously; if this dose is tolerated and no improvement in strength occurs after 45 s, another 3 mg is given; after a further 45 s, another 5 mg can be given. A positive test consists of an *objective* improvement in muscle contractility, usually lasting for 4 to 5 min. The combination of clinical findings (particularly the myasthenic fatigue of small cranial muscles and rapid recovery with rest), typical EMG response, positive Tensilon test, and presence of AChR antibodies in the serum leave little doubt about the diagnosis. Thymic tumors can be visualized by CT scan or MRI.

Treatment This varies with the severity and pattern of muscle weakness. For patients in Class I (see above), anticholinesterase drugs—neostigmine (Prostigmin) and pyridostigmine—are prescribed. The oral dose of neostigmine varies from 7.5 to 45.0 mg every 2 to 6 h and the average maintenance dose is 150 mg/day. The dose of Mestinon is twice this amount. Overdosage may cause a *cholinergic crisis* (nausea, vomiting, pallor, sweating, colic, diarrhea, coupled with increasing weakness); these symptoms should be treated by the slow intravenous injection of 0.6 atropine sulfate. Thymectomy is now recommended for all patients with thymic tumors and for all Class II and III patients. The remission rate in thymectomized patients is about 35 percent, and an equal or larger number improves to a variable extent.

In patients who fail to respond to anticholinesterase drugs and thymectomy, especially elderly patients, corticosteroids are recommended. The daily oral dose of prednisone is 40 to 45 mg, preferably given in twice this dose every other day. Corticosteroid treatment should be initiated in hospital because a slight exacerbation of myasthenic symptoms is to be expected. Anticholinesterase drugs, potassium supplements, and antacids are given simultaneously. The dose of steroids is gradually reduced as the patient improves. Plasmapheresis and immunosuppressive drugs such as azathioprine are reserved for patients with severe MG who do not respond adequately to any of the other methods of therapy and for those in crisis.

Myasthenic-Myopathic Syndrome of Lambert-Eaton

This is a special form of myasthenia in which the muscles of the shoulders, neck, trunk, and pelvic girdle gradually become weak and easily fatigable. Whereas weakness increases with activity, stamping the condition as myasthenic, there is usually a slight but definite augmentation of power during the first few voluntary contractions. The tendon reflexes are often diminished or absent, raising suspicion of a polyneuropathy. Other symptoms are paresthesias, aching discomfort, and autonomic disturbances such as dryness of the mouth, constipation, difficult micturition, and impotence.

The EMG records the augmentation in amplitude of action potentials at rapid rates of nerve stimulation (incrementing response). The basic defect is in the release of quanta of ACh at endplates, similar to the defect that occurs in botulinus poisoning. Most cases are associated with an oat-cell carcinoma or other lung tumor, which suggests that the tumor cells elaborate a substance that interferes with ACh release at the neuromuscular junctions and in sympathetic ganglia.

Guanidine hydrochloride (20 to 30 mg/kg per day) or the less toxic 3,4-diaminopyridine (20 mg, 5 times per day), in conjunction with pyridostigmine (Mestinon) or prednisone, relieves the symptoms. These drugs have been most effective in nontumoral cases.

Other Myasthenic Syndromes

Several types of congenital and familial nonimmunologic myasthenia, all of them rare, have been described by A. G. Engel and his colleagues. A deficiency of pseudocholinesterase, either genetic or acquired, may result in prolonged weakness and apnea when succinylcholine or some other depolarizing muscle relaxant is administered. Aminoglycoside antibiotics and other drugs of similar type may, in some individuals, impair release of neurotransmitters by interfering with Ca ion fluxes at nerve terminals. They pose a particular danger in patients with MG.

EPISODIC (KALEMIC) PARALYSES

At least four hereditary syndromes of recurrent muscle weakness have been identified:

1. Hypokalemic familial periodic paralysis
2. Hypokalemic periodic paralysis with hyperthyroidism
3. Hyperkalemic periodic paralysis without myotonia (adynamia periodica hereditaria of Gamstorp)
4. Hyperkalemic, cold-evoked periodic paralysis with paradoxical myotonia (von Eulenberg paramyotonia)

In each of these diseases, an otherwise normal patient develops, over a few hours, a weakness or paralysis of all the muscles of the trunk and limbs, even those of respiration. Recovery is complete in minutes, hours, or several days, depending on the type of syndrome. The hypokalemic periodic paralysis of dominant or male sex-linked inheritance is the best known member of the group. Typically, after a day of unusually heavy exercise or a meal rich in carbohydrate, the patient retires, only to awaken unable to move. Diurnal attacks also occur. The muscles most likely to escape are those of the eyes, face, tongue, pharynx, larynx, diaphragm, and sphincters. Attacks tend to occur every few weeks.

During the attack serum K levels fall as low as 1.8 meq/L without increase in urinary K excretion. Presumably, K enters the muscle fibers which in biopsy specimens are markedly vacuolated with increase in water (hydropic change). The serum K returns to normal with recovery. Muscle action potentials virtually disappear during the paralysis.

The daily administration of 5 to 10 g of KCl orally in aqueous solution prevents attacks in many of the patients. If it does not, a low-carbohydrate, low-salt, high-K diet may be effective. In an attack, 10 g of KCl or other K salt will restore power.

In hyperkalemic periodic paralysis the attacks tend to be brief, a half hour to an hour, to be more frequent than in other forms of periodic paralysis, and to occur when the serum K rises above a certain critical point (6.0 to 6.5 meq/L). Giving 2 g of KCl orally will provoke an attack. Keeping the level of serum K below this critical point, by giving hydrochlorothiazide, 50 to 100 mg daily, prevents the attacks. The addition of acetazolamide (250 to 1000 mg daily) may be beneficial.

Some of the cases of hyperkalemic periodic paralysis are sensitive to cold and have myotonia evoked by cold, overlapping the von Eulenberg and Gamstorp forms of the disease. The same measures to reduce serum K should be utilized. Procainamide and tocainide in doses of 400 to 1200 mg daily are useful in the treatment of myotonia.

Hypokalemic weakness may also be a manifestation of aldosteronism and of renal disease.

For a more detailed discussion of this topic, see Adams and Victor: *Principles of Neurology*, 4th ed, pp 1150–1167.

ADDITIONAL READING

Engel AG: Periodic paralysis, in Engel AG, Banker BQ (eds): *Myology*. New York, McGraw-Hill, 1986, pp 1843–1870.

Engel AG: Acquired autoimmune myasthenia gravis, in Engel AG, Banker BQ (eds): *Myology*. New York, McGraw-Hill, 1986, pp 1925–1954.

Engel AG: Myasthenic syndromes, in Engel AG, Banker BQ (eds): *Myology*. New York, McGraw-Hill, 1986, pp 1955–1990.

Osserman KE: *Myasthenia Gravis*. New York, Grune and Stratton, 1958.

52 Disorders of Muscle Characterized by Cramps and Spasm

In addition to the commonplace states of spasticity and rigidity, which are due to a disinhibition of spinal motor mechanisms, there are forms of muscle stiffness and spasm in which the basic abnormality can be traced to a disturbance of function of the lower motor neuron or the sarcolemma of the muscle fiber and its intrinsic conducting apparatus. Muscles may go into spasm because of an unstable depolarization of motor axons, sending volleys of impulses across neuromuscular junctions—as occurs in myokymia (waves of seemingly spontaneous contractions), hypocalcemic tetany, pseudohypoparathyroidism, and so-called stiff-man syndrome. In other cases, the innervation is normal, but there is persistence of contraction despite attempts at relaxation, as in myotonia congenita. In the physiologic contracture of McArdle disease, the muscle lacks the energy to relax so that once contracted, it is locked into a shortened state.

In each of these conditions the complaint is one of cramp or spasm, which is variably painful and interferes with free voluntary activity. Morphologic study provides little or no clue as to the nature of the altered contractile process. The best evidence comes from electrophysiologic study of nerve and muscle activity. Each of the aforementioned hyperactive muscle states may sometimes be the main characteristic of a particular nerve or muscle disease, for which reason clinical recognition is important.

MUSCLE CRAMPS

Everyone has at times experienced muscle cramps, usually in the foot or leg, after a period of strenuous activity or sometimes after a strong voluntary or postural contraction. The muscle is knotted and extremely painful, and one seeks relief by rubbing and stretching the muscle. Extremely hard cramping can injure muscle, leaving it tender for days.

The mechanism is obscure. Low levels of myoadenylate deaminase or release of some unknown metabolite into perineural spaces are current hypotheses. Quinine, in doses of 300 mg, diphenhydramine (Benadryl) 50 mg, or procainamide 0.5 to 1.0 g reduce the tendency to cramp and, if taken at bedtime, may prevent nocturnal cramping. Maintenance of adequate salt and fluid intake prevents the type of cramping that occurs in athletes.

Repeated cramping during all manner of physical activity should always suggest hypocalcemia (tetany) or hypomagnesemia. The total Ca level may be nomal, but the amount of ionized Ca may be lowered in nervous individuals by hyperventilation. There are also instances of unexplained *malignant cramp syndrome* where strong contraction of any muscle group induces cramp (pseudotetany). This disorder may run in certain families. In patients with peripheral nerve disease (and in some normal persons), there may be a sensation of muscle cramping without palpable muscle contraction (illusory cramp). Here the EMG is helpful, for during a true cramp there are bursts of high-frequency action potentials.

STATE OF PERSISTENT FASCICULATION, CONTINUOUS MUSCLE ACTIVITY, MYOKYMIA, NEUROMYOTONIA, AND THE STIFF-MAN SYNDROME

A few random fascicular twitchings occurring in muscles that are otherwise normal are very common and nearly always benign. Only if there is associated weakness and atrophy of muscle should fasciculations be considered as manifestations of motor system disease. Fasciculations that persist for hours or days in one muscle (''live flesh'') is a benign state that appears and disappears without explanation, as a rule. A state of extremely marked generalized fasciculations, often associated with fatigue and slight weakness, represents a real syndrome. Slowing of distal motor latencies in some cases suggests a distal motor axonopathy of obscure origin. Eventual recovery can be expected. Phenytoin and carbamazepine have been beneficial in some cases.

A state of *continuous muscular activity* has been described; the entire musculature, even when the patient is fully relaxed, is continuously twitching. It is not abolished even by spinal anesthesia and procaine block of nerves. Presumably motor axons and their terminal endings are persistently hyperexcitable. A continuous rippling and more or less tonic contraction of muscles, called *myokymia*, is closely related to the state of continuous muscular activity as well as to cramps and fasciculations.

Neuromyotonia is the term given to the stiffness, fasciculatory activity, and delayed relaxation of muscle which are sometimes observed in patients who are recovering from a polyneuropathy. Apparently, the regenerating motor neurons pass through a stage of hyperexcitability. The EMG distinguishes this state from a true myotonia.

In tetanus, the toxin suppresses spinal inhibitory neurons (Renshaw cells), leaving anterior horn cells overactive. Activities that normally excite these neurons—reflex postural and volitional movements—evoke violent involuntary spasms, which are especially prominent in jaw muscles (trismus), facial muscles (risus sardonicus), and extensors of the neck and back. The EMG shows the expected interference pattern of fully contracted muscles.

In the so-called *stiff-man syndrome*, a condition similar to tetanus gradually develops during adult life and may persist for years, partially or totally disabling the patient. No explanation has been found. Diazepam or other benzodiazepine drugs, in large doses, control the condition.

CONGENITAL MYOTONIA (THOMSEN DISEASE)

This is a remarkable hereditary disease beginning in early infancy and persisting throughout the patient's lifetime. Tonic spasms develop after every forceful muscular contraction and are most pronounced after a period of inactivity. Blinking is normal, but a strong voluntary closure of the eyelids initiates a myotonic contraction of the orbicularis that takes seconds to overcome; the same is true in taking the first step after sitting or in making a fist. Repeated contractions of the same muscle alleviate the spasm. During rest the muscles are soft. In advanced cases, all the musculature is involved. Tapping with a reflex hammer throws the entire muscle into a contraction that persists for several seconds (percussion myotonia). The muscles may undergo work hypertrophy and reach herculean size.

Microscopic sections of muscle reveal only the hypertrophied fibers filled with myofibrillae. Central rowing of sarcolemmal nuclei, so prominent in myotonic dystrophy, is not seen. The EMG exhibits high-frequency repetitive discharges and a characteristic "dive-bomber" sound on the audio monitor. Electron microscopy reveals no change in any of the organelles. Reduction in chloride conductance and, to a lesser degree, in potassium conductance has been found in myotonia congenita of both the dominant and recessive types but not in myotonic dystrophy.

For a more detailed discussion of this topic, see Adams and Victor: *Principles of Neurology*, 4th ed, pp 1168–1178.

ADDITIONAL READING

Adams RD, Kakulas BA: *Disease of Muscle: Pathological Foundations of Clinical Myology*, 4th ed. Philadelphia, Harper & Row, 1985.

Banker BQ, Chester CS: Infarction of thigh muscle in the diabetic patient. *Neurology* 23:667, 1973.

Meinck H-M, Ricker K, Conrad B: The stiff-man syndrome: New pathophysiological aspects from abnormal exteroceptive reflexes and the response to clomipramine, clonidine, and tizanidine. *J Neurol Neurosurg Psychiatry* 47:280, 1984.

Streib EW: Successful treatment with tocainide of recessive generalized congenital myotonia. *Ann Neurol* 19:501, 1986.

VI | PSYCHIATRIC DISORDERS

In the three remaining chapters we shall consider several diseases that fall mainly in the specialty of psychiatry. The justification for their inclusion in a manual of neurology has been set forth in the *Principles*. In brief, we state that neurologic medicine embraces all conditions that are based on a pathologic process in the nervous system—whether the lesion is obvious, like a tumor or infarct, or impossible to detect with the light or even the electron microscope, like manic-depressive disease or the encephalopathy of delirium tremens. In all instances the pathologic process is traceable to some genetic, chemical, or structural factor acting on the brain and deranging its function. The visible pathologic change represents only the most advanced and irreversible stage of a dynamic morbid process.

We take pains to separate these neurologic cerebral diseases from peculiarities of personality and from a patient's reactions to troubling life experiences—disorders that fall almost exclusively in the domain of psychiatry. Tracing these reactions to the circumstances that evoked them and teaching the patient how better to cope with them are the more practical aims of psychotherapy.

It is of interest that contemporary psychiatry has gradually adopted this point of view. Schizophrenia, endogenous depression and manic-depressive disease, childhood autism, the anxiety states and hysteria, and even the sociopathies and paranoia are being given the status of diseases of the nervous system. As with all diseases, the neuropsychiatric ones are increasingly being defined by explicit criteria, without which there can be little accuracy of diagnosis and prognosis. With the discovery of more or less specific drug therapies, accurate diagnosis becomes a matter of prime practical importance.

In the following discussion, we emphasize the biologic aspects and particularly the diagnostic features of the common neuropsychiatric diseases, ones that should be known to every neurologist.

53 The Neuroses and Personality Disorders

Included under this heading is a group of mental disorders, traditionally designated as anxiety states, neurasthenia, phobic neurosis, obsessive-compulsive neurosis, hysteria, hypochondriasis, neurotic depression, and depersonalization. Originally, Freud referred to these states as the *psychoneuroses*, and their presumed genesis was woven into psychoanalytic theory. Subsequently, biologically oriented psychiatrists abbreviated this term to the *neuroses* and more recently replaced it by the term *neurotic disorder*. The latter includes any mental disturbance with the following characteristics: (1) symptoms that are distressing to the patient and regarded by him or her as unacceptable or alien; (2) intactness of reality testing, i.e., rational analysis of one's reactions; (3) behavior (in relation to symptoms) that does not seriously violate social norms, although social functioning may be considerably impaired; (4) disturbances that are enduring, not transitory reactions to stress; and (5) absence of a recognizable organic cause.

Each of the syndromes described below is clinically identifiable and separable from others when occurring in pure form. However, many patients experience symptoms of more than one type, i.e., "mixed neurosis." Currently, these syndromes are grouped roughly into two categories, as was done in the most recent revision of the Diagnostic and Statistical Manual of Mental Disorders (DSM IIIR): (1) anxiety disorders (which include panic states and the phobic and compulsive neuroses) and (2) the somatiform disorders (comprising hysteria, conversion disorder, hypochondriasis, and somatization disorder).

Anxiety Neurosis

This term and its many synonyms (neurocirculatory asthenia; soldier's heart; panic disorder, etc.) refer to a syndrome consisting of general irritability, anxious expectation, frank anxiety attacks (panic attacks), and the autonomic-visceral accompaniments of anxiety. The syndrome may occur in relatively pure form or be a part of another psychiatric disease—such as depression, schizophrenia, hysteria, and phobic neurosis. Its closest link is with depression, which it resembles in another respect, viz., a strong hereditary factor. The family history in patients with anxiety neurosis discloses a similar illness in first-degree relatives in 50 percent of cases, but the mode of transmission has not been defined. The average age of onset is 25 years (range 18 to 40), and it occurs twice as frequently in women as in men.

Anxiety neurosis is a chronic disease punctuated by attacks of more intense anxiety with or without attacks of panic. In the periods of anxiety, which may appear without warning and last for weeks, months, or a year or more in varying intensity, the patient has feelings of dread and foreboding. The patient feels strange and the world seems unreal (depersonalization or derealization). There is a sense of apprehension and fear of imminent death (angor animi) or of losing one's mind or self-control. In an acute panic attack, the heart races, breathing comes in rapid gasps, the pupils are dilated, and the patient sweats and trembles. A cardiologist may be called because of the prominence of palpitation and feeling of suffocation. Consciousness is fully retained. After 15 to 30 min the symptoms abate, leaving the patient shaken, tense, perplexed, and embarrassed.

Hyperventilation is a prominent feature of an anxiety attack. Hyperventilation itself, by reducing P_{CO_2}, will reproduce the giddiness, paresthesias of lips and fingers, and at times even frank tetany, but these symptoms constitute only the last part of the attack.

Such attacks, which are as stereotyped and unique as a faint or seizure, may be the opening phase of a period of illness or come on a background of chronic worry, easy fatigue, hypochondriasis, and mild depression. Once they appear, they may recur infrequently or several times a day or during the night. There is poor tolerance of exercise in the chronic phase of the illness, with dyspnea and palpitation. The physical examination of such patients yields only a few nonspecific findings: slight tachycardia, sighing respirations, frequent yawning, tremor, and brisk tendon reflexes. Intolerance of hyperventilation is another manifestation.

A 20-year follow-up study of a large group of patients with anxiety disorder showed that symptoms were still present in over 80 percent, but there had been long periods of relative freedom from symptoms. Severe disability had occurred in only 15 percent (Wheeler et al).

Figuring prominently in the differential diagnosis are hyperthyroidism, menopausal symptoms, temporal lobe seizures, adrenal tumors, myocardial disease, pulmonary insufficiency, and depression. In the endocrine conditions, many of the autonomic manifestations appear without the mental components of anxiety. A variety of drugs including psychostimulants, xanthines, and sympathomimetics may also induce anxiety symptoms.

Treatment consists of reassuring the patient and teaching tolerance of the symptoms until a remission occurs, as it will within 6 months in over half of the patients. Antianxiety drugs such as propranolol and lorazepam, and, if depressive symptoms are present, amitriptyline, nortriptyline, or a monoamine oxidase (MAO) inhibitor may be useful.

Phobic Neurosis

In this condition there is a preternatural fear of some situation, disease, animal, or object. While acknowledging that there are no rational grounds for this fear, the patient is powerless to suppress it and becomes panic stricken and incapacitated when put in a situation that evokes the phobia. The resulting symptoms are those of panic. The condition develops in adolescence or early adult life. Many patients are able to intelligently adjust their affairs so as to avoid the phobic reaction and in this way may be able to function quite well. For example, one accedes to a phobia of leaving one's neighborhood or city by living and working near home. Depression may periodically decompensate the adjustment, and antianxiety or antidepressive medication are then required to restore the patient to a functional state. In some patients, behavioral modification techniques are helpful in ameliorating the condition.

Obsessive-Compulsive Disorder

Like phobic states, the obsessive-compulsive disorder begins in adolescence and early adult years, and often there is a family member with an obsessional personality. Obsessions are imperative and distressing thoughts and impulses that intrude themselves in the patient's mind despite a desire to resist and be rid of them. Most disturbing are obsessive fears of harming a family member. Compulsions are single acts (e.g., hand washing) or series of acts (rituals) that the patient feels compelled to carry out.

Antidepressant medications similar to those listed above, in the treatment of anxiety, have been helpful in allaying symptoms, especially during periods of despondency and depression.

HYSTERIA (Hysterical Neurosis, Conversion Disorder, Briquet Disease)

The terms *hysteria* and *hysterical* have several different meanings, and one must be certain as to how they are being used.

One use of the term is to designate a *personality disorder* of special type, characterized by immaturity, excitability, emotional instability, and histrionic and "seductive" behavior. Such a personality disorder may be a lifelong source of difficulty in social functioning, but there is no evidence that it is determinant in the development of a hysterical neurosis (Briquet disease, see below). Even the occurrence of certain unexplained ("conversion") symptoms, such as amnesia, paralysis, aphonia, etc., which mimic neurologic disease, should not in itself be equated with the disease hysteria. In the authors' opinion, the term hysteria should be reserved for a *disease* with a distinctive sex predilection, age of onset, natural history, characteristic somatic symptoms and signs (which typically include "conversion" symptoms), and prognosis.

There are two main types of the *disease hysteria*: In one, the patient, practically always a young woman, presents with a variety of simulated manifestations of disease (usually of neurologic type), often with variable degrees of anxiety; in the other (malingering), which occurs in either sex, various symptoms and signs of disease are feigned for the purpose of obtaining compensation, influencing litigation, avoiding military service, etc. Cases of both types are seen regularly in hospitals and are found more often on neurologic than psychiatric wards.

Classic, or Female, Hysteria (Briquet Disease)

Onset is usually in late childhood, adolescence, or young adult life. Once started, various symptoms recur intermittently, though with lessening frequency in adult years. Schooling and later social life, work, and marriage are interrupted repeatedly by violent headaches, simulated seizures, trance-like states, paralyses, intractable vomiting or regurgitation, unexplained fever, blindness, urinary retention, aphonia, and unsteadiness of gait. Typical examples are young women who appear on emergency wards with complete amnesia for the past, even of personal identity. Most cases of so-called multiple personalities are examples of classic hysteria. Often the illness that is adopted is one that has recently been observed in some member of the family or in a friend. Many of the complaints center around sexual difficulties—claims (often unsubstantiated) of childhood sexual abuse, severe dysmenorrhea, frigidity, dyspareunia, and vomiting throughout pregnancy. Symptoms of anxiety may be prominent as well.

Some of the more common syndromes are hysterical pain (abdominal, back, atypical facial); hysterical trances, fugues, and pseudoseizures; hysterical paralyses (monoplegia, hemiplegia, paraplegia) and tremors; and hysterical amnesia. Nonneurologic manifestations of hysteria include unexplained hyperpyrexia, factitious ulcers and dermatitis, repeated hospitalizations and surgical operations for imprecise reasons, and the excessive use of drugs prescribed by physicians.

Compensation Neurosis (Hysteria in Men and Women, Malingering)

As stated above, hysterical-type symptoms do occur in men, practically always in those trying to avoid legal difficulties or military service or to obtain disability payments, veteran's pensions, or compensation following injury. Unless such a factor is present, the diagnosis of hysteria in the male should be made with great caution (although a sociopath, for unexplained reasons, may sometimes present with such an illness). The symptoms may be much the same as those listed under female hysteria, but often the patient is monosymptomatic, complaining only of "seizures" or of chronic pain that is confined to the low back, neck, head, or arm.

The *differential diagnosis* of both types of hysteria includes a host of neurologic and medical diseases. A past history of repeated illnesses of this type is helpful, but often the patient appears to have forgotten the main illnesses and hospital admissions of the past. More often one must depend on the "discrepancy method"—one is unable to elicit the usual neurologic abnormalities that characterize a genuine paraplegia, hemiplegia, or seizure state. This method may mislead the novice who has limited experience with neurologic and medical disease. Lack of laboratory corroboration is a third criterion, e.g., normal EEG during a frank seizure or normal sedimentation rate and WBC count with high fever.

There has been much debate concerning *etiology*. In Briquet disease, there is a high incidence of hysteria in other female relatives (20 percent of first-degree relatives) and an increased incidence of sociopathy in male relatives. This suggests that female hysteria is the equivalent of male sociopathy, neither of which is fully understood.

In *treatment* one is faced with two problems—the correction of the long-standing basic personality defect and the removal of the recently acquired physical symptoms. In our experience, little can be done about the former. Possibly the personality disorder can be modified by long-term psychotherapy and reeducation. However, the acute symptoms of a particular attack nearly always subside with firm reassurance that recovery is imminent and kindly persuasion (with the help of a physiotherapist) that hour by hour, day by day, function is returning.

No success is to be gained by attributing the disease to nerves, neurosis, or stating that "it's all in your imagination." Compensation hysteria is managed best by determining the degree of injury, confidently stating the prognosis, urging the settlement of litigation problems, and using simple medical measures.

HYPOCHONDRIASIS

The term *hypochondriasis* refers to a morbid preoccupation with bodily functions and with physical sensations and signs. In most instances it is a manifestation of an underlying depression and will be discussed further in the next chapter. Many neurotic individuals become depressed at some time, and opinion differs as to whether the hypochondriacal symptoms are a reaction to the neurosis or are endogenous (see Chap. 54).

ANTISOCIAL PERSONALITY (SOCIOPATHY)

This disorder, known long ago as "moral insanity" and later as psychopathic personality or constitutional psychopathy, is the best defined of all abnormal personality types and the one most likely to lead to trouble in the family and community. Sociopathy is a chronic state that affects mainly males and, unlike most psychiatric disorders, is fully manifest by the age of 12 to 15 years. The most frequent antisocial activities are theft, incorrigibility, truancy, running away from home, associating with undesirable characters, physical aggression and assault, abuse of drugs and alcohol, precocious and indiscriminate sexual activity, and vandalism. Repeatedly apprehended, the sociopath exhibits no remorse, profits little or not at all from discipline or past experience, and is unable to empathize with family and friends. Restlessness and impulsivity are prominent. School and work performance is erratic and failure almost invariable. This deviant behavior naturally places the sociopath in trouble with the law, and many such persons end up in reform school or jail. The female sociopath differs only in having a higher incidence of hysterical symptoms.

Little is known about the cause. Alcoholism or sociopathy in the father and a lack of parental discipline are the most closely related factors but cannot be regarded as causal. In the classic study of L. N. Robins, more than half of the deviant children lost most of their sociopathic traits in adult life. However, of those who did not become adult sociopaths, the large majority developed other psychiatric illnesses, particularly alcoholism.

Psychotherapy has been unsuccessful.

For a more detailed discussion of this topic, see Adams and Victor: *Principles of Neurology*, 4th ed, pp 1185–1203.

ADDITIONAL READING

Diagnostic and Statistical Manual of Mental Disorders (DSM IIIR). Washington, DC, American Psychiatric Association, 1987.

Goodwin DW, Guze SB: *Psychiatric Diagnosis*, 4th ed. New York, Oxford University Press, 1989.

Nemiah JC: Psychoneurotic disorders. In Nicholi AM Jr (ed): *The New Harvard Guide to Psychiatry*. Cambridge, MA, Belknap Press, 1988, pp 234–258.

Purtell JJ, Robbins E, Cohen ME: Observations on clinical aspects of hysteria. *JAMA* 146:902, 1951.

Robins E, Purtell JJ, Cohen ME: Hysteria in men. *N Engl J Med* 246:677, 1952.

Robins LN: *Deviant Children Grown Up: A Sociological and Psychiatric Study of Sociopathic Personality*. Huntington, NY, Kreiger, 1974.

Wheeler EO, White PD, Reed EW, Cohen ME: Neurocirculatory asthenia (anxiety neurosis, effort syndrome, neurasthenia). A twenty-year follow-up of one hundred and seventy-three patients. *JAMA* 142:878, 1950.

54 Grief, Reactive Depression, Endogenous Depression, Manic-Depressive Disease, and Hypochondriasis

The illnesses listed in the title have one trait in common—a depressed or dysphoric mood. However, the different settings in which the depressive illness occurs, certain variations in the clinical picture, and the fact that each requires somewhat different management make their separation important. Taken together, they constitute the most frequent of all mental illnesses, accounting for an estimated 50 percent of psychiatric admissions and 12 percent of all medical admissions to one tertiary referral center. It has been stated that of the adult population of the United States, 20 percent of women and 10 percent of men will have a major depression at least once in their lifetime.

There are four main depressive illnesses with which every physician should be familiar:

1. Grief reaction
2. Reactive or secondary depression in relation to some medical or neurologic disease
3. Dysthymia
4. Endogenous or primary depression (with or without agitation and anxiety) and manic-depressive disease

Grief Reaction

This is the affective state that follows the loss of someone who is particularly close and dear to the patient. It is a natural response in every thoughtful and sentient person. The grief reaction consists of an intense subjective sensation of mental pain accompanied by a feeling of exhaustion, which interfere with the usual pattern of conduct. Often there is a preoccupation with the image of the deceased person, a sense of guilt concerning the relationship to the deceased, and sometimes an unwarranted hostility toward friends and relatives. The mood disturbance and the sense of exhaustion and disorganization of daily activities are the elements for which the authors can vouch.

As a rule, the grief reaction begins to abate after 4 to 12 weeks, but there are wide individual variations in its duration and intensity. It tends to be prolonged in the elderly. Also, patients who have had a previous depression may remain in mourning for a year or more, and it is then impossible to distinguish between a grief reaction and an endogenous depression.

In treating a grief reaction, one attempts to help the patient to a realistic acceptance of the loss and the changes that may be required as a result of it. Sedative-hypnotic drugs may be prescribed for anxiety and insomnia—flurazepam, 15 to 30 mg at bedtime; diazepam, 5 mg tid; oxazepam, 10 mg tid. The latter drugs can be used for daytime sedation and, by doubling the dose at bedtime, for sleep.

If the grief reaction is abnormally prolonged or severe, the assistance of a psychiatrist should be sought to determine the correctness of the diagnosis and the proper management.

Reactive Depression

Often a medical or neurologic disease will be compounded by complaints of undue weakness and fatigue, a loss of interest and pleasure from the patient's usual activities (anhedonia), inability to concentrate, or inexplicable pain. The presence of nervousness, irritability, and poor appetite and sleep may be admitted only on questioning. These should be recognized as the symptoms of depression, and any one of them may complicate the medical illness or be the source of a new line of medical investigation (masked depression).

Certain diseases, more than others, are known to be associated with reactive depression. These are myocardial infarction, hypothyroidism, pernicious anemia, carcinoma of all types, Parkinson disease, chronic hepatitis, and infectious mononucleosis. Also, there appears to be an increased incidence of depressive reaction with left frontal strokes. A large array of drugs, particularly reserpine, methyldopa, propranolol, cimetidine, and the phenothiazines, may evoke a depression reaction.

The first step in management is recognition of the depressive symptoms, and this is followed by assuring the patient that such reactions are to be expected and are medically treatable. Most patients with a reactive depression ultimately recover, even without medical assistance or pharmacologic intervention, but the toll taken by the depression in terms of mental suffering and prolongation of convalescence may be significant, in which case one can safely use tricyclic antidepressants or fluoxetine (Prozac).

Dysthymia

A depressive state that persists for years ("all my life I have been depressed") is now usually classed as dysthymia. Prevailing opinion is that it responds only to psychotherapy, if at all, and that antidepression drugs are of little use. We believe that this generalization does not hold in all cases and that dysthymic patients may respond to antidepressant therapy. Psychologic support, i.e., explanation and reassurance, are helpful but probably do not alleviate the illness.

Endogenous Depression and Manic-Depressive Disease

These are hereditary diseases that occur in cycles of several months or longer. Current nomenclature recognizes two types of these diseases: *unipolar or depressive disorder*, in which only endogenous depression occurs, and *bipolar disorder*, in which mania occurs, often alternating with depression.

A *depressive episode* may occur without provocation, but often there is a history of some stressful situation or loss in the preceding months. The patient feels low in spirits, sad, or depressed and expresses feelings of deep pessimism or hopelessness. With this affective disturbance there is a loss of interest in one's affairs and capacity for enjoyment, a lack of energy, mental and physical fatigue, disturbed sleep (often early morning wakening), loss of appetite, weight loss, waning of sexual interest, and pain. These latter are called vegetative symptoms. Agitation and anxiety are present in many patients, especially the elderly. Psychomotor retardation characterizes others. Self-deprecation, feelings of worthlessness or guilt, suicidal ideation, and somatic delusions may impart a psychotic aspect to the illness.

A *manic attack* expresses itself by an elevation of mood and hyperactivity (excess in amount and speed of speech, excess of all activities). With the euphoria, little sleep is required. When severe, thought may become incoherent. One plan after another is initiated and abandoned. Judgment is faulty. The patient lacks insight into his problem and may embark on impractical schemes that jeopardize his social and financial condition. Despite the lively and expansive state, frustration is often tolerated poorly and euphoria is mixed with irritability. Some patients are frankly paranoid and hostile.

As to *etiology* of this disease, most neurologists and psychiatrists agree that genetic factors are most important. While stress and other environmental changes may be provocative, studies of families show a high coincidence of either unipolar or bipolar disease and a concordance rate of 75 percent in monozygotic twins, clear evidence of a genetic factor. Attempts to investigate the mechanism by measurements of serotonin, norepinephrine, dopamine, or their metabolic products have not yielded consistent results.

Depression is now being managed with reasonable success by pharmacotherapy, electroconvulsive therapy (ECT) being reserved for patients who do not respond or cannot tolerate antidepressant drugs. For unipolar disease, one of the tricyclic antidepressants, such as amitriptyline or norpramine, is the usual first line of therapy, in gradually increasing doses to 150 mg/day. If unsuccessful, one of the MAO inhibitors or fluoxetine is tried. In the patient with a manic attack, a neuroleptic agent may be necessary in the acute episode and lithium carbonate may afford relief from future attacks. In using these drugs, one should be familiar with all the side effects and cross-reactions with other drugs. Some 20 percent of such patients respond poorly to drugs in current use.

Suicide

Manic-depressive psychosis, endogenous unipolar depression, reactive depression that complicates life-threatening disease, pathologic grief, and depression in an alcoholic or schizophrenic—all carry a significant risk of suicide. One of every five suicidal persons with one of these conditions will commit suicide without having made medical contact. In many of the remaining patients, the presence of a depressive illness and potential for suicide will not be recognized by the physician at the time the patient ends his or her life. Between 20,000 and 35,000 suicidal deaths are recorded annually, and about 10 times this number attempt suicide. The incidence rises with age.

In evaluating the risk of suicide, a previous suicide attempt or a history of suicide in a parent are important warnings. Chronic illness, alcoholism, cancer, heart disease, and progressive, incurable neurologic disease all contribute to the risk. Declared fear of death, devout Catholicism, and devotion to family are deterrents. The only rule of thumb is that all depressed patients should be asked about their intentions and all suicide threats should be taken seriously. If there is suspicion of risk, the family should be warned, a bed should be obtained in a general hospital (preferably in a locked psychiatric ward), and a psychiatrist should be consulted. Precautions against suicide should be taken, with the help of the nursing staff. If the patient has already attempted suicide, hospital admission is imperative and the patient should be placed under constant surveillance.

Hypochondriasis

This disorder is defined as a constant preoccupation with matters of health and an excessive concern about real or imagined symptoms of illness. The most common complaints are of pain in the lower abdomen, chest, and head. It is estimated that in over 85 percent of such patients hypochondriasis is part of another psychiatric syndrome, chiefly depression. The remaining 15 percent of patients, referred to as "primary hypochondriacs," are the habitues of medical clinics and are passed from one specialist to another in accordance with their major symptomatology.

In the management of such patients one must first reach a diagnosis. If the symptomatology is part of a depression or anxiety state, this should be treated. If primary, the use of symptomatic therapies and maintenance of a supportive role for the patient and his family are all that can be offered.

Anorexia Nervosa and Bulimia

Anorexia nervosa (AN) is a disease of unknown cause occurring almost exclusively in previously healthy adolescent girls and young women. Anorexia in boys and men is often linked genetically and clinically to an endogenous depression; hence there is no impropriety in appending the description of the anorexic states to this chapter.

AN is culturally linked, being more prevalent is social groups with free access to food and deeply embedded ideas about body habitus. Many of the patients are depressed, impatient, and irritable. Often as much as 30 percent of the patient's body weight will have been lost by the time medical help is sought. Menses cease. To hasten weight loss, the patient may resort to exercise and purging. The cachexia may reach such proportions as to end fatally. For this reason treatment is mandatory. Effective management requires hospital admission, gaining the patient's cooperation, and strict supervision of food intake, which is increased gradually to 3500 to 4000 calories per day. Tube feedings are needed if the patient resists. Once weight is gained, the loss of appetite tends gradually to correct itself. Imipramine, 150 mg/day, has been a helpful adjunct in the therapeutic program, even though patients do not exhibit the typical picture of depression. A relationship between depression and AN is suggested by the unusually high incidence of depression in first-degree relatives of patients with AN. Relapse is frequent and the therapeutic program in most cases needs to be continued for 3 to 4 years.

Bulimia is an eating disorder characterized by massive binge eating followed by induced vomiting and the use of laxatives. It is probably a variant of AN. The authors are attracted to the view that bulimia, like AN, is a manifestation, peculiar to the female, of a deranged appetite-satiety mechanisms in the hypothalamus. At present, proof of this hypothesis is lacking.

For a more detailed discussion of this topic, see Adams and Victor: *Principles of Neurology*, 4th ed, pp 1204–1219.

ADDITIONAL READING

Anderson AE: *Practical Comprehensive Treatment of Anorexia Nervosa and Bulimia*. Baltimore, MD, Johns Hopkins University Press, 1985.

Cassidy WL, Flanagan NB, Spellman M, Cohen ME: Clinical observations in manic-depressive disease. *JAMA* 164:1535, 1957.

Diagnostic and Statistical Manual of Mental Disorders, 3rd rev ed (DSM IIIR). Washington, DC, American Psychiatric Association, 1987.

Goodwin DW, Guze SB: *Psychiatric Diagnosis*, 4th ed. New York, Oxford University Press, 1989.

Hamilton M: Mood disorders: Clinical features. In Kaplan HI, Sadock BJ (eds): *Comprehensive Textbook of Psychiatry (5th ed.)*, Baltimore, MD, Williams & Wilkins, 1989, pp 892–913.

Robins E: *The Final Months: A Study of the Lives of 134 Persons Who Committed Suicide*. Oxford, Oxford University Press, 1981.

Schildkraut JJ, Green AI, Mooney JJ: Affective disorders: Biochemical aspects, in Kaplan HI, Sadock BJ (eds): *Comprehensive Textbook of Psychiatry*, 4th ed. Baltimore, MD, Williams & Wilkins, 1985, pp 769–778.

Starkstein SE, Robinson RG, Price TR: Comparison of cortical and subcortical lesions in the production of poststroke mood disorders. *Brain* 110:1145, 1987.

Winokur G, Clayton PJ, Reich T: *Manic-Depressive Illness*, St. Louis, Mosby, 1969.

55 The Schizophrenias and Paranoid States

The schizophrenias and the depressive illnesses are the two major psychiatric disorders, and together they rank among the most important unsolved medical problems of the twentieth century.

The historical events that led to our present view of schizophrenia and the epidemiology of the disease are elaborated in the *Principles* and are omitted here for lack of space. Uncertainty of diagnosis has thwarted efforts to accumulate vital statistics, since there is no way of proving that a patient is schizophrenic except by the use of clinical criteria. Schizophrenia is defined in DSM IIIR as an illness that has lasted at least 6 months, that had begun during adolescence and early adult life, and that consists of delusions, hallucinations, and disordered thought (looseness of associations and tangential thinking) and verbal communication, all of which result in a deterioration from a previous level of functioning. Important negative criteria are absence of depression, mania, dementing brain disease, and mental retardation. To these criteria, we would add a positive family history of a similar disease.

Often, eccentricity of personality and behavior (a tendency to be solitary and withdrawn socially) and academic difficulties precede frank psychosis by many years. Then, usually during adolescence and practically always before the age of 40, the patient becomes disturbed and is unable to continue school or work. When first seen, he or she expresses bizarre fears and ideas and suspicions of the motives of family members or of others. Often the patient is hallucinating and deluded—relating fantasies about controlling the thoughts of others or having one's own thoughts controlled. Notably absent are primary disturbances of memory, perception, orientation, etc., which are so common in dementing brain diseases and confusional-delirious states. Such outbreaks of illness occur repeatedly until the patient finally settles into a condition in which delusions and hallucinations are denied but for unclear reasons continuation of education and effective work are impossible. Some patients recover but always in such cases there is the question of reliability of diagnosis.

The subdivision of schizophrenia into simple, hebephrenic, catatonic, and paranoid types has not been particularly helpful. Catatonia, in which the patient lies in a dull stupor—mute, resistant, and apathetic—is a syndrome more closely related to a retarded form of depression than to schizophrenia, and paranoid schizophrenia is considered by many European psychiatrists to be a mental illness of diverse etiology; some cases are clearly not schizophrenic. Acute psychosis in a previously well-adjusted person is probably not a form of schizophrenia (called "brief reactive psychosis" in DSM IIIR). In 75 to 80 percent of such patients the illness is reversible within a few months; there is a family history not of schizophrenia but of manic-depressive disease, and the patient responds to antimanic-depressive medication. Thereafter, the mental illness pursues the course of manic-depressive disease. Also, brief illnesses (2 weeks or less) with schizophreniform symptoms often have the characteristics more of a confusional state than of schizophrenia; probably an illness of this type lasting less than 6 months is also an illness other than schizophrenia (possibly hypomania or metabolic disease). There is still much debate about childhood schizophrenia, which is rare and must be distinguished from partial autism (Asperger syndrome).

Even in the group of patients conforming to the DSM IIIR diagnostic criteria for schizophrenia, not all patients are alike. Some have suggestive thalamic–frontal lobe signs such as inattentiveness, difficulty in shifting cognitive set from one task to another, poor function on continuous-performance tasks, and poorly sustained initiative and drive. Also, smooth ocular pursuit movements, paroxysmal saccadic eye movements, episodic lateral deviation of the eyes, reflex asymmetries, and slight lowering of IQ are recorded in some. The EEG is abnormal in 5 to 80 percent of cases. Finally, some patients have slightly enlarged third and lateral ventricles, unrelated to the duration of the illness and medication. Studies of cerebral blood flow have revealed an inability to increase flow to the frontal lobes during demanding psychologic tests. These findings have led to the notion that schizophrenia is a syndrome, not a single disease, and that within the syndrome there is a genetic core disease, which might be called true schizophrenia and other diseases that simulate schizophrenia, i.e., schizophreniform.

Search for a consistent neuropathology has been singularly elusive. Crude neuronal destruction and gliosis have not been found. Yet quantitative studies are beginning to reveal decreased neuronal populations in certain structures such as the nucleus accumbens, globus pallidus, and limbic system. Whether these data apply to the core syndrome or to other diseases of schizophreniform type is unsettled.

Etiology Here the evidence favors a genetic factor. The siblings of schizophrenic patients have a higher incidence of schizophrenia (11 percent) than is expected in the general population (0.9 percent). The concordance rate in monozygotic twins is three to six times greater than in dizygotic twins, whether raised with their biologic or adoptive parents. The pattern of genetic transmission is unsettled. The two suggested possibilities are that schizophrenia is due to a dominant gene with incomplete penetrance or to a polygenic mode of transmission. Again the problem is whether we are dealing with a homogeneous disease or a group of heterogeneous diseases.

The major pathophysiologic hypothesis, advanced by Carlsson and by Snyder, is that an abnormal gene or genes cause a hyperfunctional dopamine system. Supporting this concept is the observation that drugs blocking dopamine receptors are potent therapeutic agents.

Treatment Frank psychotic episodes usually require that the patient be admitted to a psychiatric hospital, especially if there is danger of injury to self or others. In the florid stage of the disease, antipsychotic medication (either a phenothiazine, such as thioridazine or fluphenazine, or haloperidol) is routinely administered. Anxiety and insomnia, if present, should be controlled by anxiolytic and hypnotic drugs, and antipsychotic drugs are usually reserved for patients with delusional-hallucinatory symptoms. When the latter drugs are used, there is always the danger of developing tardive dyskinesia, parkinsonian rigidity, or the neuroleptic malignant syndrome (Chap. 40).

Paranoia and Paranoid States

Patients who have fixed suspicions, persecutory delusions, or grandiose ideas that are false but logically elaborated are said to be paranoid. They often display other traits that are indicative of schizophrenia and are then classified as paranoid schizophrenics. However, there is a group whose conduct is formally correct, whose emotional reactions are adequate, and whose train of thought is entirely coherent. To them the term *pure paranoia* is applicable. Mild degrees of the latter are found among the eccentric people of every community. Only when their behavior becomes overly bizarre or socially obnoxious, annoying others, do they come to the attention of legal authorities or a physician. In some cases, neuroleptic drugs have been helpful.

A few of our alcoholic patients have developed a chronic delusional-hallucinatory state as a sequela to an attack of acute auditory hallucinosis. Acute or chronic drug intoxication (amphetamines, cocaine) accounts for episodes of paranoid behavior in others.

Puerperal (Postpartum) Psychoses

This is a complex problem. Postpartum depression of mild degree and short duration is a frequent and well-known phenomenon. Severe prolonged depression in this setting differs in no particular way from a monophasic endogenous depression and should be treated as such. It is of interest that some patients with depression have lapsed into this state only in the postpartum period, being normal at all other times.

An acute confusional-delusional psychosis, unlike any of the previously described psychiatric illnesses, may also appear during the postpartum period. Here major affective changes are mixed with delusional ideas, disorientation, and clouding of the sensorium. The new mother may reject or even kill her baby. Recovery takes weeks or months, but the outlook in general is better than for schizophrenia. Careful exclusion of drug psychosis and diseases such as postpartum cerebral venous thrombosis is part of the neurologic investigation. In some instances a frank schizophrenic break can occur in the postpartum period. The treatment of this type of syndrome must be undertaken in a psychiatric hospital, and antipsychotic medication is usually needed.

The *endocrine psychoses* are also difficult to classify, for they vary widely in symptomatology. An acute onset of confusion, insomnia, mood elevation or depression, and delusional thinking in some combination has been reported with large doses of steroids or ACTH, Cushing disease, and hyperthyroidism. Control of the endocrine disease usually restores the patient to normality.

For a more detailed discussion of this topic, see Adams and Victor: *Principles of Neurology*, 4th ed, pp 1220–1235.

ADDITIONAL READING

Carlsson A: Antipsychotic drugs, neurotransmitters, and schizophrenia. *Amer J Psychiatry* 135:164, 1978.

Kety SS, Matthysse S: Genetic and biochemical aspects of schizophrenia. In Nicholi AM Jr (ed): *The New Harvard Guide to Psychiatry*. Cambridge, MA, Belknap Press, 1988, pp 139–151.

Lehmann HE: Schizophrenia: Clinical features, in Kaplan HI, Sadock BD (eds): *Comprehensive Textbook of Psychiatry*, 4th ed. Baltimore, MD, Williams & Wilkins, 1985, chap 15.4, pp 680–713.

Snyder SG: Dopamine receptors, neuroleptics, and schizophrenia. *Amer J Psychiatry* 138:460, 1981.

Winokur G: Delusional disorder (paranoia). *Compr Psychiatry* 18:511, 1977.

Index

Page references followed by *f* or *t* indicate figures or tables, respectively.